A Pregnancy Roadmap for First-Time Moms and Dads

A Compilation

Elizabeth Benson

Pregnancy From Conception to Birth

The Essential Roadmap for First-Time Mothers

Book 1

© Copyright 2023 - All rights reserved.

The content contained within this book may not be reproduced, duplicated or transmitted without direct written permission from the author or the publisher.

Under no circumstances will any blame or legal responsibility be held against the publisher, or author, for any damages, reparation, or monetary loss due to the information contained within this book, either directly or indirectly.

Legal Notice:

This book is copyright protected. It is only for personal use. You cannot amend, distribute, sell, use, quote or paraphrase any part, or the content within this book, without the consent of the author or publisher.

Disclaimer Notice:

Please note the information contained within this document is for educational and entertainment purposes only. All effort has been executed to present accurate, up to date, reliable, complete information. No warranties of any kind are declared or implied. Readers acknowledge that the author is not engaged in the rendering of legal, financial, medical or professional advice. The content within this book has been derived from various sources. Please consult a licensed professional before attempting any techniques outlined in this book.

By reading this document, the reader agrees that under no circumstances is the author responsible for any losses, direct or indirect, that are incurred as a result of the use of the information contained within this document, including, but not limited to, errors, omissions, or inaccuracies.

Table of Contents

INTRODUCTION 1

TRIMESTER 1: NEW ADVENTURES 4
    CHAPTER 1: MONTH ONE 5
    CHAPTER 2: MONTH TWO 33
    CHAPTER 3: MONTH THREE 43

TRIMESTER 2: THE HONEYMOON PERIOD 49
    CHAPTER 4: MONTH FOUR 50
    CHAPTER 5: MONTH FIVE 65
    CHAPTER 6: MONTH SIX 85

TRIMESTER 3: WAITING IMPATIENTLY 95
    CHAPTER 7: MONTH SEVEN 96
    CHAPTER 8: MONTH EIGHT 117
    PRESENTATION AND POSITION OF BABY FOR DELIVERY 119
    CHAPTER 9: MONTH NINE 129

TRIMESTER 4: THE STORK HAS ARRIVED 139
    CHAPTER 10: LABOR 140
    CHAPTER 11: DELIVERY 153
    CHAPTER 12: POSTPARTUM 167
    CONCLUSION 199
    GLOSSARY 201
    REFERENCES 205
    IMAGE REFERENCES 225

INTRODUCTION 229

CHAPTER 1: FACING YOUR FATHERHOOD FEARS 233
    RESPONSES TO PREGNANCY NEWS 234
    THE COMMON WORRIES OF NEW DADS 236
    THE COMMON WORRIES OF NEW MOMS 241
    FATHERHOOD AND MASCULINITY 242
    ARE YOU READY TO BE A DAD? 245

WHAT TYPE OF DAD DO YOU WANT TO BE? 247

CHAPTER 2: THE FATHERHOOD EFFECT 251

DAD BRAIN: IS IT A THING? 253
MORE ON PATERNAL INSTINCT 256
PREGNANCY SYMPTOMS IN FATHERS 259

CHAPTER 3: NAVIGATING THE EXPECTANT PATH—PREPARING THE PERFECT PREGNANCY PLAN 263

CREATING A BIRTH PLAN 264
THE FINANCIAL ELEMENTS OF THE BIRTH PLAN 299
KNOWING YOUR RIGHTS 306
BIRTH PLANS: A COMPREHENSIVE TEMPLATE 310

CHAPTER 4: INITIATING DAD MODE 313

CAR SEAT INSTALLATION 315
KEEPING MOM SAFE AND HEALTHY 317
BABYPROOFING YOUR HOME 323

CHAPTER 5: THE LOWDOWN ON PRENATAL CHECK-UPS 327

WHY YOU SHOULD BE PRESENT DURING PRENATAL VISITS 327
HOW OFTEN SHOULD THEY BE? 328
WHAT HAPPENS DURING A PRENATAL VISIT? 329
THE IDEAL PRENATAL VISIT SCHEDULE 330
QUESTIONS TO ASK DURING PRENATAL APPOINTMENTS 335
FAMILY HISTORY AND GENETIC TESTING 337
HOW TO BE THE BEST SUPPORT PERSON FOR YOUR PARTNER 342

CHAPTER 6: A PEEK INTO THE WOMB 345

A WEEKLY BREAKDOWN OF WHAT'S UP WITH BABY AND MOMMY... AND WHAT YOU CAN DO TO HELP 346
WHEN YOUR BABY'S DUE DATE HAS PASSED 366
YOUR SEX LIFE DURING AND AFTER PREGNANCY 368

CHAPTER 7: OVERCOMING THE CHALLENGES OF PREGNANCY 373

PREGNANCY COMPLICATIONS 374
POSTPARTUM DEPRESSION 376
MISCARRIAGE 378
PROBLEMS AND STRESS RELATED TO RELATIONSHIPS 380

CHAPTER 8: REMEMBERING THE OTHER PERSON IN YOUR PREGNANCY JOURNEY 383

POSTPARTUM DEPRESSION IN MEN 383
COPING WITH MISCARRIAGES AND LOSS 386

SUPPORT GROUPS FOR FATHERS	387
SELF-CARE TIPS	389

CHAPTER 9: PREPARING FOR YOUR FIRST DAY AS A DAD... AND BEYOND 391

WHY YOU SHOULD ATTEND THE BIRTH	391
D-DAY HOSPITAL BAG PACKING CHECKLIST	392
HOW TO HELP DURING LABOR AND DELIVERY	394
WHAT HAPPENS IF YOU DON'T MAKE IT OUT OF THE HOUSE	396
THE APGAR SCORE	398
THE NEWBORN SCREENING TEST	399
TAKING YOUR BABY HOME	402
NEW DAD PARENTING HACKS	412

CONCLUSION..............415

REFERENCES..............417

IMAGE REFERENCES	448

"Your children are not your children.

They are sons and daughters of Life's longing for itself.

They come through you but not from you.

And though they are with you yet they belong not to you.

You may give them your love but not your thoughts,

For they have their own thoughts.

You may house their bodies but not their souls,

For their souls dwell in the house of tomorrow, which you cannot visit, not even in your dreams.

–Kahil Gibran

Introduction

Motherhood is a journey that begins with love and curiosity, and transforms into a never-ending story of learning, growth, and pure joy.

Pregnancy is a lot of things, but I think the overarching theme throughout those nine months is anticipation. It's like being in a constant state of wonder. From the day you find out you're pregnant, you'll be wondering what your baby will look like. As you progress, you'll be anticipating what's to come in the next month. When you eat, you might be subconsciously asking yourself if you've made a good meal choice. When you work out, you may ask yourself whether you're doing so at a safe enough pace for your baby. You're always going to want to know something.

If I were to ask you what you think the most important thing to have for a safe and happy pregnancy is, what would you say?

Would you say a healthy diet? A positive mindset?

The answer is: information. When you're clued up or reading up on pregnancy, you get to know what's happening in your body, what's normal and what's not, and how well your baby should be developing. You also get to know all the things you can do to ensure a healthy baby with ten fingers and toes.

But most importantly, you'll be able to recognize potential risks and have the confidence and knowledge to ask questions and seek prompt intervention if needed.

If you've got a litany of anxious questions, here are all the reassuring answers you need. As well as all the physical and emotional symptoms you might experience.

Most of the things that are happening to you are completely normal, but it's still nice to feel reassured and like you're on the right track.

The *journey* into parenthood has already begun. This book is a roadmap to tell you where you are, how long it takes to reach the finish line, and what happens in between. You're already a great mom.

I'm going to walk you through your pregnancy, from the time you find out, until a month and a half after your special bundle has arrived.

You'll learn more about:

- What's going on in your body?
- How your baby is developing month by month.
- The effects of certain foods and drinks on your baby and how to keep healthy throughout the pregnancy.
- The benefits of exercise, the kinds that are harmful, and the ones you should incorporate into your routine.
- How to comfortably change your lifestyle for the duration of pregnancy to ensure a healthy, bouncing baby.
- What could potentially go wrong, signs to look out for, and the recommended course of action.
- Statistics on ailments, the percentage of women they affect, and how you can either prevent or prepare for such things.
- Ways to maintain your relationships through this period and once the baby's born.

As a bonus, you'll feel like you have one more person celebrating with you.

I'm a mother myself. I've got grandchildren too, and I remember what I felt during my first pregnancy. I cherished it. I wanted to know what was going on every step of the way, and there was only one comprehensive book around at the time. I read that thing until it fell apart.

I also recall my own daughters and daughter-in-law experiencing pregnancies and exchanging some very conflicting information. It's what inspired me to seek out accurate information and put it all in one book.

Any pregnancy is beautiful, but a first pregnancy is especially wonderful. I wish I could experience it again. What you learn in this book will help to eliminate some of the anxieties that will inevitably accompany your journey into new territory. I hope it will help make a wonderful experience even better.

TRIMESTER 1: New Adventures

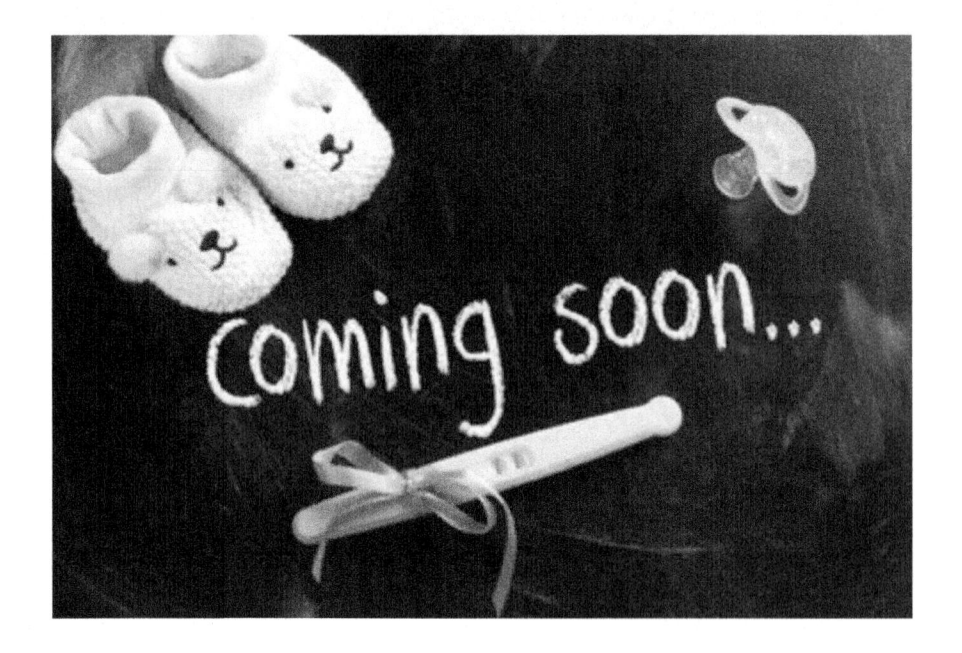

Chapter 1: Month One

You're Pregnant!

A very big congratulations to you! Here's wishing you every bit of joy that comes with being a parent—and then some!

If this news comes as a surprise and you're feeling a little unprepared, don't worry. You've got about eight more months to figure some things out. I say some because there are moms with kids in college who are still figuring things out!

There's a lot that goes on in a really short space of time when you're pregnant. As time goes on, it becomes apparent that you're sharing your body. This means you'll have to start making some changes in order to accommodate your new guest and…

It's Never Too Late to Change Your Habits

As far as changing habits go, I say the earlier the better, but better late than never. There are some vices that pregnant women and women trying to conceive should avoid. These include alcohol, smoking, marijuana, and caffeine.

Alcohol

We've all heard the myth that a glass of red wine a day is okay to have when you're pregnant, but this couldn't be further from the truth. There is just no safe level of alcohol consumption during pregnancy, despite all the conflicting information you may find online or hear in passing. Alcohol should be absolutely avoided by expectant mothers and those attempting to conceive until after the baby is born.

Fetal alcohol spectrum disorders (FASD), are a group of developmental, emotional, mental, and physical problems and illnesses that can affect the fetus should the expectant mother decide to imbibe throughout the pregnancy. Similar to any liquid or food consumed by a pregnant woman, alcoholic beverages will pass to the fetus through the umbilical cord and into the placenta. So, if a pregnant woman drinks heavily, her high blood alcohol levels can prevent vital nutrients from reaching the baby, which is harmful for the baby's development. It takes around 2 hours for a fetus' blood alcohol level to be on par with that of its mother, and the alcohol ends up staying in its system for longer because their metabolisms are slower than ours. So, if one chooses to drink frequently or to excess, their fetus will be exposed to alcohol for longer.

That's why it's always better for women to quit drinking and abstain from it from the moment they suspect they're pregnant.

Can Alcohol Cause Birth Defects?

Birth defects are physical abnormalities that are present in the body before birth. They're caused by teratogens, which include alcohol.

Birth malformations caused by alcohol's impact on physical and structural development include:

- height and weight that are below average.
- issues with hearing and vision.
- bone, heart, and renal issues.
- small head circumference.
- abnormal facial features that might include:
    - a smooth ridge between the nose and upper lip.
    - an upturned nose.
    - a flat nasal bridge.
    - a thin upper lip.

Caffeine

Caffeine is a natural substance found in fruits, leaves, and seeds like cocoa beans and coffee beans. It also ends up in a lot of man-made foods like chocolate, ice cream, and the like.

There's no way to completely avoid it, but if you can keep your intake down to 200 milligrams per day, you'll be okay. It may sound far-fetched, but according to studies, more than 200 milligrams of caffeine per day while pregnant can cause harm. Caffeine consumption has been associated with a higher risk of miscarriage and low birth weight.

The precise amount of caffeine in a cup of coffee is difficult to determine because it can vary depending on the brand, preparation method, and cup size.

Here are some ways you can cut back on caffeine:

- Limit your coffee intake to a cup or two a day (be sure to pay attention to the size of the cup).

- Mix your regular coffee with some decaf.

- Start to phase out your regular coffee until you're only drinking decaf.

Keep in mind that green tea and other soft drinks also have caffeine. You can switch to decaffeinated versions. There are still trace amounts of caffeine, but nowhere near the amount that would be harmful to you and your baby.

You can still have chocolate in moderation, because the caffeine content in a chocolate bar varies from 5 to 30 milligrams.

Smoking

Smoking and pregnancy don't go together. Smoking during pregnancy is dangerous for both the mother and the unborn child. Nicotine, tar, and carbon monoxide are among the harmful chemicals found in cigarettes. Smoking greatly increases the chance of difficulties during pregnancy, some of which can be deadly.

Here are seven dangers one can encounter while smoking during pregnancy:

Birth Defects

Smoking increases the likelihood that a baby will be born with defects. Congenital cardiac abnormalities—abnormalities with the structure of the heart—and cleft lip and palate are among the most prevalent.

Ectopic pregnancy

See page. 35

Low birth weight

Smoking can contribute to low birth weight in newborns, but it goes beyond simply giving birth to a smaller baby. Other health issues and disabilities can occur too. Thankfully, the number of deaths caused by low birth weight has decreased tremendously because of medical advancements. However, it's still a severe condition, and it can lead to:

- delayed development
- hearing and vision impairment
- cerebral palsy

Miscarriage and stillbirth

Smoking increases the risk of miscarriages and stillbirths because cigarettes contain hazardous compounds that are harmful to babies.

Placental abruption

Smoking increases the risk of numerous placenta-related problems, the main one being placental abruption.

Placenta previa

See page. 110

Preterm labor

See page. 109

Marijuana

Marijuana is the most widely used illicit substance among pregnant women in the United States. A lot of pregnant women consider it a secure, all-natural cure for morning sickness, nausea, and vomiting. However, using marijuana while pregnant has significant, even fatal, risks.

Marijuana (even in small doses) has not been proven safe to use during pregnancy. The American Academy of Pediatrics issued its first set of official guidelines in 2018, recommending pregnant and breastfeeding women abstain from using marijuana since it poses risks to both mother and child.

Studies indicate that marijuana usage during pregnancy can result in:

- Low birth weight
- A higher chance of stillbirth
- Fetal growth restriction
- Preterm birth
- Ongoing brain development issues that affect behavior, learning, and memory

Narcotics: What Are the Effects in the Womb and After Birth?

Unfortunately, it's not uncommon for women of childbearing age to use illicit substances. Cocaine and other illegal drugs can have terrible effects on a fetus.

An expectant mom who takes illegal substances is at risk of so many other things. She's at risk of anemia, hepatitis, skin infections, blood infections, and heart infections. Over and above that, she is more vulnerable to developing STIs.

Everything a mother ingests gets transferred to the baby through the placenta, so any drugs she takes increase the likelihood of drug dependence in the unborn child.

The use of cocaine, methamphetamine, dextroamphetamine, methadone, and other opiates has been linked to stillbirth, preterm birth, placenta detachment, high blood pressure, and miscarriage. They also might cause withdrawal symptoms in newborns, like jitteriness, difficulty falling asleep, and feeding difficulties. Later on, they may experience issues with muscular tone and tremors. They are also more vulnerable to SIDS. Some symptoms linger for a few weeks, and these babies are more likely to have apnea and struggle to feed.

Mothers who use drugs during pregnancy are more likely to have low birth weight babies who might be more susceptible to:

- growth problems
- hyperactivity
- behavioral issues
- learning issues

A woman's chances of having a healthy baby increase if she stops using illicit drugs during the first trimester.

When the subject of pregnancy is brought up, the first thing that comes to mind is being more mindful about what you put into your body. Something we rarely talk about is our environment and how it needs to be healthy too. So...

Let's Talk Toxoplasma

Toxoplasma is a parasite that can be found in unwashed fruits and vegetables, raw or uncooked meat, soil, contaminated water, and anywhere that cat feces are present. Should you come into contact with it, you can develop toxoplasmosis, which is dangerous for you, and your unborn child.

Ways You Can Get It

- Consuming contaminated water.
- Using contaminated utensils or a cutting board that has come into contact with raw meat.
- Consuming undercooked or raw meat, or putting your hands in your mouth after handling uncooked meat.
- Accidentally consuming cat feces by touching your mouth after handling the litter box, touching soil, or anything else that's been in contact with it.

How It Affects You and Your Baby

Toxoplasmosis isn't always immediately detectable and can be hard to diagnose. People can be infected without having any noticeable symptoms, which means a pregnant woman could easily expose her fetus without even being aware of her condition. That's why it's so important to prevent it.

Symptoms include

- Headaches
- Swollen glands
- Muscle pain
- Fever
- A stiff neck

Visit a medical professional right away if you suffer from any of the aforementioned symptoms.

Toxoplasma in babies can cause blindness, intellectual impairment, and hearing damage. Even years after birth, some children may experience difficulties with their eyes or brains.

Babies born with the infection may also need years of specialized care, like special education and ophthalmology care.

In order to lessen the impact of the parasite, it's crucial to identify and treat the infection as soon as possible.

How You Can Prevent It

Cook

- Don't taste-test meat until it's cooked.
- Always make sure the meat is completely cooked. It should be cooked internally to a temperature of 160° F (71° C). To check, use a food thermometer.

Clean

- After handling raw meat, cat litter, soil, or unwashed produce, wash your hands with soap and warm water.

- Always wash your utensils and cutting board with warm, soapy water after use.

- All fruits and vegetables should be thoroughly washed and/or peeled before consumption.

Separate

- Separate raw meat from the other food in your fridge. Also, keep raw meat away when you're handling or preparing other food.

Always make sure that any water you consume has been treated. Should you travel to a less developed country while you're pregnant, be vigilant and mindful, or just stick to bottled water.

If you have a cat, you don't have to get rid of it. Just bear in mind that toxoplasma infects virtually all cats that spend any time outdoors. They get it by consuming contaminated raw meat or small animals. The parasite is subsequently spread via the cat's droppings. A pregnant woman might not be aware that her cat has it because toxoplasma doesn't make cats appear ill.

Here are some tips you can follow to prevent or lessen the chances of contracting it from your cat:

- Avoid stray cats (especially kittens).

- Feed your cat dry or canned food; avoid letting them near raw meat.

- Have someone else change the litter box if at all possible. If you must clean it, put on disposable gloves and then thoroughly wash your hands with warm water and soap.

- The parasite takes one to five days to become contagious, so changing your litter box daily can help prevent contraction.

- Wear gloves when tending your garden in case there's any excrement in the soil. When you're done, wash your hands.

Now that your environment is safe for YOU, let's see how you can ensure that your body is a safe environment for babies.

Keeping Fit While Pregnant

For some, pregnancy's a breeze. For others, it's months of discomfort and feeling like you're no longer in charge of your body. Exercising regularly can offset some of that discomfort and keep you healthy throughout your pregnancy. It can also minimize some common aches, pains, and exhaustion. Exercise also helps alleviate stress, lessens your chances of developing gestational diabetes, and helps you build the endurance you need for labor and delivery.

If you exercised regularly before pregnancy, you can keep it up, just at a slower rate, and with less intensity. Always listen to your body and do what you can handle. If you didn't previously exercise, you can speak to your doctor about starting a nice and safe regimen. A good place to start would be about 30 minutes of mild to moderate exercise once daily. Keep in mind that exercise doesn't have to be taxing on the body to be beneficial.

Exercise Tips

- Drink plenty of fluids, especially water.

- Never work out without warming up beforehand, and always cool down afterward.

- Should you decide to join a class, make sure the instructor has experience with pregnant women.

- Try and exercise daily; even a walk is okay. Avoid strenuous exercise, especially in the heat.

- Given that water will sustain your increasing weight, you might want to give swimming a try. Aqua-natal sessions are offered at a few local swimming facilities with trained instructors. Find a pool in your area.

- Do your best to avoid exercises where there's a possibility you'll fall. For example, horse riding or cycling.

Exercises to Avoid

- After 16 weeks, avoid lying flat on your back for prolonged periods since the pressure from your bump on the main blood vessel transporting blood to your heart can cause you to feel dizzy.

- Avoid engaging in contact sports like kickboxing, martial arts, or squash, where there is a chance of getting hit.

- Avoid scuba diving because your baby won't be protected against gas embolism (gas bubbles in the bloodstream) and decompression sickness.

- Never exercise at 2500 meters above sea level because altitude sickness is a concern for both you and the baby.

Who Shouldn't Exercise While Pregnant?

If you have a preexisting condition like diabetes or asthma, exercise is not recommended. Exercise can also be harmful when you've got pregnancy-related conditions like:

- A weak cervix

- Continual or imminent miscarriage

- Low placenta

- Past preterm births or a history of premature labor

Which Exercises Are Safe?

As long as you work out carefully and don't overdo it, most exercises are safe to do while pregnant.

Here's a list of workouts you can incorporate into your routine. They will strengthen your muscles enough to help you carry any added weight. They'll also strengthen your joints, increase circulation, relieve back pain, and generally make you feel good.

Abdominal Exercise

As your pregnancy progresses, you may notice a dip in your lower back deepening, which can cause back pain. These exercises can help with that while strengthening your abdominal muscles:

- Get onto all fours and keep your back straight, by lifting your abdominals and placing your hands beneath your shoulders with your fingers pointing forward.

- Curl your trunk and let your head softly relax forward while contracting your abdominal muscles and raising your back towards the ceiling. Try not to let your elbows lock.

- Hold for a brief moment before returning gradually to the box position.

- Keep in mind that your back should always return to its natural, straight position.

- Make your muscles work hard and carefully move your back as you repeat this motion ten times slowly and methodically.

- Only move your back in a way that's comfortable, don't strain it.

Pelvic Floor Exercises

The pelvic floor is made up of layers of muscles that extend from the pubic bone to the tailbone. It's shaped like a hammock. Our pelvic floor muscles get put under a lot of strain while we're pregnant and once we've given birth.

If your pelvic floor becomes weak, urine can escape if you cough or sneeze. It's called "stress incontinence," and there's nothing to be embarrassed about. It happens to a lot of women after birth.

Exercises that target the pelvic floor can help you develop these muscles. This aids in preventing or reducing postpartum stress incontinence. Even if you're young and don't currently experience stress incontinence, every pregnant woman should do it.

- Close up your bottom, like you're trying to hold it in a while using the restroom.
- Draw in your urethra like you're stopping the flow of pee while also drawing in your vagina like you're grasping a tampon.
- Perform this exercise quickly at first, immediately contracting and relaxing the muscles.
- Slow it down by holding the contractions for up to ten seconds at a time.
- Try to do three sets of eight daily. A good rule of thumb is to do it before or after every meal.
- For even better results, do pelvic floor exercises before and during a cough or sneeze.

Pelvic Tilt Exercises

- Stand, and put your bottom and shoulders up against a wall.
- Soften your knees.

- Draw your belly button toward your spine so that your back is completely straight, then release after 4 seconds of holding.

- Do this repeatedly, up to ten times.

Vitamins and Supplements

We get most of the vitamins we need from the food we eat, but should there be a deficit, we can supplement our intake with herbal supplements, fish oil capsules, single minerals, and multivitamins.

In order for your baby to grow and develop at a healthy rate, you need to be sure you're getting good amounts of all the nutrients you need.

In pregnancy, our need for certain nutrients increases to account for ourselves and the baby. These include folate, iodine, iron, vitamins B and D, and protein.

- Folate is vital. It prevents neural tube defects, especially when taken very early in the pregnancy.

- Iodine aids in the development of the brain and the nervous system.

- Iron helps prevent low birth weight in the baby and anemia in the mother.

- Vitamins B and D assist with the growth of the baby's skeleton and nervous system. Adding vitamin C to the mix will help you and your baby better absorb iron from your diet.

Should You Be Taking Supplements?

All pregnant women are advised to take vitamin D, iron, and folic acid supplements. All the other vitamins you need should ideally come from your diet, especially if it's a healthy one. Some pregnant women, however, do need to supplement more than the three main vitamins as well.

Your doctor may recommend more supplements for you if:

- You're vegan/vegetarian and don't get enough vitamin B12.

- You can't get enough calcium from dairy or other calcium-rich foods.

- You lack iron.

- If you eat little to no seafood and aren't getting enough omega-3 fatty acids.

Multivitamins designed for pregnant women are a welcome addition to your new routine. Keep in mind that they don't serve as a replacement for a balanced diet. It's important to keep your diet healthy and nutrient-dense even if you're taking multivitamins.

Each vitamin is only slightly necessary for your body, and larger amounts are not always advised. Overindulging has negative effects. For instance, taking excessive amounts of vitamins A, C, or E can be harmful. So, there's no need to supplement those vitamins during pregnancy. You should also stay away from foods like liver and its byproducts because they're extremely high in vitamin A.

Diet

Everything you eat and drink while you're pregnant should support your health and provide the nutrients your unborn child needs to grow and develop. That means your diet should be balanced, nutrient-dense, and low in salt, sugar, and saturated fats.

Gaining weight during pregnancy is normal, but doing so at the expense of your health or the health of your baby puts you at greater risk of experiencing complications.

Your pre-pregnancy weight affects how much weight you can gain safely. There is evidence to support using BMI as a benchmark when determining the ideal weight gain during pregnancy.

A balanced diet is more than enough for you to get all the nutrients you need, but some foods have higher amounts of specific nutrients that are especially important during pregnancy.

We've done all this talking about a balanced diet, but we haven't specified exactly what that is.

What Constitutes a Balanced Diet?

A balanced diet is a wide variety of nutrient-dense foods from the five food groups, and lots and lots of water:

1. Fruit
2. Legumes and vegetables
3. Cereals and wholegrains
4. Dairy
5. Lean meats

Nobody's perfect. There'll be days where you're on your best behavior and eating all the right things, and there'll be days where you may treat yourself a little more than usual. Cravings will definitely make it harder to stay away from sugars and saturated fats.

There's an old theory that cravings are an indicator of vitamin deficiencies in a pregnant mother's diet. There isn't much evidence to support this because our tastes change so much when we're pregnant. We start to dislike things we liked and begin to like things we disliked.

With everything happening in our bodies and our hormones going haywire, we may also start to develop food aversions. If you experience unbearable morning sickness, eat whatever you can stomach and contact a medical professional if you start to get worried.

Which Foods Should I Avoid?

Some foods contain harmful bacteria or parasites that could contribute to serious difficulties for the unborn child and raise the possibility of miscarriage. Below is a list of the types of foods to avoid while pregnant:

Seafood High in Mercury

Seafood is pretty iffy. On the one hand, it's a great source of omega-3 fatty acids, which are amazing for a baby's brain development, and on the other, some forms of seafood have so much mercury in them that they could threaten your baby's nervous system.

The likelihood of a fish containing more mercury increases with size and age. The Food and Drug Administration (FDA) recommends that you stay away from:

- Tilefish
- Swordfish
- Shark
- Orange roughy
- Marlin
- King mackerel
- Bigeye tuna

Worry not; there is seafood out there with very small concentrations of mercury that is safe to eat and is a good source of protein. You can have two to three servings per week of:

- Trout
- Tilapia
- Shrimp

- Shad
- Sardines
- Salmon
- Pollock
- Pacific Oysters
- Light canned tuna
- Herring
- Cod
- Catfish
- Anchovies

Raw, Undercooked, or Contaminated Seafood

- Don't eat raw fish or shellfish. This includes ceviche, raw oysters, scallops, sashimi, sushi, and clams.

- Steer clear of raw, refrigerated seafood. This includes: nova-style seafood; lox; kippers; jerky; or smoked foods. You can have smoked seafood if it's part of another dish or if it's canned.

- Always look at fish advisories for your area, especially if you're eating local fish.

- Cook seafood thoroughly. Fish should be cooked to a temperature of 145°F. Consider your food cooked when it flakes and becomes opaque all throughout. Cook lobster, scallops, and shrimp until they are milky white. And oysters, mussels, and clams should be cooked until their shells open. Throw the ones that don't open away.

Undercooked Meat, Poultry, and Eggs

In order to avoid foodborne illness:

- Use a meat thermometer to make sure that everything is fully cooked and ready to eat.

- Avoid eating hot dogs and luncheon meats altogether, or cook them to a boiling temperature. They may be sources of listeria infections.

- Keep chilled pates and meat spreads to a minimum. Canned and shelf-stable spreads are okay.

- Eggs should be cooked until the yolks and whites are set because raw eggs contain potentially dangerous bacteria. Steer clear of anything made with partially cooked eggs. This includes wet batter, eggnog, hollandaise sauce, or Caesar salad dressing.

Unpasteurized Foods

Unpasteurized milk products can lead to foodborne illness. Soft cheeses like brie, blue cheese, and feta shouldn't be consumed unless they're prepared from pasteurized milk or are clearly labeled as such. Avoid unpasteurized juices too.

Low-fat dairy products are the safer option. This includes: cottage cheese, mozzarella, and skim milk.

Unwashed Fruits and Veggies

All raw fruits and vegetables should be thoroughly washed to get rid of any dangerous bacteria. Steer clear of raw sprouts. This includes: mung bean, alfalfa, clover, and radish. When you eat sprouts, ensure that they're properly cooked.

Food Prep

If ever there was a time to be fussy about food safety, it was during pregnancy. Do so prudently, because contaminated food is the leading cause of food poisoning. Sometimes it's easy to spot when food smells or looks different. But sometimes it's less obvious, so to be on the safe side, you should always:

- Defrost your meat in the microwave.
- Wash your hands before cooking and again before eating.
- Have separate cutting boards for meat and veggies.
- Change dishcloths often, because once there's a smell, it's probably contaminated.
- Cook and reheat your meat thoroughly; make sure it's at least 140°F and steaming when you reheat.

Recommended Serving Size

Food Group	Servings per Day
Fruit	2
Legumes and vegetables	5
Cereals and whole grains	8
Dairy	3.5
Lean meats	3.5

(Healthdirect Australia, 2022)

Medication During Pregnancy

A lot of medications say "Not safe for pregnant or lactating women" on the packaging, so it's hard for us to know what we can and can't take. Pregnant women are not typically used in drug studies because researchers are concerned about the effects on unborn babies. There are some medications that have been around for so long that doctors can attest to their safety for pregnant women.

It's generally safe to take the following:

Over-the-counter medication

- Acetaminophen for pain and fever (like Tylenol)
- Certain antihistamines, like loratadine and diphenhydramine (like Claritin and Benadryl)

Prescription medication

- Hypertension medication
- Asthma medication
- Antidepressants
- Penicillin and other antibiotics
- HIV medication

Speaking of medication, who better to advise you than your doctor? Let's look at your first visit with them and what that may be like.

First Antenatal Visit—What to Expect—Who Will I Meet?

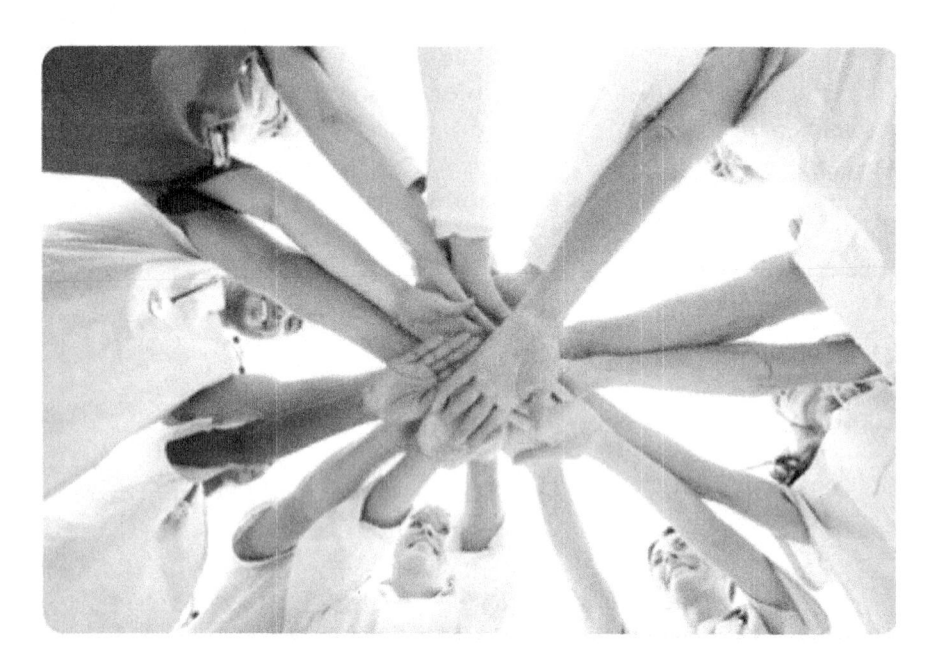

Your first visit is basically for you to find out how far along you actually are, and for your doctor to get to know about your medical history up until this point. The doctor will also run a series of standard tests just to make sure you and baby are okay.

Some things your doctor might ask about:

- Your gynecological history, any past pregnancies, and your last menstrual cycle.

- Your medical histories, both personal and familial.

- Exposure to potentially harmful substances.

- Any medication you're taking: pharmaceutical and homeopathic.

- Your lifestyle.

- Whether you've traveled in the last six months.

Your doctor will then perform a physical exam that includes a breast and pelvic exam. Depending on your general health, you might need tests of your thyroid, lungs, and heart. The doctor will also calculate your BMI to find out how much weight you need to gain for a safe pregnancy.

Then, in order to get your estimated due date, they will use the beginning of your last period, plus seven days, then go back three months. It will be roughly 40 weeks after the first day of your most recent period. Estimating the due date is important because it allows medical personnel to properly monitor your progress and the baby's growth.

Your due date doesn't necessarily indicate when you'll give birth. Very few women actually go into labor on their due date.

The blood tests your doctor may order include the following:

- A test to determine blood type
- A test to measure your hemoglobin
- A test to check your immunity levels
- A test to detect exposure to infection

Rh Factor: Why Will I Be Tested? What Happens if It's Positive?

Your blood type's Rh factor isn't an issue in general, but being Rh-negative is a problem if your baby is Rh-positive. Your body will produce antibodies that could harm your baby's red blood cells if your blood types mix. Your baby can get anemia and possibly develop other issues as a result of this.

Each person belongs to one of the four main blood types: A, B, AB, or O. The types of antigens on blood cells determine blood types.

Antigens are proteins located on the surface of blood cells that can trigger reactions in the immune system. The Rh factor is one of those proteins. Rh-positive individuals have the Rh factor, and Rh-negative people don't.

If you turn out to be Rh-negative while your baby is positive, the antibodies you produce can affect your baby. Your body may react as though you were allergic to the baby if a small amount of the baby's blood mixes with yours. As a result of your increased sensitivity, your antibodies are now able to cross the placenta and target the blood of your unborn child. Once they start to break the baby's red blood cells down, it leads to anemia. This specific type of anemia is called "hemolytic disease" or "hemolytic anemia." It has the potential to harm the fetus' brain, cause major illness, or kill them.

If you go for all your prenatal checkups and get all your blood tests; doctors can find this out in time and intervene. If your body hasn't yet produced the antibodies, the doctor can inject you with Rh immunoglobulin and prevent the development of antibodies.

If you've already developed them, Rh immunoglobulin is ineffective. All the doctors can do is closely monitor yours and the baby's conditions until you give birth. If the baby is delivered on time, they may receive a blood transfusion to replace the sick blood cells with healthy ones. In more extreme situations, the baby could need to be delivered early or get transfusions while still in utero.

Hepatitis B: Why Will I Be Tested?

An estimated 73,000 people contract the viral illness hepatitis B each year. It's carried by about 1,250,000 people in the United States. About 30% of those affected will not show symptoms, but symptoms include: (*Hepatitis B explained*, 2019)

- abdominal pain
- fatigue
- jaundice

- nausea
- vomiting
- reduced appetite

There is no treatment for it, so once you get it, you're infected for the rest of your life. It can lead to serious liver damage. Liver failure and liver cancer claim the lives of about 5,000 people annually.

Hepatitis B is spread through sexual activity, from mother to child, from contact with contaminated blood, and via IV drug use.

You can avoid it by abstain from unprotected sex, being in a monogamous relationship, and refraining from injecting narcotics. There is a vaccine, and that's by far the best way to prevent this illness.

Sickle Cell, Why Test?

Sickle cell disease is a congenital genetic disorder characterized by defective hemoglobin. It prevents the red blood cells' hemoglobin from carrying oxygen. Sickle cells have a propensity to cluster, obstructing tiny blood vessels and resulting in painful and detrimental complications. Children who inherit two sickle cell genes—one from each parent—get it. A person who has SCD can pass the trait on to their children.

Sickle cell trait is not a disease, but a gene that one inherits from a parent. SCT patients typically don't experience any SCD symptoms and have normal lives, but they can pass the sickle cell gene to their offspring as well.

As soon as a woman decides she'd like to get pregnant, she, along with her partner, should get tested for SCT. Most hospitals and medical facilities offer testing, as do many community-based organizations and regional health departments. A genetic counselor can offer further information and further explore the dangers to their children if a woman or her spouse has SCT.

What Are the Odds?

When both parents have SCT, there is a 25% probability that each pregnancy will result in a child with SCD.

When both parents have SCT, there is a 50% probability that each pregnancy will result in a child with SCT.

(CDC, n.d.)

Can a Woman Have SCD and a Healthy Pregnancy?

A woman with SCD can have a healthy pregnancy if she receives early prenatal care and has close supervision throughout her pregnancy.

Pregnant women with SCD are, however, more prone to experiencing issues that could harm both their health and the health of their unborn child. They should visit their obstetrician, hematologist, or general care physician frequently.

SCD can worsen during pregnancy, so the bouts of pain will be more frequent.

There's also a higher chance of preterm labor and low birth weight in babies born to pregnant women with SCD.

Your Baby's Development

POPPY SEED

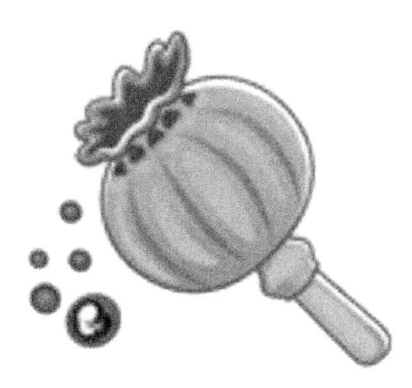

Assuming you've taken a pregnancy test because you've missed your period, you're four weeks along.

Four weeks? That probably doesn't sound right, because you likely conceived two or three weeks ago. We start measuring pregnancy from the first day of your last menstrual cycle, so technically, you're four weeks long.

Your body is starting to build the placenta and amniotic sac.

You may experience abdominal discomfort and sore breasts as the group of cells that will eventually form your baby penetrates the lining of your uterus. You may also experience some implantation bleeding. If you're not showing any symptoms, that's normal too.

Your baby is as tiny as a poppy seed at the moment. They are still a ball of cells, but they've managed to find a nice, comfy spot in your uterus and set up shop. After about 6–10 days, the ball starts dividing some more and ends up as two bundles of cells. The inner bundle of cells will become your baby, while the outer bundle will become the placenta. This is the time when your baby graduates from being a blastocyst to an embryo.

The embryo is tiny, but mighty. It has three layers that form the building blocks for your little baby:

- **The endoderm**: The innermost layer that will eventually become the liver, lungs, and digestive system.

- **The mesoderm**: The middle layer that will eventually become the heart, kidneys, bones, muscles, and sex organs.

- **The ectoderm**: The outermost layer that will eventually become the brain, skin, nervous system, eyes, and hair.

Judging by the amount of information here, a lot can happen in a month. Let's see what happens in the next one.

Chapter 2: Month Two

You've taken a pregnancy test, you've seen the positive sign, and now that it's confirmed...

You May Be Experiencing...

- **Fatigue**: During the first trimester of pregnancy, progesterone levels rise, which may cause you to feel sleepier or more exhausted than usual.

- **Frequent urination**: Your kidneys create extra fluid because they have to work harder during pregnancy since your blood volume increases. That means you'll be in the loo quite often.

- **Sensitive breasts**: Your breasts will most probably feel painful and uncomfortable when you first get pregnant. But this usually goes away as your body becomes used to the change in hormones.

- **Nausea and/or vomiting**: After a missed period, nausea is the most obvious sign of pregnancy. Some women only experience it within the first three months, others have it throughout the entire pregnancy.

- **Bloating**: Pregnancy hormones tend to make you feel bloated. You could mistake the bloating for a sign of PMS.

- **Cramping**: You may experience some uterine cramping due to all the changes in your hormonal balance.

- **Spotting**: Some women mistake spotting for a period, but it's lighter and is a good indicator that one is pregnant.

Prenatal Tests: Why They're So Important

Pregnancy is nine months of pure anticipation (and sometimes anxiety). You wake up every day wondering what your baby's going to look like, who they'll grow up to be, and most importantly, whether they'll come out with ten fingers and toes. The truth is, most babies are born healthy, but it's okay to be concerned. You have every right to do all that you can to find out whether your baby will be healthy and what steps you can take should you find out they won't be, and that's where prenatal testing comes in. The two main types are:

Screening tests: Many birth defects and genetic illnesses can be detected during prenatal screening tests. You'll also find out the likelihood of your baby having them. They come in the form of blood tests, a special ultrasound, and prenatal cell-free DNA screening. These tests are usually concluded by the second trimester. Keep in mind that they're unable to make a definitive diagnosis; they can just indicate risk. Should your doctor pick up any risk factors, you'll be scheduled for a diagnostic test as soon as possible.

Diagnostic tests: If you've had a screening test done and your age, family history, or medical history puts you at elevated risk of delivering a baby with a genetic condition, the only way to get a definitive diagnosis is via a diagnostic test. They can be invasive. The two main ones are amniocentesis and chorionic villus sampling. They have the potential to cause miscarriages.

Miscarriage

Another word for miscarriage is *spontaneous abortion*. The majority of miscarriages are unavoidable and happen when the fetus stops developing. These things happen, and nine times out of ten, they're out of our hands.

There are different types of miscarriage, namely:

Missed miscarriage: In these cases, the mother is usually unaware that a miscarriage has occurred. It can only be confirmed if the fetus is found to be without a heartbeat on an ultrasound.

Complete miscarriage: This one is obvious because there will be bleeding and the fetal tissue will pass through you. In this case, the pregnancy is completely over and your uterus is empty.

Threatened miscarriage: Your cervix remains closed, but you'll experience bleeding and have cramps in your pelvis. There usually aren't any further complications, and the pregnancy continues as normal. But for the remainder of your pregnancy, your obstetrician may keep a closer eye on you.

Inevitable miscarriage: Your cervix opens, you dilate, and you possibly leak blood and some amniotic fluid. There are high chances of miscarrying completely.

Recurrent miscarriage: Three successive miscarriages. It affects only 1% of expectant mothers.

Ectopic Pregnancy

Ectopic pregnancies usually occur in the fallopian tube; you may also know them as tubal pregnancies. But sometimes they happen in other parts of the body, like the abdominal cavity, the cervix, or the ovary. These types of pregnancies cannot develop properly because the fertilized egg can't survive anywhere other than the womb. If left untreated, the expanding tissue may result in a life-threatening hemorrhage.

Symptoms include:

- **Normal pregnancy symptoms**: In the beginning, there will be no warning signs. Everything will feel normal. A missed period, nausea, etc.

- **Vaginal bleeding and pelvic pain**: The initial warning signs are light vaginal bleeding and pelvic pain. Should your fallopian tube bleed, your shoulders could ache, and you may feel the need to urinate frequently. It all depends on which nerves become inflamed and where the blood gathers.

- **A ruptured tube**: The fallopian tube could burst if the fertilized egg is left there long enough to start growing. This then leads to bleeding in the abdomen and then lightheadedness, shock, and fainting.

Should you experience any or all of the above symptoms, contact your doctor immediately.

Multiples?

The only surefire way to know whether or not you're having multiples is via ultrasound, but there are some little telltale signs that might be clues that you've got more than one bun in the oven.

Several women who've been pregnant with twins say that even before they were certain, they had a hunch or felt they were. For others, the news comes as a great shock.

Here are some signs that seem to have popped up in lots of pregnancies:

- **Measuring ahead**: Although some women who are carrying twins claim to start showing earlier, the exact time depends on the individual and the pregnancy. Many women start to show sooner if it's their second pregnancy.

- **Increased weight gain**: Another warning sign that might not surface until later in your pregnancy. Weight gain in your first trimester of pregnancy is probably going to be minimal. If you notice rapid weight gain in the first trimester, contact your OB/GYN to discuss the possible reasons.

- **Early movement**: It's possible to feel movement a little bit earlier with two or more infants than with just one, but it's still likely to happen in the second trimester as well.

In 2018, there were 32.6 twins for every 1,000 live births, according to the CDC. The number of twin births each year is influenced by a wide range of factors. The likelihood of having twins can be increased by elements like genetics, age, and fertility treatments.

While having multiples is fantastic, there are certain risks involved. It's crucial to pay attention to your health and seek prenatal care.

Choosing Your Birth Plan

Labor and delivery seldom go according to plan, but it's normal to want some control over how you bring your child into this world. It's a really big deal, it's scary, and it's best to be as prepared as humanly possible.

A birth plan can help manage your expectations and pave the way for a seamless experience despite the overwhelming amount of decisions to be made.

Even though your plans may change as you go, mapping out your ideal labor and delivery will help you make important choices that will help your support team keep you and your unborn child safe and comfortable.

If you're unsure of your birth plan, here's a thorough list of questions that can nudge you in the right direction:

Environment

1. Do you want to give birth at home, in a hospital, or at a birthing center?

2. Would you like a specific kind of lighting?

3. Would you like photography or videography?

4. Would you like music playing in the room?

5. Would you like to be fully dressed?

People

1. Who will look after you while you are in labor?

2. Would you like a birthing coach?

3. Who is permitted to be present during the birth or to visit immediately after?

4. Would you allow medical students to be present if you gave birth in a teaching hospital?

Upon arrival

1. Would you prefer to have the hair on your pubic region shaved? Many hospitals no longer allow prenatal shaving, but it wouldn't hurt to ask.

2. What are your thoughts on getting an enema? Like shaving, they're no longer commonplace. But it wouldn't hurt to find out whether it's an expectation.

3. Are you okay with getting a routine IV?

4. Are you allowed to watch your cesarean section by mirror?

5. Would you like to eat and drink during labor? This all depends on your procedure and how everything goes on the day, but you can inquire about the policies.

Interventions

1. Would you like fetal monitoring?

2. What's your take on internal and external exams?

3. What are your feelings on induced labor and artificial membrane rupturing?

4. Is an episiotomy welcome or unwelcome?

5. Are you open to forceps and vacuum extraction?

6. Do you have any specific preferences or worries regarding having a C-section?

7. When or under what conditions would you think about having any of the above procedures?

Labor and delivery

1. Which type of pain management would you prefer—medical or natural?

2. Will you be active while giving birth? If so, how active?

3. Would you like a shower or a bath while in labor?

4. Is there a specific type of food you'd like during labor?

5. How long can you wait before cutting the umbilical cord?

6. Who would you like to cut the cord?

7. How soon and for how long will you and your partner be able to interact with the baby after birth?

8. How soon should you feed your baby after birth?

Postpartum

1. Will the baby remain in your care or in the nursery?

2. Where will your partner and other children stay while you're away?

3. Will you breastfeed or bottle-feed? Will you need assistance with either?

4. Will you consent to the baby having supplemental bottle-feeds?

5. Should you give the baby a pacifier?

6. Who will give the baby their first bath? Would you need help doing it?

7. Will you have the child circumcised? If so, when and by whom?

8. What are the rules of the NICU should your baby be admitted?

Going home

1. Will you be using a car seat?

2. Do you have pre-arranged transportation to get you home?

3. Should you prepare the first few family dinners in advance for when you get home?

4. Do you need a strategy for pet-proofing your baby's nursery or sleeping area?

5. Do you require company while you get settled at home?

Your Baby's Development

BEANS

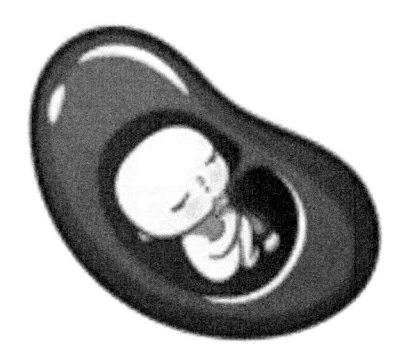

So, you may not be showing, but it's likely that your clothing is feeling a bit snug. That's because by month two, your uterus—which is typically the size of a fist—has expanded to the size of a giant grapefruit.

In the grand scheme of things, that's pretty small. So, even if you probably don't appear pregnant on the outside, you surely do on the inside.

By now, the baby is around 1/2 to 2/3 of an inch long and is about the size of a kidney bean. The baby is growing by a millimeter everyday and is developing its lips, nose, and eyelids.

The bulk of your baby is actually its head, where the brain is forming and building at an astonishing rate. The nerve cells are proliferating and connecting to create a neural network that will one day be able to pass messages from the brain to the body.

Your baby's limbs are bulking up and getting longer, thanks to their developing bones and cartilage. They're also close to developing joints, so there will eventually be elbows, shoulders, and knees to look forward to. The umbilical cord is starting to make an appearance, and get this, the intestines are inside it. They will migrate into the body when the time is right.

It's still early days, but things are getting serious. Now is a better time than any to try and start finding out if everything is going according to plan.

Chapter 3: Month Three

Emotions in Trimester One

Most of us will spend the majority of our pregnancies worrying, but nothing compares to the anxiety we might feel in the first trimester. Once month three is over, there's a bit of reprieve because that's known as the "safe zone," where the chance of miscarriage is significantly reduced.

Now, it's everything else as well. You worry about your future child's health, the delivery process, your connections with friends and family, how having a baby will impact those relationships, and the financial strain of adding to your family. These concerns are all reasonable, and a certain level of anxiety is actually protective for us. It's there to push us so we can see ourselves through different phases of our lives.

Coping With Mood Swings

Your fast-changing hormones, particularly estrogen and progesterone, are a major contributing factor to mood swings throughout pregnancy. In the first 12 weeks, your estrogen levels rise by more than 100 times.

Estrogen and serotonin (the *happy* hormone) go hand in hand. Even though serotonin boosts feelings of happiness, it's not a shortcut to happiness. So all the imbalances and variations in that neurotransmitter (serotonin) can lead to emotional dysregulation.

Progesterone levels also rise quickly, particularly in the first three months. Progesterone is linked to relaxation, whereas estrogen is linked to energy (and too much of it is linked to neurotic energy).

Relaxing hormones sound appealing, but some progesterone can cause *too much* relaxation. It can lead to lethargy and sometimes even feelings of sadness. It's actually what makes you cry at the sight of seemingly normal things. It's no wonder you're so up and down. You've got estrogen making you excitable and progesterone making you teary.

Should your mood swings become unmanageable or sway more towards feelings of depression, consult your GP or healthcare professional. Getting in front of it before it gets bad will really help. You can look for support groups in your area or online.

First Trimester Mood Swings

Besides hormones, the physical changes of pregnancy can cause emotional distress. The main one is nausea. The faintest hunger pangs or the aroma of food cooking can cause nausea and perhaps vomiting. The urge to puke at inopportune times may cause you to feel anxious.

You may also start to feel anxious because you don't know when you'll start to feel sick, and there's always the threat of passing out in public or without warning. Another symptom that contributes to mood swings is fatigue. When you're exhausted, it can be hard to function well emotionally, and because you'll experience extreme fatigue in the first couple of months, you're more likely to feel dysregulated a lot of the time.

Last but not least, women who have lost pregnancies before may worry that it'll happen again because of the higher chances of miscarriage in the first three months.

With all these changes happening, it's easy to feel like you're not in control of a lot of things. You may want to do some of the things you used to do—the things that could help you feel *normal*.

Grooming is one of those things. It's okay to wax, dye your hair, use fake tan, and get a massage as long as you do so safely. You might want to wait until you're at least in your second trimester before attempting these things.

So, what can't you do?

Botox: Is It Okay?

Botox is the brand name, despite the widespread misunderstanding that all cosmetic neurotoxins are Botox. There are other neurotoxins that are also injected to reduce wrinkles and fine lines in a similar way. They consist of Xeomin, Jeauveau, and Dysport.

Botox is classified as being in the pregnancy category X, which means it's unsafe to use while pregnant. When a drug or a treatment has dangers that far outweigh the benefits, the FDA classes it under X. There is also evidence of fetal abnormalities associated with Botox.

Since the risks far outweigh the benefits, it's best to reschedule your Botox appointment after you've given birth.

Despite our best efforts, we can never fully prepare for all of life's tiny surprises. What if you already had Botox and then discovered you were pregnant? Your initial reaction can be one of dread, which is understandable. No adverse effects have been documented in studies on pregnant women who received Botox injections before discovering they were pregnant. It's unlikely to cause problems because it has very limited bioavailability in the bloodstream. If you find yourself in this situation, you can breathe; it's unlikely that anything bad will happen, but you should contact your doctor just in case.

Your Baby's Development

LIME

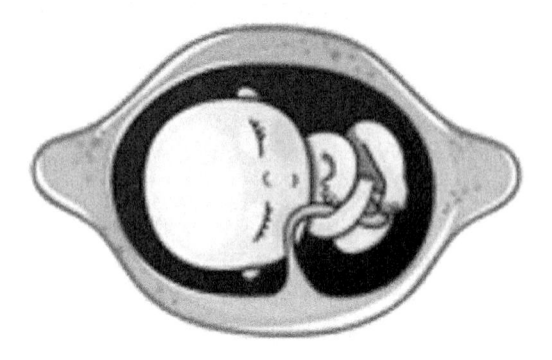

Your uterus, which is still roughly the size of a big grapefruit, starts to move from the bottom of your pelvis to the front and center of your abdomen.

If you're lucky, this will stop you from having to urinate all the time.

Some of the early pregnancy symptoms, like nausea, painful breasts and nipples, food aversions, and fatigue, are also expected to lessen considerably now that you're approaching the end of your first trimester. Your digestive system is starting to slow down now, so you'll absorb more nutrients, but you'll probably also experience bloating, gas, and constipation.

A lot has happened in the past month. Baby has doubled in size, measuring two to two and a quarter inches. The size of a small lime. All of the baby's vital organs and key body systems are fully formed. The brain structure is also complete, so brain matter will start to grow as the weeks' progress. The thyroid is fully functional, the pituitary gland has started producing hormones, and the pancreas is producing insulin. Lastly, a baby's bone marrow is starting to produce white blood cells to protect them against infection, and the muscles in their digestive tract are starting to contract so they'll be able to process food once they're born.

You should be able to hear your baby's heartbeat at your 12-week checkup, so you've got something really exciting to look forward to.

TRIMESTER 2: The Honeymoon Period

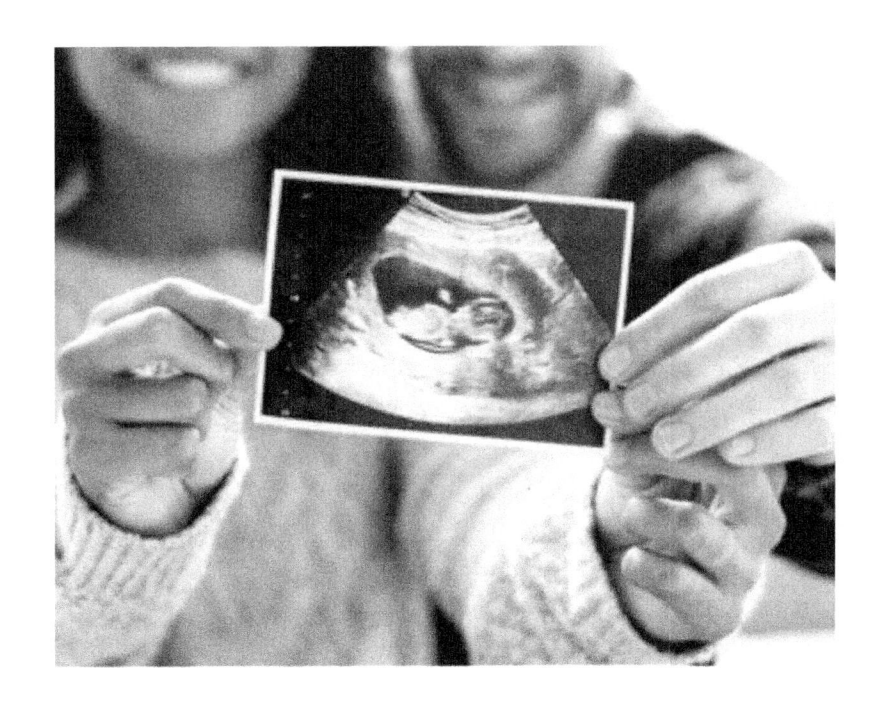

Chapter 4: Month Four

Emotions in the Second Trimester

The second trimester is often referred to as the "honeymoon" period. Although they are fluctuating far less than they were during the first three months, hormones are still fluctuating. Most women report having more energy and experiencing less morning sickness than before.

It's more comfortable, but it's not without its triggers. The main one being the changes in the body. In trimester one, you can get away with wearing your old clothes and essentially *hiding* your pregnancy. But in trimester two, you start to show, and you have to start considering maternity wear and sharing the news with people. Some women experience excitement at their physical changes. Some, though, may experience anxiety. This is especially true for women who've struggled with their body image.

Other emotional anguish you may experience could be due to prenatal testing throughout the second trimester. When recommended, amniocentesis is typically performed early in the second trimester. You could feel anxious while deciding whether to get tests done or not, and then start stressing over the results and what they might reveal.

It's not all negative, though. Some women report a spike in libido. This may be a result of their physical health beginning to improve as well as increased blood supply to the pelvic area.

Figuring Out Your Ideal Weight

We gain weight to ensure we have enough nutrients for the fetus' development and to store enough nutrients to get ready for breastfeeding. Weight gain is completely normal, and needed during pregnancy, but research has revealed that specific weight gain ranges depending on BMI have better overall effects on the expectant mom and her baby.

The rule of thumb is to gain one to four pounds in the first trimester and then a pound every week thereafter. This can be done by eating an extra 300 calories per day.

Here is the recommended weight gain range:

Pregnancy BMI	Category	Total Weight Gain Range	Total Weight Gain Range for Pregnancy with Twins
<18.5	Underweight	28–40 lbs	
18.5–24.9	Normal weight	25–35 lbs	37–54 lbs
25.0–29.9	Overweight	15–35 lbs	31–50 lbs
≥ 30	Obese	11–20 lbs	25–42 lbs

(*Pregnancy Weight Gain Calculator*, 2009)

Potential Complications of Suboptimal Weight Gain

Both inadequate and excessive weight gain during pregnancy have their drawbacks. Inadequate weight gain can endanger the fetus' health and result in preterm labor or premature birth. Excessive weight gain can complicate labor, result in larger than normal babies, cause postpartum weight retention, and raise the chance that you'll have an emergency C-section.

Heartburn

When you're pregnant, the rise in progesterone causes several parts of your body to relax, so the lower esophageal sphincter (LES) fails to close properly, and the acid is able to move up into your esophagus.

Other causes include:

- **Changes in hormone levels**: Throughout pregnancy, your hormone levels fluctuate, which impacts how you absorb and digest food. Your digestive tract slows down, then food moves slowly, resulting in bloating and heartburn.

- **Uterus enlargement**: Your uterus grows bigger as your child develops, so all the organs surrounding it (including the stomach) become constricted. This ends up forcing stomach acid into your esophagus.

For relief from heartburn, you can eat yogurt or drink milk. Warm your milk and add a teaspoon of honey to it.

Over-the-counter antacids tend to be high in salt, and that could make you retain water. Several of them also include aluminum, which is unsafe during pregnancy. A pregnancy-safe antacid can be suggested by your doctor.

How to Prevent Heartburn

There are steps you can take to prevent heartburn without harming your baby.

Dietary changes

- Instead of three big meals, spread your meals out throughout the day.

- Eat slowly.

- Don't drink with your meals, but between them.

- Steer clear of fried, hot, or greasy foods.
- Don't consume citrus fruits or juice.

Other tips
- Sit up straight while eating.
- Avoid eating after midnight.
- Don't lie down immediately after a meal.
- Keep the foot of your bed lower than the head of your bed, or put pillows under your shoulders.

Stretch Marks

Stretch marks are a normal side effect of your skin expanding to accommodate the growing baby and uterus. Depending on your skin color, they can either be red, purple, pink, or brown. They can develop on your breasts, tummy, arms, hips, thighs, and buttocks.

Not everyone gets them, but if they do appear during pregnancy, they eventually fade... but never really go away. If you get them, blame genetics and your mom.

On the upside, they serve as a constant reminder of your adorable child and a stamp of pride for all the labor that goes with being pregnant!

There isn't anything in particular that you can do to prevent them. Topical or exterior treatments aren't effective since they form deep within your skin, primarily in connective tissues. It's also largely out of your hands because hormones and heredity play a role.

There are some things you can do to lower the likelihood of developing stretch marks and/or lessen their visual impact. It's important to start these precautions before your tummy starts to grow and continue them throughout your pregnancy:

- Apply cream or lotion to your skin every day to keep it hydrated. Even if you don't see stretch marks, do it anyway; it helps with itching too.

- Drinking plenty of water will help you stay hydrated and keep your skin smooth and less susceptible to stretch marks.

- Avoid coffee when pregnant, as it may increase the likelihood of getting stretch marks.

- Maintain a nutritious and healthy diet. Skin health can be supported by a balanced diet high in protein, zinc, and vitamins A, C, and D.

To many, stretch marks are natural and beautiful, but we have to acknowledge that there are people who just don't like the look of them and want to be able to lessen their appearance. Here are some treatments that may minimize their appearance:

- **Creams**: The easiest and most cost-effective solution. Some creams contain ingredients like tretinoin and other retinoids, which are derived from vitamin A. These assist with collagen production on the skin's surface.

- **Light and laser therapy**: Similar to cream, light, and laser therapy can increase elasticity and stimulate the creation of collagen.

- **Hyaluronic acid, micro-needling, and microdermabrasion**: These are more invasive procedures that can also stimulate collagen production. Additionally, they minimize the appearance of stretch marks by helping them integrate with the surrounding skin. Applying hyaluronic acid to the skin everyday can also treat stretch marks.

Like with most medical procedures, talk to your doctor before attempting any of these.

Second Trimester Visits

Every time you see your doctor, they'll check your vitals (weight and blood pressure). Use your visits as a chance to express any concerns you might have. Besides looking out for your well-being, every visit is special because it's a chance for you to see the baby move and hear their heartbeat. Ideally, these moments should be shared with both parents, but it's not always possible. If the father has to miss out for some reason, invite a friend, your mom, or your sister to share in the celebration because every time you see your baby on the screen or hear their heartbeat, that is what it feels like.

With regards to the baby, your doctor will:

- **Assess fetal movement**: Try and take note of how much your baby's moving as soon as you start to feel flutters or kicks, and let your doctor know.

- **Listen to baby's heartbeat**: A Doppler device may be used to detect your baby's heartbeat. It perceives motion and then conveys it as sound.

- **Track baby's growth**: Size can be determined by measuring the distance between the pubic bone and the top of your uterus. This is called "fundal height." This measurement is in centimeters, and usually corresponds with the number of weeks you've been pregnant, give or take 2 cm, after 20 weeks of pregnancy.

Other tests you can look forward to:

- **Genetic tests**: These tests are conducted to check for chromosomal or genetic disorders like Down syndrome or spina bifida. Should your results be a cause for concern, your doctor will suggest an amniocentesis.

- **Fetal ultrasounds**: Imaging that allows you to see images of a developing baby inside the womb using high-frequency sound waves. A thorough ultrasound can assist your doctor in assessing the fetal anatomy, and give you a chance to learn the baby's gender.

- **Blood tests**: Between weeks 24 and 28, you might get tested to ascertain your blood count, iron levels, and to check for gestational diabetes. You may also need a test to look for Rh-antibodies if you've got Rh-negative blood. It's a genetic condition that refers to a particular protein located on the surface of red blood cells. If your baby's blood is Rh-positive and it mixes with yours, antibodies can form. Without treatment, the antibodies can cross the placenta and destroy the developing baby's red blood cells.

You're getting to a stage in your pregnancy where you're almost *settled in*. You've had a couple of doctor's visits, you're feeling a little better, and this is around the time you'll potentially start to show. It's time to start thinking about how and when to let people know.

Making the Announcement: When Is the Best Time?

Pregnancy has many milestones, but a really important one is sharing the news with friends and family. There's always the possibility that you could run into problems early on in the pregnancy, so choosing when to share the news is a delicate thing. Different moms are ultimately going to decide what's best for them and when to share, but there are a few things to consider.

A lot of couples prefer to postpone the announcement until after the first trimester. This is because miscarriages generally occur in the first 12 weeks.

There are some mothers, however, who choose to share the news early because they've had miscarriages before and prefer to have the support of friends and family should it happen again.

These are some of the milestones you should hit before announcing:

- First ultrasound

- Baby bump development

- First anatomy scan

You should feel supported regardless of when you decide to announce your pregnancy. Whether you're expecting your first or fourth child, being pregnant can be a difficult journey. Always discuss any worries you have with your doctor, who may then direct you to a local support group where you can meet other expectant moms in person.

Worker Rights: Should I Tell My Boss?

Women make up 50% of the labor market, and 85% of them will have children throughout their working years. Despite this, finding the ideal time and way to let your employer know you're expecting is daunting. It can get pretty convoluted because letting them know right away seems like the professional thing to do, but doing that might end with you being passed up for opportunities. Your professional growth and the likelihood of receiving raises and promotions may be impacted by your sharing as well.

What Are My Rights and the Legal Requirements for Notice?

When to reveal your pregnancy is not subject to any legal requirements. All you need to do is ask for leave at least 30 days before your planned delivery date if your firm is covered by the Family and Medical Leave Act.

That said, it would be wiser to disclose earlier because women who conceal their pregnancies for extended periods have been found to experience more anxiety while engaging with coworkers than their counterparts who are upfront about it.

I'd suggest letting your employer know towards the end of the first trimester, because your chances of miscarriage are lower, and you may start showing at this time. This way, there'll be enough time to discuss your absence and develop a suitable transition plan for your replacement. There are times when it's necessary to reveal your pregnancy sooner, like if you get sick often and need to schedule doctor visits more frequently.

Also, you have legal protection against discrimination: Pregnancy-based discrimination is illegal under the Pregnancy Discrimination Act (PDA). It prohibits it in all areas of work, including hiring, firing, salary, job assignments, promotions, layoffs, training, and fringe benefits like leave and health insurance.

Even though the law protects us, discrimination still happens. In the last ten years, more than 50,000 accusations of pregnancy discrimination have been leveled against employers.

If you believe you're being victimized, there are steps you can take, like reporting any incidents to the Equal Employment Opportunity Commission and Fair Employment Practices Agencies.

With work sorted, there are things at home that need tending to.

Your Sex Life in Trimesters Two and Three

Some couples believe that sexual activity during pregnancy raises the possibility of miscarriage. But, unless your doctor or midwife has specifically advised against it, it's completely safe.

Sex in the Second Trimester

Throughout the second trimester, women's sexual preferences and habits change. Couples may discover that they revive their sex life at this point in the pregnancy because the expectant mom might be embracing the changes in her body. This could lead to an increase in libido.

But for a lot of couples, it's the opposite. They experience what's called a "five-month crisis." This might happen because some women tend to withdraw into themselves, which makes their partners feel isolated.

Some couples opt to abstain when pregnant because they don't feel comfortable. Despite not engaging in direct sexual activity, they employ various strategies to feel sexually satisfied in their relationship.

Sex in the Third Trimester

Even in the third trimester, your partner will still be very interested in sex, but naturally, there will be a decline in activity because of discomfort. Many women in their third trimester worry that orgasms will cause their uteri to contract. Some also start to feel less attractive, become less willing to engage, and then start to feel anxious about their partners' sexual gratification.

A good compromise for a lot of couples is rear or side entry positions as opposed to the ones that need anybody to be on top.

Potential Risks and When to Avoid Sex in Pregnancy

Sexual activity may increase your chance of developing an infection or bleeding before giving birth if you have a placenta praevia.

Penetrative sex should be avoided while pregnant if:

- You have placenta previa.
- You're bleeding heavily.
- Your waters' broken.
- You have cervical issues.
- You're having multiples or are very late in your pregnancy.

Should you or your partner be engaging in sexual activity outside of the relationship, always use condoms to prevent yourself or your unborn child from contracting any STDs.

Depression During Pregnancy

We've all heard about postpartum depression, but have you heard about antenatal depression?

We go through so many emotions while we're pregnant. Most are positive, but according to research, roughly 7% of pregnant women experience depression (Mayo Clinic, 2019).

Depression is the most common mental illness, and it affects women more than it does men, especially during our reproductive years.

Sometimes It Goes Unnoticed

The symptoms of depression can be mistaken for normal pregnancy symptoms because they're so similar. Low energy levels, increased sleeping time, and changes in appetite. It's very easy for your doctor to miss.

We're in the 21st century, but there's still a stigma attached to depression, so some women may be hesitant to discuss changes in their mood during pregnancy with their doctors. Also, there is a propensity to prioritize a woman's physical health during pregnancy over her mental health.

Risk Factors
- Anxiety
- Stress
- Prior depression
- Inadequate emotional support
- Unplanned pregnancy
- Intimate partner violence

Signs and Symptoms

- Extreme anxiety regarding your baby
- Low self-esteem, and feeling like you won't be a good parent
- Not enjoying activities you once did
- Being unresponsive to reassurance
- Not complying with prenatal care
- Using drugs
- Poor weight gain due to insufficient diet
- Suicidal thoughts

Treatment Options

Untreated depression may lead to you not being receptive to prenatal care, eating the nutritious meals your baby needs, or having the motivation to take care of yourself. Moreover, you are more likely to have postpartum depression and trouble bonding with your child in the future.

Your options are psychotherapy or medication like antidepressants; this all depends on the severity of your depression.

Your Baby's Development

TOMATO

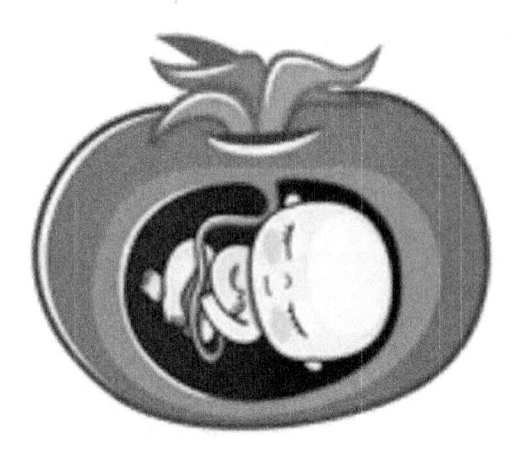

This is the start of the *honeymoon period*. Your uterus is expanding very quickly, roughly at the same rate as your baby, and it's moving higher up into your abdominal cavity, so you may start to notice your belly becoming a little pudge.

In contrast to trimester one, you are probably feeling more energized and somewhat "normal." It's around this time that you'll be a lot more peckish, and eating more means more gas, indigestion, and bloating.

Baby is around 4–5 inches in length and weighs around three ounces. Roughly the size of a tomato. They're also starting to gain a bit of muscle mass and back muscles, so their body will start to straighten out more and look less bean-like.

Due to the increase in muscles, they can actually make facial expressions. Baby's eyes are no longer on the sides of their heads, and they have eyelashes and brows.

Baby's heart is working really hard, pumping about 25 quarts of blood everyday.

Chapter 5: Month Five

Fetal Movements

Monitoring your unborn child's movement is an excellent idea, especially during the third trimester. This way, you can alert your doctor for further investigation if you feel a decrease in movement.

When Does It Start?

Some people refer to those initial, fluttery sensations as "quickening." You might feel something initially, and then question whether you actually did, because those early movements may feel like bubbles or like a gentle flutter. Some people even mistake them for gas.

You will start feeling movement in your second trimester. It can start anywhere between 16 and 22 weeks, but if it's your first pregnancy, it can happen later on—possibly between 20 and 22 weeks. If you've been pregnant before, you might be more aware of them a little earlier, possibly at the 16-week mark. Every pregnancy is different, though, and there's no specific time to feel movement.

What's It Like in the Second Trimester?

During the second trimester, your baby's movements can be a little erratic. It will start off with the flutters, and then the actual fetal movements will start to happen a little more regularly and intensely because the baby's warming up for the Olympics. Eventually, you may start to feel some stretches and possibly even some punches and kicks as your baby grows, and its movements become more intense.

What's It Like in the Third Trimester?

You might begin to recognize certain patterns in your baby's movements at some point during this final trimester. Maybe there are specific hours of the day or night when he/she is more active.

The movements will become bigger and more forceful, and occasionally you might feel a particularly ferocious kick or punch. If your baby is moving beneath your skin, you might be able to see it.

Unfortunately, by this time, your baby is beginning to run out of room to move about. But that just means they're becoming stronger, gaining weight, and gaining some of that healthy baby fat. Since the baby can't stretch and move around as freely, they may start to move less, but you should still feel some sort of movement. If you become worried, your doctor might suggest a kick count.

Kick Count

You choose a time of day and count how many times your baby kicks or moves throughout that period. It's also called a "fetal movement count" (FMC). There are apps you can download to keep track of things.

For the most accurate comparison, it's best to perform a kick count at the same time every day. Keep an eye on the baby's movement and time how long it takes to get to ten kicks.

Try having a snack, shifting positions, and then continuing your count for another hour if your baby doesn't kick, wriggle, or poke you ten times in that period. You can stop the count if you get to 10 before the second hour is up.

So if you keep track of your baby's kicks and notice a day when they stop, tell your doctor as soon as you can.

What Causes a Decrease in Movement?

There are many reasons why your baby's movements might slow down. Most of them aren't alarming, but sometimes not feeling your baby kick could be an indication that something's wrong. If you see a dramatic decrease in activity over several hours, you should call your doctor.

Benign causes:

- Your baby is too little for you to feel anything. This is normal early on in the second trimester.

- You engaged in sexual activity. After intercourse, some babies become more active and others become less active. Your baby may fall asleep if you reach orgasm or because of the sexual motions. It can go either way in both the second and third trimesters.

- You've been physically active. If you move around a lot, your baby may fall asleep, or you might be too busy moving around to notice anything that's going on with the baby.

- Your baby has dozed off. Babies normally sleep for 20- to 45-minute intervals all throughout the day. They can spend up to 95% of their time asleep by 38 weeks of gestation.

- Your baby's too big to be mobile. As your due date draws near, your baby is approaching their birth weight and size.

- Your baby's preparing for birth. They may be less active if their head has sunk into the pelvis in preparation for delivery.

How to Increase Movement

If you're feeling uneasy and want to encourage your baby to say hello, here are some things you can do to get them moving:

- Move around.

- Have a snack or a sugary beverage, like orange juice.

- Speak to your baby.

- Light up your tummy with a flashlight.

- Try to feel your baby in your belly by pushing or poking at it gently.

Once your baby starts kicking, you'll probably start to look forward to it, and it'll be the highlight of most of your days. On the other hand, the kicking might keep you awake at times.

Trouble Sleeping?

Sleep can be so elusive during pregnancy. You start off sleeping all the time and end up hardly getting any at all. Many sleep issues are caused by physical discomfort, hormonal changes, excitement, and worry related to becoming a new mother. In fact, it's estimated that at least half of pregnant women have trouble sleeping.

Sleep is a really important part of prenatal care, but it escapes many of us. Let's delve into sleeping issues, the best sleeping positions, and some tips on how to maximize your sleep during pregnancy.

Common Sleep Disorders and Problems During Pregnancy

- **Obstructive sleep apnea**

    Many women start to snore once they fall pregnant because of weight gain and nasal congestion. Should you experience snoring, gasping, and periodic breathing pauses that impair sleep quality, you've developed obstructive sleep apnea. It can obstruct the flow of oxygen to your fetus and raise the risk of preeclampsia, gestational diabetes, and C-sections. It is estimated that one in five pregnant women experiences this, so consult your doctor if you notice any signs.

- **Gastroesophageal reflux disorder**

    GERD for short. It's like ongoing acid reflux, and it can really affect your sleep across all trimesters. It affects about half of pregnant women in the third trimester and a quarter in the first. If left untreated, it can damage the esophagus.

- **Restless leg syndrome**

    People with RLS have uncontrollable urges to move their legs due to sensations that are best described as crawling, tickling, or itching. The symptoms tend to be more severe when one is at rest, and that makes it difficult to fall asleep. Up to a third of pregnant women may get RLS during the third trimester.

Why Is Sleep Such a Big Deal?

Getting quality sleep is crucial for both mom and baby. Sleepless nights eventually result in exhaustion and daytime sleepiness. Sleep aids memory, learning, appetite, mood, and decision-making—all of which are imperatives while getting ready to welcome a newborn home.

Your immune system suffers when you're deprived of quality sleep on a regular basis. It's why sleep has such a profound effect on maternal and fetal health. Sleep also helps manage your blood sugar, so if you're not getting enough, you run the risk of developing gestational diabetes.

Women with unbalanced sleeping patterns in early pregnancy are prone to developing high blood pressure in their third trimester. This can lead to preeclampsia, which in turn raises your risk of preterm delivery and long-term complications for the kidneys, heart, and other organs.

There is new evidence that poor sleep during pregnancy is a precursor to babies with sleep problems who cry incessantly.

Treatment for Pregnancy-Related Sleep Issues

There are several methods for reducing sleep issues without needing medication. The key to having better sleep is controlling pregnancy-related sleep disturbances and practicing good sleep hygiene. Try some of these methods before opting for medication.

Best Sleeping Positions

The ideal position is on your left side with your legs slightly curled. This way, your baby's oxygen and nutrients are distributed nicely, and there's more blood flow to the uterus, heart, and kidneys. The right side is okay too; it's just not as ideal.

If you're not used to sleeping on your side, you can use a couple of extra pillows to help you feel comfortable. If you'd like to ease pressure on your lower back, put a lightweight pillow between your knees or tuck a wedge pillow under your tummy for support. Body pillows are also really good and less complicated to navigate.

Sleeping on your back can give you back pain and put a strain on your vena cava as the uterus expands. It's one of your main veins, so if it's obstructed, you could start to feel lightheaded. You're not expected to avoid sleeping on your back altogether; you can do it in short bouts. Just try your best to avoid it as much as humanly possible.

Once your belly grows past a certain point, it will be impossible to sleep on your tummy.

Sleep Hygiene

The following practices may help minimize insomnia and enhance overall sleep quality:

- Maintain a calm, quiet, dark bedroom, and only use the bed for sleeping and sexual activity.

- Make sleep a priority, maintain a regular bedtime, and plan naps earlier in the day to avoid disturbing your nocturnal sleep.

- Prepare your body for sleep by reading a book, taking a bath, or engaging in another activity you find peaceful.

- Consider getting a nightlight to make those nighttime bathroom breaks easier to navigate.

- To lower your risk of GERD, stay away from coffee, spicy foods, and big meals too close to bedtime.

- Turn off all screens at least an hour before bedtime and avoid bringing electronics into the bedroom.

- Workout regularly, and try to do so earlier in the day.

- While it's important to stay hydrated throughout the day, cutting back on liquids a couple of hours before bed will help you avoid nighttime trips to the bathroom.

- If you have trouble falling asleep, get up and do something else until you're tired.

- If you're feeling stressed, seek help from your partner, friends, or doctor. You may also find it helpful to get a journal you can jot your thoughts down in before bed.

Oral Health Conditions During Pregnancy

- Hormonal changes that intensify the body's response to microorganisms in the gum tissue can cause gingivitis.

- Cavities can develop as a result of dietary changes, like increased snacking, which increases mouth acidity. They can also come from vomiting, dry mouth, or poor oral hygiene brought on by nausea and vomiting.

- Pyogenic granuloma, or granuloma gravidarum, is a spherical growth that typically has a thin cord of tissue connecting it to the gingiva. It may form as a result of hormonal changes.

- Due to all the vomiting, erosion could occur. Avoid brushing the teeth immediately after vomiting, because the teeth can become exposed to stomach acids. To neutralize the acid, rinse with a water and baking soda solution. You can make it with 1 cup of water and a spoonful of baking soda.

Good daily oral hygiene is so important because you're at an increased risk of getting gingivitis and developing cavities. Brush twice daily with a soft-bristle toothbrush and fluoride toothpaste. Flossing would be helpful too.

High Blood Pressure and Preeclampsia

Gestational hypertension develops when a woman experiences high blood pressure during pregnancy without any other cardiac or kidney issues, or protein in the urine. It's usually discovered after 20 weeks of pregnancy or just before delivery. It normally subsides once you give birth, but some women are more likely to develop chronic hypertension.

Preeclampsia is basically gestational hypertension paired with proteinuria. Proteinuria is the presence of protein in the urine, which can be a sign that there is some kidney damage and, in some cases, multiple organ damage.

In the US, preeclampsia affects roughly one in every 25 pregnancies. Once a woman starts experiencing seizures, her condition worsens, and she develops eclampsia, which is a medical emergency.

Symptoms include:

- Difficulty breathing
- Unusual weight gain

- Nausea and vomiting
- Pain in the upper stomach
- Face and hand swelling
- Cloudy vision, seeing spots, or experiencing changes in eyesight
- Persistent headaches

Preeclampsia can set in after birth. It's called "postpartum preeclampsia." The symptoms are the same, and it can happen to women who didn't experience preeclampsia while pregnant. Your healthcare team can usually tell if it's happening a couple of days after birth, but sometimes it can take up to six weeks to manifest.

If you experience symptoms, call 911 right away or inform your healthcare professional. You might need immediate medical attention.

Gestational Diabetes

Gestational diabetes is diagnosed during pregnancy. It's the same as other forms of diabetes in the sense that it affects your blood sugar. Elevated blood sugar can be harmful to you and your baby.

You can manage it by eating well, working out, and taking medication if necessary. If you have it during pregnancy, your blood sugar should go back to normal very soon after delivery. You would, however, be at risk of developing type 2 diabetes and have to undergo testing more often.

Gestational diabetes has no apparent indications or symptoms apart from increased thirst and more frequent urination. You will most likely find out through testing, as that's part of your prenatal care.

Causes

It's still unknown why some women develop gestational diabetes and others don't. Weight gain is usually the main suspect, though.

Normally, your hormones control your blood sugar levels. So when you're pregnant and your hormones are out of whack, your body has a tougher time effectively processing the sugar in your blood. This causes a spike in your blood glucose levels.

Risk Factors

- Overweight/obesity
- Not engaging in physical activity
- Being pre-diabetic
- Having Polycystic Ovary Syndrome (POCS)
- Having immediate family with diabetes
- Having delivered a baby over 9 lbs in the past
- Ethnicity. Namely: Asian American, American Indian, African American, Hispanic

Complications

- **Breathing difficulties**: Early babies may develop respiratory distress syndrome, which makes breathing extremely hard for them.
- **C-section**: Uncontrolled diabetes increases a woman's likelihood of needing a C-section to deliver the baby.
- **High birth weight**: Your baby may become too big if your blood sugar levels are above the recommended range. Babies

who weigh 9 pounds or more are more likely to experience delivery injuries, become trapped in the birth canal, or require a C-section.

- **Hypoglycemia**: Some babies born to moms with GD can suffer hypoglycemia just after birth. Their low blood sugar may lead to them experiencing seizures. The baby's blood sugar level can be brought back to normal by early feedings and, occasionally, an intravenous glucose solution.

- **Obesity and type 2 diabetes**: Babies born to moms with GD may experience obesity or type 2 diabetes later in life.

- **Preterm birth**: Moms with diabetes are more likely to experience preterm labor, especially if the baby is already very big.

- **Stillbirth**: If left untreated, gestational diabetes can lead to the baby's passing away either before birth or soon after.

Prevention

- Eat nutritious food
- Be physically active
- Start your pregnancy off at a healthy weight
- Avoid gaining more weight than is advised
- Attend all antenatal checkups

Anemia

When you're iron deficient, your red blood cells aren't healthy enough to carry enough oxygen to your body's tissues. Your body needs more iron when you are pregnant because of the increased blood volume. If your iron levels are insufficient and you don't supplement, you could develop anemia.

Risk Factors

- Having two consecutive pregnancies
- Expecting multiples
- Frequent vomiting
- Having insufficient iron in your diet
- Heavy menstrual flow before pregnancy
- A history of anemia

Symptoms

- Headache
- Pale skin
- Difficulty breathing
- Craving ice (PICA)
- Dizziness
- Weakness
- Fatigue

Symptoms of severe anemia:

- Low blood pressure
- Rapid heartbeat

- Trouble concentrating

Treatment and Prevention

Iron is usually present in prenatal vitamins, but in some instances, your medical practitioner may advise you to take an additional iron supplement. You need at least 27 milligrams of iron per day while you're pregnant.

Maintaining a healthy diet that includes iron-rich foods helps a lot. You can get iron from fish, poultry, or lean red meat. You can also get it from breakfast cereals, leafy green veggies, peas, or dried beans.

Your body absorbs iron from meat and other animal products a lot easier. So if you're a vegetarian or if you're opting to get your iron from non-animal products, combine them with other elements high in vitamin C. You can use juices like tomato and orange or have some strawberries on the side. Refrain from drinking fruit juices that have been fortified with calcium because they make it harder to absorb iron.

Skin Discoloration

Most of the changes that happen to your skin are harmless, but some could irritate you and cause you discomfort. Here are some changes you can anticipate and some advice on when to consult your midwife or doctor:

- changes in skin tone (pigmentation), like darkening of the neck, inner thighs, breasts, nipples, and parts of the face

- moles, freckles, and birthmarks becoming more pigmented

- blemishes or acne

- varicose veins

- spider veins

- skin tags
- crimson or darkened palms
- skin sensitivity
- itchy skin

Pregnancy-related skin changes are harmless to both you and your unborn child.

Skin issues might occasionally be an indication of an underlying condition that a doctor should examine. Keep in mind that these illnesses are quite rare:

- **Intrahepatic cholestasis**

Almost everybody itches during pregnancy, but a small percentage of women struggle with severe itching due to a liver condition called "intrahepatic cholestasis." Your body begins to accumulate bile acids as a result of the illness.

There's no visible rash, and you might notice that the itching is more pronounced on the soles of your feet and palms of your hands. It's usually worse at night. Thankfully, things tend to improve shortly after delivery.

See your doctor or midwife if you are experiencing these symptoms so they can order some blood tests to determine how well your liver is functioning.

To stop the itching, your doctor may recommend lotions or medications.

- **Pemphigoid gestationis**

A rare illness that causes an itchy rash that turns into blisters during pregnancy.

This occurs when your body mounts an immunological reaction, which may be brought on by tiny amounts of placental material getting into your bloodstream. It usually happens in the second and third trimesters.

It's crucial to see your doctor or midwife if you get an itchy rash, because the itching can be lessened, and sore regions soothed with lotions and ointments they prescribe.

If you observe any changes in the color, size, form, or thickness of a mole or birthmark, always talk to a doctor.

Why Does Your Skin Get Darker?

Your skin will get darker during pregnancy. It might be all over, or it might be in little patches. You may also observe the following:

- Dark patches on your face (pigmentation). This is referred to as melasma or the pregnant mask. Hormonal changes that occur may cause melasma by temporarily increasing the amount of melanin your body generates. It is estimated that this happens to up to 75% of expectant mothers (*Melasma: Treatment, Causes & Prevention*, 2020).

- Your neck, inner thighs, genitalia, and areolas turn darker.

- Your birthmarks, moles, freckles, and recent scars start to darken.

- The region surrounding your belly button, as well as your armpits and inner thighs, may darken if you have brown or black skin. After birth, these areas will gradually become lighter again, but some may remain a little darker than before.

Your patches might become darker in the sun, making them more visible. Wear a wide-brimmed hat outside, use sunscreen with an SPF of 50 or higher, and try to stay as much as you can in the shade to protect your skin.

It's normal to feel self-conscious about your patches, but they will probably go away within a year of the birth of your child. Concealer, foundation, and tinted moisturizer can all help even out your skin tone in the interim.

After the birth of their children, one in ten mothers discovers that their black spots persist. If this is the case, your doctor may suggest some treatment options.

What is the Dark Line Running Up Your Bump?

Linea nigra is the scientific term for the vertical line that runs down the center of your belly. Normally, it extends from the top of your pubic bone to the center of your belly, but it can occasionally cross over to end just below your breastbone.

It starts to show in the second trimester, and it's a normal aspect of pregnancy. But if you don't get one, it's not a cause for concern.

It's located on the abdominal muscles, so it expands and widens as your baby grows, but it's just due to hormone-related pigmentation.

Once you give birth, it starts to disappear and should be gone within a few months.

Does Pregnancy Glow Exist?

There are some upsides to all the changes happening in your body, you get a luminous, slightly flushed glow that makes you look so good during pregnancy. It's due to fluctuating hormone levels, increased sebum (oil) production, and increased blood flow throughout your body.

The only drawback is that when your body retains moisture, your legs and ankles may swell. Also, if you have any spots on your face, neck, or chest, the blood flow to your skin may make them more obvious. Like most things, a few months after giving birth, these things will stop happening.

Drinking plenty of water can really aid your body in eliminating extra water. Maintaining good hydration will also be amazing for your skin.

Why Are My Veins More Pronounced on My Cheek?

- Acne: It results in broken blood vessels, often known as "spider veins." When they are swollen or dilated just beneath the surface of your skin, you get tiny, red lines that spread out into the shape of a web.

- Rosacea: This condition results in swollen veins that cause the skin to flush and turn red. Spider veins are usually present in people with rosacea.

How Can I Look After My Skin?

- Avoid over-cleansing because this can make your skin dry. Use a fragrance-free makeup remover or gentle soap to wash your face twice daily. This will be plenty to keep your skin clear and young-looking.

- Go for pore-clearing water-based solutions rather than oil-based ones. Search for products with the designations "noncomedogenic" or "pH-balanced."

- Avoid picking or squeezing your pimples to prevent scarring on your skin.

- Use acne creams and treatments only on your doctor's recommendation. Certain acne remedies should not be used during pregnancy because they could harm the developing fetus.

- Keep up a balanced diet.

Your Baby's Development

MANGOSTEEN

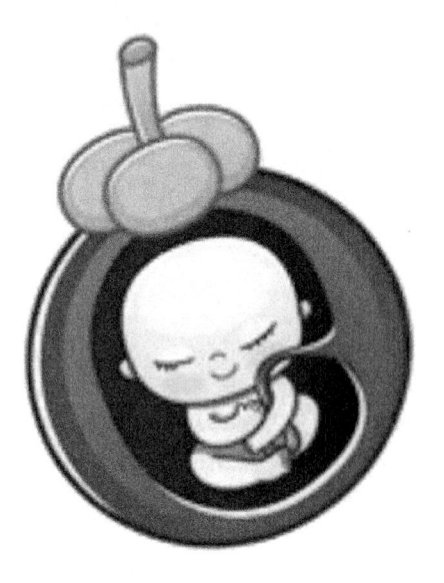

You are officially halfway through your pregnancy at 20 weeks along! Take a deep breath if you're not too congested to do so. Your hormones are working in your favor this month, as they're triggering an uptick in circulation. This means your nails will grow faster, and your hair will be thicker and longer.

Baby measures 6.5 inches long and weighs about 10 ounces, like a mangosteen. If you haven't already found out the baby's gender, now would be as good a time as any.

If you're carrying a boy, his testicles have developed in his abdomen this month and will begin to descend into the scrotum. If you're carrying a girl, her genitals may not be as clear on an ultrasound, but they're there, and her vaginal canal is slowly developing. She's got a fully formed uterus and ovaries with millions of eggs inside.

This is a really nice time for baby in the pregnancy because there's still lots of space to move around. Speaking of kicking, if you haven't felt any yet, it should start soon.

Chapter 6: Month Six

This is quite a good month for most women. You're relatively far along in the pregnancy, but you're not experiencing extreme discomfort like you would in trimester three. Your baby bump is probably nice and round now, and you may love the look of your cute belly.

Something that couples enjoy doing is having a babymoon—one last holiday to connect as a couple before the baby comes. It takes a bit of extra planning, though, because you're carrying precious cargo.

Is It Safe to Travel By Air?

A lot of women travel while pregnant, but it's still important to consider any issues that can arise when traveling abroad. Moreover, consider how you would access high-quality medical care in the nations you are visiting. Instead of waiting to get the necessary vaccinations while pregnant, get them all before.

According to the American College of Obstetricians and Gynecologists, the safest time to travel is in the second trimester—between 14 and 28 weeks—because it's when you feel your best. Moreover, your chance of spontaneous abortion and early labor is at its lowest. It's advised that you stay within a 300-mile radius of your home during the third trimester, or from 25 to 40 weeks. This is due to issues like phlebitis, elevated blood pressure, and false or preterm labor. For domestic flights, women are often prohibited from flying after 36 weeks, and for international flights, after 28 to 35 weeks. But the final decision should be between you and your doctor or midwife.

There are a few conditions under which you are likely to be prohibited from flying to countries with pre-travel vaccines:

- Incompetent cervix

- Pregnant with multiples

- History of early labor or early membrane rupture

- Cardiomyopathy or congestive heart failure
- Severe anemia
- History of blood clots
- Gereatric pregnancy
- Prior reproductive issues or difficulties getting pregnant
- History of toxemia, hypertension, or diabetes during any pregnancy
- Past or present placental anomalies
- History of ectopic pregnancy or miscarriage
- Threatened miscarriage or vaginal bleeding

Tips for Traveling While Pregnant

- Prior to your trip, try to prepare for any problems or emergencies that might arise. Verify that your health insurance is still in effect while you're traveling. In the event that you give birth while away, make sure the plan will cover your child as well. Consider getting supplementary travel and medical evacuation insurance.

- Look into the local hospitals before you go. Women who are in their third trimester of pregnancy should seek out facilities that can handle cesarean sections, toxemia, and other pregnancy-related problems.

- Make arrangements for prenatal care in advance if you'll need it while traveling.

- Know your blood type and confirm the places you'll be visiting to screen blood for hepatitis B and HIV.

- Verify that safe foods and drinks like pasteurized milk and bottled water are available where you're going.

- When traveling by air, request an aisle seat at the bulkhead. That way, you'll have more space and comfort. If you experience morning sickness, make travel arrangements for a time of day when you typically feel good.

- On a calm flight, try to move your legs every 30 minutes. Avoid blood clots by frequently flexing and extending your ankles (thrombophlebitis).

- To stay hydrated, consume lots of liquids because the humidity in aircraft cabins is minimal.

As amazing as month six is, it's not without its discomforts. These are some things you may start to experience:

Hemorrhoids

These are inflamed veins around your anus that can make going to the bathroom a very painful experience. They typically go away once you give birth.

When hemorrhoids are external, they're on the anus, and when they're internal, they're in your rectum. Your rectum is the portion of your large intestine that connects to your anus. They are an uncomfortable but typical aspect of pregnancy, but the good news is that they're relatively easy to cure at home.

Symptoms

You can actually have hemorrhoids and not exhibit any symptoms, but the most common ones are:
- Discomfort while passing a stool.

- Your anus and its surrounding area itch.

- An internal hemorrhoid that causes excruciating pain outside of your anus (prolapsed hemorrhoid).

- Blood in your stool, on the toilet, or on the toilet paper you used after relieving yourself (usually from an internal hemorrhoid).

Treatment Options

Relieve constipation: Regular bowel movements might relieve some of the pressure on your hemorrhoids. The less time you spend straining yourself, the less pressure you apply to these veins. You can:

- Drink 8–12 cups of water per day.

- Eat up to 30 grams of fiber everyday.

- Take a pregnancy-safe laxative.

Use home remedies:

- To relieve mild pain or discomfort, apply pure aloe vera or food-grade coconut oil.

- To relieve the itch and pain, apply witch hazel.

- To relieve itching, apply dry or wet baking soda directly onto your hemorrhoids.

- Sit in a tub with 2 to 3 inches of warm water, or take a sitz bath. The tense muscles surrounding your anus will start to relax, and your blood flow may be improved in the water.

Medication: If constipation is the main problem, ask your doctor to recommend a laxative, hemorrhoid cream, or fiber supplement. It's better to consult with your doctor on this before opting for any over-the-counter medication. Your doctor or midwife is your best bet at ensuring that you get solutions that are both safe and effective.

Failing these, your doctor might be able to recommend a procedure to remove them that's safe for both you and your baby.

What Are Anal Fissures?

Same ballpark, just a little different. Anal fissures are tears in the anus.

Hemorrhoids and fissures share similar symptoms and can both be uncomfortable and painful. They can also result in bleeding, which you'll see either in your stool or on the toilet paper you use after wiping. The bleeding is harmless, but if you're really worried, don't hesitate to call your doctor. They'll be able to confirm the source of your bleeding and whether or not it's from a more serious condition.

Belly Button Protrusion

We don't usually give our navels much thought, but once we fall pregnant, our belly buttons are one of the many changes we'll see on our bodies.

You're likely to notice the change in your second trimester. Your abdomen moves forward as your uterus continues to grow, and then your belly button eventually protrudes because of your expanding abdomen.

It's completely harmless, but some women have noted that clothing rubbing against it irritates it. If it bothers you, you can wear a belly button cover or a support tool like a tummy sleeve.

Some ladies do experience pain, but there's no universally accepted medical explanation for why some women do. Some people think it has to do with the belly button's location at the thinnest part of the abdominal wall.

Like a lot of things, it usually goes back to normal a couple of months after you've given birth.

What's an Umbilical Hernia?

Sometimes your protruding belly button can actually be an umbilical hernia. It happens when a small hole in your abdominal wall allows abdominal tissue, like the small intestine, to protrude. It can be very uncomfortable.

Symptoms

- A soft lump near your navel that is more pronounced when you are laying down.
- A nagging pain near your navel.
- Some discomfort when you cough, sneeze, or lean over.

Causes

Most umbilical hernias are congenital. They just go unnoticed until your abdomen starts stretching.

Treatment

It's best to leave it alone if it's not causing discomfort. Some ladies rub the lump until the bulge goes inward, and to prevent them from expanding even more, some ladies use belly bands.

After your pregnancy, the hernia will probably start to heal. Your doctor might suggest certain exercises you can do to help it along.

Surgery may be advised by your doctor in some circumstances, but it won't be done until after you've given birth.

Stillbirth

The untimely loss of a pregnancy in any trimester is heartbreaking. Miscarriages usually occur within the first three months, but they can occasionally happen after 20 weeks. Those cases are referred to as stillbirths.

Even though you might never know what led to your loss, it's important to understand that it's highly unlikely that anything you did or didn't do contributed to it. Most miscarriages are the result of issues with the baby's development.

Other causes include:

- **Chromosome or genetic abnormalities**: these occur by chance, but sometimes they're passed down by parents. You can request blood tests to check your chromosomes and assess the likelihood of the same issue arising again.

- **Infection**: some infections affect the baby directly, and others are in the amniotic fluid. Sometimes bacteria from the vagina gets into the womb.

- **Structural abnormalities**: these occur when there's a problem with a baby's development. One example is a congenital heart defect.

- **Problems with the uterus or cervix**: An oddly shaped uterus or a weakened cervix can result in a late loss.

Dealing With Loss

It's normal to experience a great deal of grief and other feelings like guilt, anger, despair, and shock. Those feelings will feel real, but it's never your fault. Everyone reacts differently, so it's important to be honest about your feelings with your spouse and keep in mind that you might not both be processing the loss in the same way. Give yourself time to recover, rely on your loved ones, and think about attending a support group for miscarriage or stillbirth.

Healing

Sometimes you may feel distant, moody, and unable to focus or sleep.

Don't put pressure on yourself to get over your unhappiness. If you can handle your grief as it manifests, your healing will be more thorough. The pain may come back on special occasions like your due date, but with time, things will improve and you'll feel better.

You may be okay physically, but it would help to take a bit of time out. You need time to process, and it may be easier to embrace everything you're going through if you take a break from your usual routine.

Talking

Sharing your story can help you feel less alone and put you on the path to healing. It may seem unpleasant or taboo, but you'll start to see how many people you know have experienced loss and found recovery.

You may find comfort in the most unlikely people, and being transparent about your story, might liberate someone else from the loneliness associated with pregnancy loss and provide them with the strength and confidence to do the same.

If you don't get the response you expected from certain people, bear in mind that people who haven't experienced such a loss can't possibly understand how it feels. Most people actually want to offer comfort but lack the words. If someone says something you deem inappropriate or nothing at all, try not to take it personally.

Support

You won't need to do much Web searching to be reminded that you're not alone. You might find it easier to deal with loss through internet forums. Sometimes it just helps to know you're not the only one going through something.

Ask your ob-gyn or midwife about local pregnancy-loss support groups if you prefer to be face-to-face with people.

Don't give up if you don't enjoy the first one you try; it could take some time to find a group that suits you. Try to learn as much as you can in advance about the group's members to determine whether you'll fit in. (Do they deal more with miscarriages or with stillbirths?)

If a group feels like too much, a counselor might be able to assist you in navigating the feelings you're having and ultimately help you accept your loss.

Your Baby's Development

ARTICHOKE

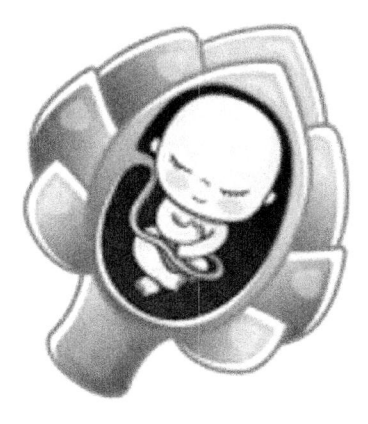

Your belly button may be popping out now, and you could be experiencing round ligament pain. Your ligaments are stretching to support your growing baby.

Baby is measuring in at 11.5 inches and weighs in at around 1.3 pounds. The same as an artichoke. Your baby's bones, muscles, and organs continue to grow and develop. They even have some body fat now.

At this stage, your baby's facial features are starting to take shape. If anything, baby is ready for his/her photo opp. They haven't yet developed pigment. So the baby has white eyebrows, hair, and eyelashes.

Their auditory system develops quickly, so if you play a certain song often enough, they may recognize it and find it calming after birth.

TRIMESTER 3: Waiting

Impatiently

Chapter 7: Month Seven

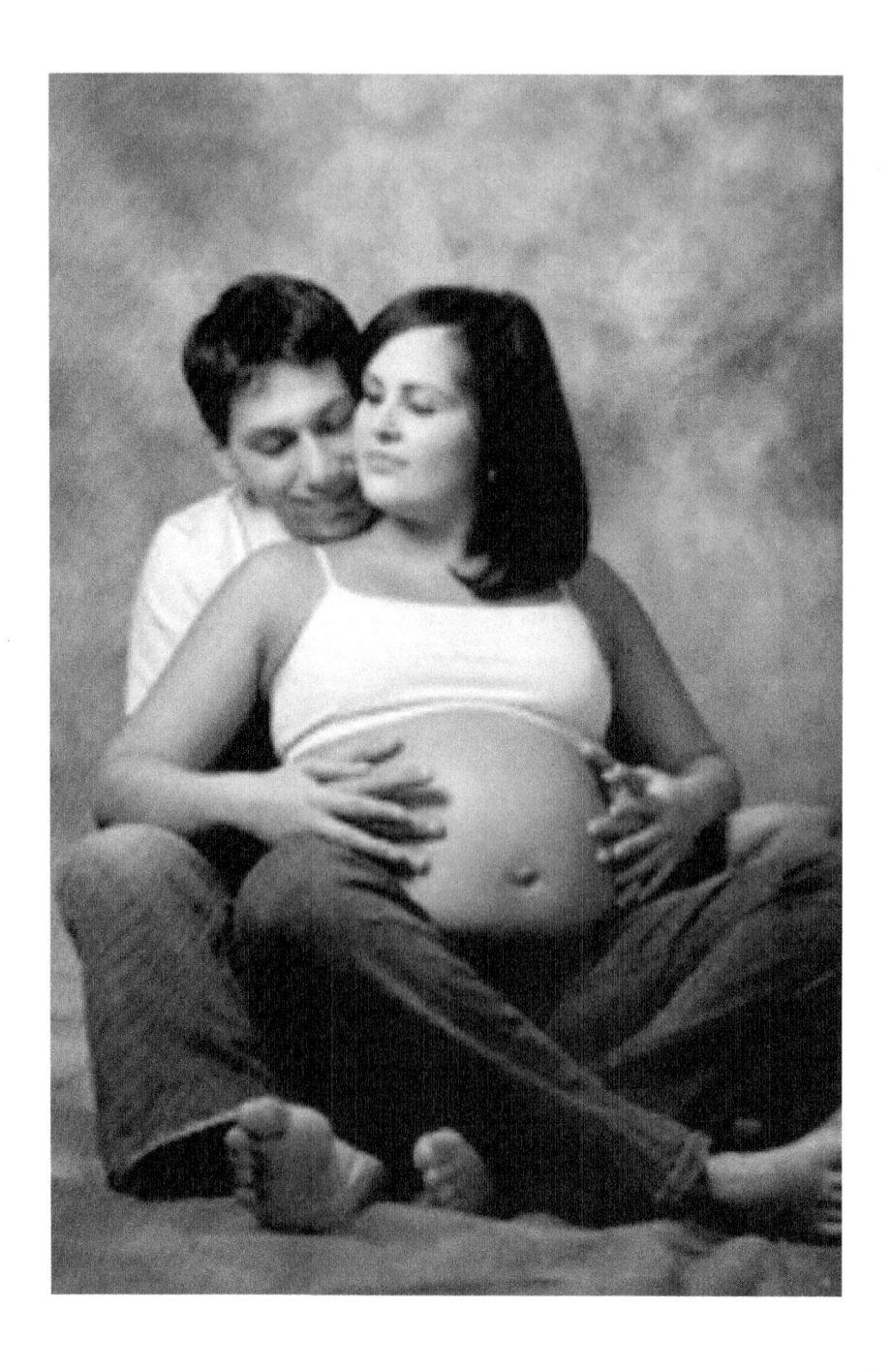

Two months may seem like a long time, but this is the final stretch, and it's getting closer to delivery time. There are things to start thinking about, things to start planning, and things to start implementing.

Birthing Partner: Why Have One?

A birth partner can offer you much-needed support throughout your labor.

You can decide to choose both your partner and a close friend or relative. Just take some time to really consider who you want in the room. If, for any reason, family and friends aren't an option, you can hire a professional like an independent midwife or a doula.

What's important is that you feel at ease with the person you choose. Over and above that, you should have faith in their capacity to keep you at ease and reassured when you are in labor.

Partners

For a lot of dads, witnessing the birth of their child was easily one of their most emotional experiences. But there are some dads who are anxious about being the only support partner.

Likewise, some women worry about their partners' ability to cope, while others don't want them to see them go through labor at all. A good idea is to have two birth partners. That way, they can alternate or take turns looking after you without feeling burned out.

Family and friends

Women have been helping other women give birth since the beginning of time, so it's no wonder a lot of moms-to-be go with female family members in place of their partners. Some women have female family members there in conjunction with their partners.

Your mom is probably the best option because she can let you know what to expect, and since she has firsthand knowledge of the labor process, she can offer you solid support.

Professionals

Independent midwives are a good option if you're planning a homebirth. They can deliver your child and provide you with antenatal and postnatal care. If you choose to deliver at a birthing center, they can support you throughout labor but won't actually deliver the baby.

A doula provides emotional support during labor and delivery. There will be a bit of a rapport because they will get to know you beforehand and will be there to help you emotionally in the days and weeks following the birth of your child. The only thing they can't do is deliver the baby.

Birthing Classes vs. Lamaze

Birthing courses have different philosophies and objectives, but they all offer helpful guidance for labor, delivery, and postpartum issues. Some are focused on how to manage labor pain without drugs. Others start early in a woman's pregnancy and concentrate on the changes that take place for the whole nine months.

Lamaze Technique

Probably the most popular birthing method—it's in all the movies!

Lamaze classes view delivery as a natural and healthy process. They don't encourage or discourage the use of drugs or standard medical procedures during labor and delivery. Instead, they educate expectant mothers about their choices so that they can plan their own labor and delivery. The Lamaze program includes instruction on confidence-building and safe, easy childbirth techniques.

The classes are small, and there are about 12 hours of instruction that provide you with knowledge on:
- A healthy lifestyle
- Assistance during labor

- Breastfeeding
- Breathing exercises for labor
- How to communicate effectively
- Medical procedures
- Pain relief with massage and relaxation techniques
- Positioning yourself in various ways for labor and delivery
- Standard birth, delivery, and early postpartum care
- Using both internal and external focal points to help practice relaxation

Alexander Technique

Your balance, flexibility, coordination, and freedom of movement can all be enhanced by the Alexander Technique. Ideally, you should participate in weekly classes while pregnant, because it's more of an educational process. So, the more you practice, the more you'll gain. Anyone can take these classes, but the objectives for pregnant women include:

- Aid with postpartum healing
- Boost comfort levels during pregnancy
- During delivery, increase the effectiveness of pushing
- Reduce breastfeeding discomfort

HypnoBirthing

Hypnobirthing, also known as the Mongan method, is a laid-back educational approach to natural childbirth. It teaches you self-hypnosis techniques. Instructors place a strong emphasis on prenatal care, parenting, and the consciousness of the unborn child. It's delivered in a series of either four or five classes, each lasting three hours.

The Bradley Method

The Bradley method, also known as husband-coached delivery, gets mom ready to give birth without painkillers and gets dad ready to be mom's birth coach. Although this strategy gets you ready to give birth without drugs, it also gets you ready for unforeseen events like an emergency C-section.

This 12-session program covers:

- Advice for the coach regarding support for the mother
- Breastfeeding
- How to give birth vaginally
- Postpartum care
- Pain management techniques based on relaxation
- The significance of diet and exercise
- Labor rehearsals

If you're unsure about the type of class you want to enroll in, take some time to explore the ones close by, and talk through your options with your doctor. You should also ask where you can find local childbirth classes. Failing that, search online.

Pain Relief in Labor

Labor is hands-down the most painful experience a woman will go through in her lifetime. So learning about all the ways you can ease the pain is so important. Your birth partner/s should also be well informed so they can step in if you need help.

Gas and Air (Entonox) For Labor

It contains both nitrous oxide and oxygen. Although gas and air cannot completely alleviate pain, they can help to lessen it and make it more tolerable. It is simple to use, and you are in complete control.

You hold the mask or mouthpiece while inhaling gas and air through it. You breathe it in just before a contraction starts, since it takes the gas around 15–20 seconds to start working. You should breathe deeply and slowly for the best results.

Side effects:

- There are no adverse effects for you or the child.

- It may cause you to feel dizzy, ill, sleepy, or unable to concentrate, but you can stop using it if this happens.

You might also request an injection of painkillers if gas and air do not sufficiently relieve your discomfort.

Epidural

An epidural is a local anesthesia that numbs the nerves that transmit pain signals from the birth canal to the brain. It doesn't make you feel sick or drowsy. It typically provides total pain relief, so it's really helpful if your labor is protracted and painful.

It can only be administered by an anesthesiologist, so it's not available for home births. Find out if anesthetists are always available at your hospital if you believe you might need one.

Bear in mind that the baby's heart rate must also be remotely (through telemetry) monitored at this time, but many hospitals lack the necessary equipment. Find out from your midwife whether your hospital of choice offers mobile epidurals.

It works most of the time, but it's not always successful. According to the Obstetric Anaesthetists Association, one in ten women who have an epidural during labor end up needing additional painkillers.

Side Effects

- Depending on the local anesthetic used, it may cause your legs to feel heavy.

- It's possible for your blood pressure to drop (hypotension), but it rarely happens because the fluid you get via the drip in your arm aids in maintaining healthy blood pressure.

- The second stage of labor may be prolonged in the event that you're unable to feel your contractions anymore. Your midwife will have to instruct you on when to push, and then she may need the assistance of forceps or a ventouse (instrumental delivery).

- As long as the baby is not displaying any signs of distress, your midwife or doctor will wait longer for the baby's head to drop before you begin pushing. This lowers the likelihood that you'll require an instrumental delivery. They also start weaning you off the anesthesia toward the end of labor, so the effects wear off and you can feel the contractions.

- The epidural may make it difficult for you to urinate. If so, a catheter might be inserted into your bladder to assist you.

- It may cause a headache. But that's only roughly 1 in 100 cases.

- Your back could be a little sore for a day or two, but epidurals don't result in chronic back pain.

- After giving birth, you might have tingling or pins and needles down one leg. This happens in about one out of every 2000 cases. It may not be the epidural though, it's probably labor itself.

Spinal Block

A spinal block is a back injection that offers speedy anesthesia during surgery. It can also be used in conjunction with an epidural, to relieve labor pain quickly. You get a single injection of a numbing chemical that acts fast to help you feel comfortable. It's different from an epidural, in that it doesn't keep a plastic tube in place on your back so you can receive medication.

It's mostly used for C-sections, forceps deliveries, and all other surgical operations performed during pregnancy and childbirth. Believe it or not, it's the most popular option.

It takes about five minutes to carry out, and then another two to ten minutes for the anesthesia to start working. After the first minute, you'll feel warmth swiftly spread across your lower body and legs; it's comparable to stepping into a warm bath.

Following anesthesia, your and your baby's vital signs will be monitored.

Possible Reasons I Can't Have a Spinal

- Major blood coagulation abnormalities that make you bleed more than usual (including some anti-clotting medications).

- A back infection that affects the skin or tissue where a spinal would normally be placed.

- A severe sensitivity to the medicines used in spinal surgery (local anesthetics, opioids).

According to your doctor's assessment, the following conditions could make a spinal more difficult or dangerous but still feasible:

- Sepsis (Infection)

- Significant scoliosis or other modifications to the spine's form.

- A history of spinal surgery.

- Spina bifida

Side Effects and Risks

The likelihood of major issues for either mom or baby after receiving a spinal block is incredibly minimal. The key dangers and adverse effects of spinal blocks are listed here, and your anesthetist should go over them with you before inserting one.

The Epidural Information Card (2008), which you can find on the website of the Obstetric Anaesthetists' Association, served as the inspiration for the following list of spinal risks.

Risk/Side Effect	Chances
Accidental unconsciousness	1 in 100 000 women
Abscess	1 in 50 000 women
Haematoma	1 in 170 000 women
Meningitis	1 in 100 000 women
Nerve damage (numb patch on foot, or weak leg) lasting less than 6 months.	1 in 1000
Nerve damage (numb patch on foot, or weak leg) lasting over 6 months.	1 in 13 000
Paralysis or severe injury	1 in 250 000
Severe headache	1 in 500
Significant drop in bp	1 in 5
Spinal not working well enough for surgery	1 in 100

(Ridgeon, 2021)

Hydro—Water Birth

Water births take place in a warm water bath. Some women stay in the water during labor and then get out when it's time for delivery. Other women choose to deliver their babies in the water.

The theory is that after spending nine months in amniotic fluid, giving birth in a comparable environment is easier on the baby and less stressful for mom.

What Are the Risks?

- You or your child could contract an infection.
- It's possible for the umbilical cord to snap before your baby emerges from the water.
- The baby's temperature may be either too high or too low.
- Some water could go into your baby's lungs.
- Your baby might experience seizures or be unable to breathe.

What Precautions Can You Take?

If you're considering a water birth, find out early on in your pregnancy if the hospital offers the service. You also need to find out who's going to oversee your labor and delivery if they do. A midwife can help, but they will require medical support from a doctor.

If it's not offered at the hospital, you can either opt for a birthing center or your home.

Here are some things to look for:

- Your healthcare provider should be skilled and certified, so they're able to properly assist you with labor and delivery. But there should also always be a doctor present as a backup.
- The tub is clean and well-maintained.
- There are effective infection control procedures in place.
- While in the tub, you and your child are being appropriately monitored.

- There's an exit strategy in place to get you out of the tub as soon as your doctor, nurse, or midwife says so.
- The temperature of the water is always kept between 97 and 100 °F.
- You drink enough water throughout to avoid dehydration.

Are You a Good Candidate?

Don't attempt a water birth if:
- You have an infection.
- You have preeclampsia or diabetes.
- You're under 17 or over 35.
- You're pregnant with multiples.
- Your baby's breech.
- You're going into early labor.
- Your baby is large.
- There is severe meconium.

What Are the Costs?

It usually costs the same as a vaginal birth in a hospital, if it's covered by insurance. The tub may need to be rented, which might cost an additional $200 to $400.

Depending on your preferences, the cost of a tub or pool for a home birth might range from $65 to $500.

If a midwife or nurse-midwife comes to your home, they'll charge anywhere between $2,000 and $6,000. It's pretty much the same as a normal birth.

The midwife's fee may be covered by the facility if you give birth at a hospital or birthing center where they're employed. They charge anything between $3,000 and $4,000.

One major study conducted in 2020 found that women who completed a hypnobirthing program had significantly lower stress levels and pain ratings than those who did not. Also, there were reported benefits in terms of shorter labor, fewer interventions, and improved feelings of control over the birthing experience (University of Michigan, 2020).

Emotions in the Third Trimester

One thing that seems impossible during the third trimester, is getting a good night's sleep. Slumps in your mood may be caused by fatigue and sleep issues.

Anxieties about the impending birth, being a mother, or worrying about raising a human being can become very overwhelming.

On the positive side, nesting can be considered an emotional thing. When you suddenly feel the need to clean, arrange, and actually get ready for the baby, you are nesting. Not everybody experiences it, but for the moms who do, it can really feel like a positive experience.

At this stage in the pregnancy, we may start to interpret little things as big things, so it's important for us to know that not all pain is bad.

Braxton Hicks

Braxton hicks contractions are in all the movies. They're practice contractions that usually happen in the last few months of your pregnancy.

A Braxton hicks contraction might make your tummy feel hard. It will feel soft once again following the contraction.

Each contraction lasts between 30 and 60 seconds. They can occur throughout the day, but they might disappear when you workout and reappear when you relax.

Actual labor contractions are stronger and more frequent than Braxton Hicks. If you're a first-time mom, it might be challenging to distinguish between Braxton hicks and the real thing. Contact your midwife if you feel worried or anxious. Better safe than sorry.

What to Do if You Have Them

- Remain calm, do some breathing exercises, or go for a quick walk.
- A warm bath can ease some of the discomforts.
- Ask nicely for a shoulder or back rub from your partner.
- Stay hydrated and eat at regular intervals to maintain your energy levels.

Vaginal Bleeding in the Third Trimester

These are some potential reasons for vaginal bleeding in the second or third trimester:

- Uterine rupture: A rare but potentially fatal condition where the uterus ruptures along the scar from a previous C-section.
- Cervical issues: Like an infected or inflamed cervix or growths on the cervix
- Preterm labor: Light bleeding or spotting is common, as the fetal membranes can rupture (known as water breaking) before or during preterm labor.

- Placenta previa: The placenta typically develops at the top of the uterus during pregnancy. This is so that the cervix is unobstructed for delivery. Placenta previa occurs when the placenta is closer to the bottom of the uterus, partially or sometimes completely covering the cervix. In this position, the placenta often ruptures, leading to uncontrollable bleeding and the deprivation of essential nutrients and oxygen to the fetus.

- Placental abruption: This happens when the placenta detaches from the uterus before childbirth. It can result in serious bleeding and endanger both the mother and the unborn child's lives. There isn't medication or surgery to reconnect it, but prompt medical intervention may help raise the likelihood of a healthy birth after an abruption.

- Intrauterine fetal death: If the fetus remains in the body, the mother may have blood clots, infection, discomfort, fever, vomiting, diarrhea, and severe bleeding.

At the end of your pregnancy, you may notice light bleeding, usually mixed with mucus. It's normally pink in color, but it's called "bloody show." It's a sign that labor is starting.

Packing Your Bag for the Hospital

Once you've given birth, you'll be tired, disoriented, and hopefully on cloud nine. So your birthing partner or healthcare team should easily be able to find everything they need once the baby's born.

Being practical and having everything organized in different bags that you will bring in with you, is the best approach to preparing for a hospital stay:

A large bag (preferably a weekend bag)

A hospital bag for your baby

A separate bag for your birthing partner

To better keep track of the smaller items you've packed, you can use freezer bags or old shopping bags. Clear is better—this way you can label them.

We've got the bags down; let's get into their contents.

What to Pack

It's best to have your bag fully packed before you hit the 37-week mark. Pack the things you'll need later on in your stay first, so they're at the bottom of the bag. This will make finding everything so easy.

Main Bag

This will be your biggest bag; it should have space for 3 toiletry bags—your labor bag, post-birth bag, and baby's bag.

Checklist:
- Gadgets and chargers
- Breast pads and nipple cream
- Maternity pads
- Two light-weight dressing gowns (preferably dark in color)
- Two nightdresses (preferably with front button openings to facilitate skin-to-skin contact and breastfeeding)
- Three pairs of socks
- Five dark pairs of sweatpants (one will be in your post-birth bag)
- Three nursing bras
- A dark towel

- A change of clothes

Labor Bag

Put this bag at the very top of your main bag.

Checklist:

- A flannel
- A hand-fan
- Hair-ties
- A water bottle
- Massage oil

Post Birth Bag

This bag should include the things you'll need just after giving birth and for your first time in the bathroom post-birth.

Checklist:

- One pair of pants
- One nightdress
- Two maternity pads
- Flip flops (good for swollen feet)

Baby's Bag

Checklist:

- Ten nappies
- Four baby grows

- Four baby vests
- Five muslin cloths
- A blanket
- Two sets of hats and mitts
- Wet wipes
- Diaper cream

Birthing Partner's Bag

Checklist:

- Money
- A change of clothes
- Food and drinks
- Gadgets to pass the time (if need be)
- Power banks to charge their gadgets in case the hospital doesn't allow for them to use their power points.

After this month, things start to get a bit uncomfortable. Sometimes to the point where you start googling ways to induce labor. It might be too early for that, but it's never too early to start thinking about and weighing delivery options.

Your Baby's Development

GRAPEFRUIT

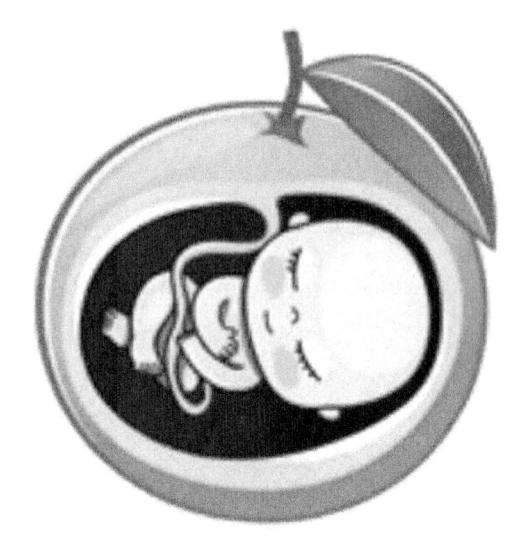

Congratulations on the beginning of the third trimester!

It may be a bit hard to celebrate, considering the back pain you might be experiencing. When your little one kicks at night, it probably keeps you awake, and if they don't kick during the day, you're probably not napping either.

Your child's head and your expanding uterus tend to rest on the sciatic nerve in the bottom part of your spine as baby prepares for delivery.

This may result in sciatica—a sharp, shooting pain, tingling, or numbness that begins in your buttocks and spreads down the back of your legs. The pain can at times be severe, only subsiding if the baby switches positions.

Your baby is measuring in at a whopping 15 inches long, and weighing in at 2.4 pounds. The same as a grapefruit. Your baby can now blink.

That's just one of the many reflexes they've developed so far. Others include: hiccuping, sucking, coughing, and taking practice breaths.

Your baby has also started dreaming. When you move throughout the day, your baby becomes relaxed and falls asleep. Then, when it's your turn to sleep, baby is wide awake.

Chapter 8: Month Eight

Shower vs. Bath

A lot of women stick to showering once they find out they're pregnant because they're avoiding immersing themselves in tubs of hot water. But to a pregnant woman, a nice long bath probably sounds like a dream. It's so nice on the skin, and it can help alleviate some of those aches and pains.

It's perfectly safe to bathe, so long as you follow a few safety precautions.

As long as the water is warm, you're good to take a bath. Beyond that, what you have to think about is whether you're physically able to take that bath.

It can be challenging just getting into the tub, let alone reaching all the body parts that need washing and rinsing because of your expanding belly and declining energy. Keep in mind that you'll need to heave yourself out before you can towel off.

Hot Baths

As you near the end of your pregnancy, things start getting really uncomfortable, and you've probably said, "I want this baby out!" countless times.

Naturally, you'll start to look up natural ways you can induce labor. One method that pops up quite a lot is taking a hot bath.

Unfortunately, hot baths are potentially dangerous to unborn babies, and there is no irrefutable proof to back up the theory that hot baths can jumpstart labor.

A baby may become distressed if the blood flow to their body is reduced. That can happen if the expectant mom sits in hot water. This is because the water can potentially raise your body temperature to over 101 °F. The temperature of the bath water should not exceed 98 °F. Also, sitting in the water for extended periods increases your risk of infection.

Speaking of infection…

Strep B

Group B strep is a common type of streptococcal bacteria found in the body—usually in the vagina or rectum. It's also referred to as GBS or strep B. Although carrying group B strep is mostly safe, it can occasionally infect a baby while you are in labor. The GBS infection can make your baby very ill, but with prompt treatment, most babies recover completely.

GBS causes sepsis, pneumonia, or meningitis. One in 14 newborns who recover from it will have a long-term disability of some kind. Tragically, 1 in 19 infants with an early-onset GBS infection passes away.

There are rare instances where it can affect the baby in utero. Those babies tend to fall ill within their first week of birth, and in other cases, it can take up to 3 months to manifest.

As GBS is not a sexually transmitted illness, the majority of carriers will not exhibit any symptoms.

During the third trimester of your pregnancy, you can request to undergo a group B strep screening test. Antibiotics can be prescribed to safeguard your baby if you have it during delivery.

At your doctor's appointment this month, you want to hear that the baby is finally head down. But there are actually an array of positions they could be in.

Presentation and Position of Baby for Delivery

Early on in your pregnancy, your baby moves around freely in the womb because there's an abundance of space. However, as they grow, they have less wiggle room.

What Is Fetal Position?

Fetal positioning refers to how your unborn child, or fetus, is laid out in the womb, whether that means on its back, with its head down, or any other way. The *fetal position* refers to the traditional curled-up baby position.

With the head down, a curved spine, and the arms and legs drawn close to the body, it resembles the shape of a C. Your baby will stretch, kick, and move around from time to time, but this is usually the position they'll choose to stay in most of the time.

It's the most comfortable position for your baby in the womb and for a while after birth. It actually helps your baby get into the optimum position for birth and reduces the possibility of difficulties.

Types of Fetal Positioning for Birth

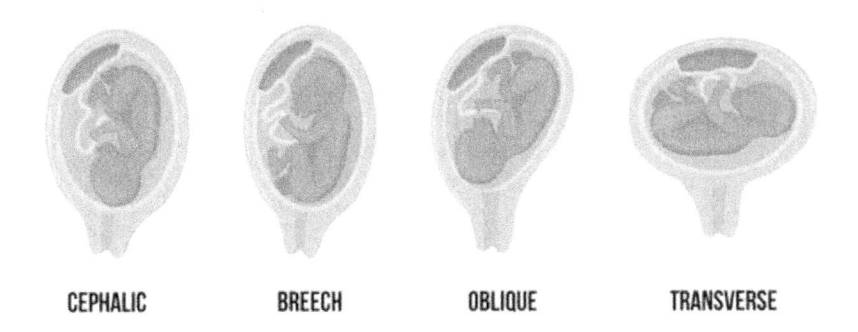

CEPHALIC   BREECH   OBLIQUE   TRANSVERSE

Most babies can position themselves head down by 36 weeks for an easy exit. Others decide they're completely at ease and have no intention of leaving.

Breech position

Just 3 to 4% of babies born at full term choose to remain in the breech position, head up and bottom down. There are different types, and they all raise the possibility that you might need a C-section (*Movement and Positions during Labour*, n.d.)

- **Complete breech**: Baby's knees are bent, and their feet are close to their bottom, which is near the birth canal.

- **Footling breech**: Baby has one or both legs near or in the birth canal.

- **Frank breech**: Baby is shaped like a V, with its feet close to its head, legs up, and bottom near the birth canal.

Oblique position

Oblique means your baby is sitting diagonally or is slanted across the womb. It's quite uncommon, but not impossible.

Because the head isn't properly aligned with the birth canal, there is a higher risk of umbilical cord compression during delivery. If the umbilical cord enters the birth canal first, pressure from the head may compress the cord, impeding blood flow and creating a crisis.

If medical personnel can't turn your baby into a head-down position, you might need to have a C-section.

Occiput Anterior

This is the ideal fetal position for delivery. Baby is feet up, head down, facing your back, with their back resting against your tummy. The back of their head is close to your pubic bone, and they can exit the birth canal with ease.

It's also called the "vertex position" or "cephalic position."

There's really no *easy* way to give birth, but this position makes it easier for your baby to descend and for you to deliver. Your baby has the best chance of passing through the birth canal this way.

Occiput Posterior

This position is almost identical to the OA, with the exception that the baby is now facing your belly rather than your back. Other names for it are the back-to-back and sunny-side-up positions.

Your baby can't tuck their chin down to easily pass through the birth canal in this position. Labor could take longer if your baby is unable to turn over. A C-section might be recommended by your doctor for safety.

Transverse Position

When a baby is transverse, they're in the fetal position while resting sideways across the womb. In this position, you never know whether their back, shoulders, hands, or feet could be closest to the birth canal.

The most dangerous thing about this position is that the placenta could be damaged during delivery or when trying to turn the baby over. Your doctor will make the call on whether a C-section is the most prudent course of action.

Cesarean Section

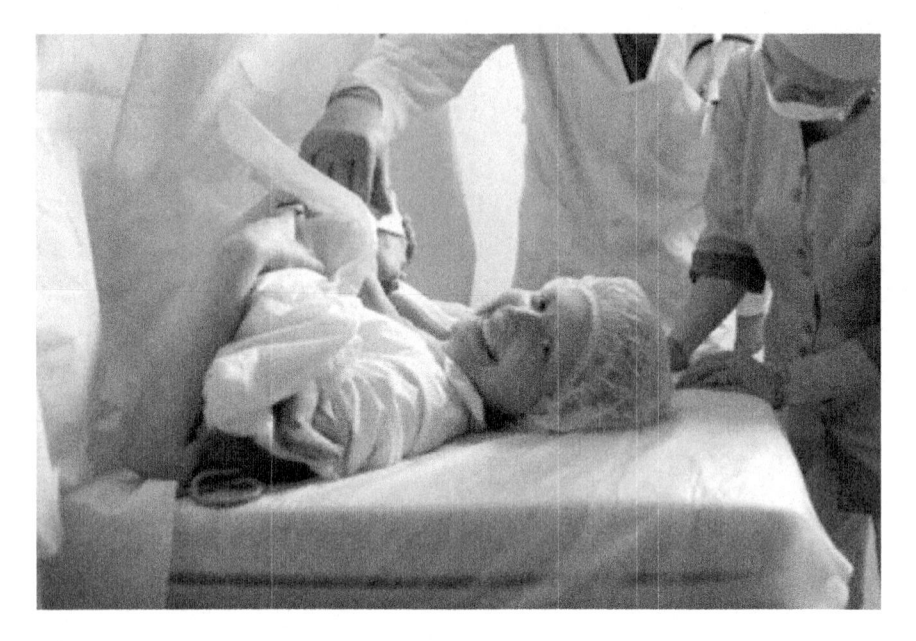

A cesarean section is a surgical operation that's employed to deliver a baby when a vaginal delivery can't be performed safely. It's usually done in an emergency, but it can also be an elective surgery that's scheduled ahead of time. It has a somewhat longer recovery time and a higher risk than a vaginal delivery.

Reasons to Have One

- Breech presentation

- **Cephalopelvic disproportion (CPD)**: Your baby's head or body is too large to fit through your pelvis, or your pelvis is too small to birth an average-sized baby.

- Expecting multiples

- **Health issues**: Labor can exacerbate health issues like cardiovascular disease. If you have a venereal disease like herpes, vaginal birth is not an option.

- **Obstruction**: You might need a C-section if you have a large uterine fibroid, a pelvic fracture, or if you're expecting a child with any congenital abnormalities.

- Placenta previa

- Previous C-section

- Transverse lie

What Are the Risks?

- Fetal injury

- Problems with general anesthesia

- Abnormalities of future placentas

- A weakened uterine wall

- Damage to the bladder or bowel

- Embolism

- Hemorrhage

- Infection

Recovery

You'll start to feel the pain from the incisions when the anesthetic wears off. It creeps up on you at first and then becomes a bit more pronounced, but it's nothing painkillers can't fix. Also, it might be difficult to take deep breaths, and you may feel gassy. For the first few days after surgery, make sure you have assistance getting out of bed from an adult. C-section moms usually stay in the hospital for up to three days after giving birth.

It can take anywhere from four to six weeks to fully recover. Medical professionals advise abstaining from stairs, lifting, and strenuous activity, for several weeks. So that you can relax and heal nicely, ask your friends, family, or partner to help with errands. This includes driving.

For those six weeks, you can anticipate cramps, bleeding, and some discomfort near the incision. For pain, over-the-counter painkillers like acetaminophen or ibuprofen can help. For at least six weeks—or until your doctor gives the all-clear—avoid engaging in any sexual activity.

As your uterine lining sheds following the procedure, you will have vaginal discharge—called "lochia." It starts out crimson and progressively turns yellow. If you encounter severe bleeding or a bad odor coming from your discharge, make sure to contact your healthcare professional right away. Use sanitary pads rather than tampons until all of your bleeding has stopped.

Vaginal Birth After Delivery

A lot of women who've had C-sections think about the possibility of vaginal delivery in their subsequent pregnancies. The odds of having a vaginal birth after a cesarean (VBAC) are higher if you meet the following requirements:

- Your first C-section was not an emergency one.
- You're not carrying multiples.
- Your pelvis is not too narrow to support a baby of typical size.
- Your doctor made a small transverse incision.

Is It Safe?

When you've had surgery on your uterus, it leaves a scar. Doctors fear that the strain of labor can cause that scar to rupture.

But after years of research, it was found that 60% to 80% of women who had cesarean births also had healthy vaginal births in their subsequent pregnancies. The National Institute of Child Health and Human Development released figures that lend credence to the safety of VBAC. They found that 75% of VBAC attempts are successful. (*Vaginal Birth after Cesarean (VBAC): Facts, Safety & Risks*, 2021)

Am I at Risk of a Uterine Rupture?

The probability of a ruptured uterus after a previous C-section with a horizontal (transverse) cut is around 0.9%, or little less than 1 in 100, according to the American College of Obstetricians and Gynecologists (2021).

Risks associated with a ruptured uterus include:

- Damage to the bladder
- Infection
- Blood clots
- Blood loss
- Hysterectomy

Natural vs. C-Section

Natural Pros

- Vaginal births often need shorter recuperation and hospital stays.
- The dangers of major surgery, like hemorrhaging, scarring, infections, reactions to anesthesia, and intense pain, are often avoided with vaginal births. Also, moms are able to start breastfeeding earlier because they've avoided surgery.

- A baby who is born vaginally will be able to interact with their mother more quickly since she can start breastfeeding right away.

- The muscles used in a vaginal delivery are more likely to press out the fluid in a newborn's lungs, which is good since it reduces the likelihood of breathing difficulties at birth.

Natural Cons

- A vaginal delivery is a long, physically taxing process. First-time mothers often have active labor for four to eight hours on average.

- The skin and surrounding tissues of the vagina are in danger of stretching and rupturing once the fetus passes through the birth canal. Stitches may be needed for severe tears and stretching. The pelvic muscles that regulate bowel and urinary movements may become weak or suffer an injury as a result of the stretching and tearing.

- Studies found that women who gave birth vaginally were more likely to develop pelvic organ prolapse, which is when one or more organs drop into the pelvis. They were also at risk of developing urinary incontinence, which causes urine to leak when a person laughs, sneezes, or coughs.

- Moreover, the perineum, which is located between the vagina and the anus, may continue to hurt indefinitely after a vaginal delivery.

- Newborns can sustain injuries during the birth process itself, resulting in a bruised scalp or a fractured collarbone. It mostly happens if a woman has had a long labor or if the baby is large.

Cesarean Pros

- If a woman has extreme anxiety around giving birth vaginally, she may decide to have a C-section and save herself from a negative experience.

- Women who undergo C-sections are less likely to get pelvic organ prolapse and suffer incontinence.

- Compared to natural labor, a surgical birth can be planned in advance, making it convenient and predictable.

- A C-section can save both mom and baby's lives in emergency situations.

Cesarean Cons

- The average hospital stay following a C-section is two to four days. Moreover, there may be increased abdominal pain and discomfort during the healing time.

- Due to the various potential complications, women are three times more likely to die with a cesarean delivery than with a natural birth.

- A woman is more likely to get a C-section in the future if she has already had one.

- Infants delivered through C-section may be more susceptible to respiratory issues both at birth and later in life.

- There is a slight possibility that a baby could be cut by the scalpel during a surgery and get hurt.

Your Baby's Development

EGGPLANT

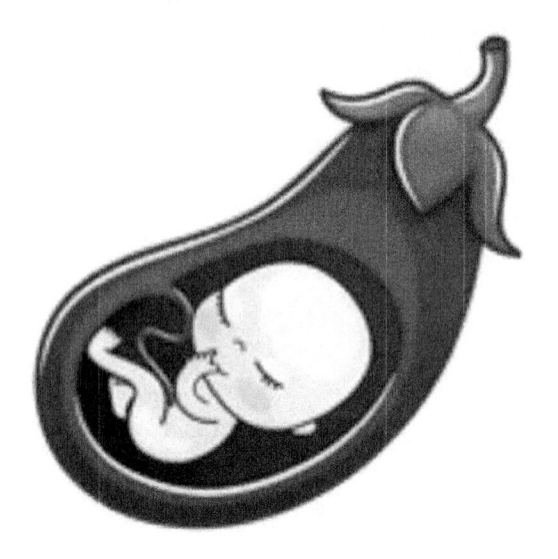

This month, your uterus is just inches above your belly button, so some of your organs up THERE are really feeling it. It's crowded up there. This means you'll experience some shortness of breath as your lungs and diaphragm are a bit squished.

Something to look out for is Braxton hicks. Chances are, you're starting to experience them now.

Baby is weighing in at 3.5–4 pounds and measuring in at 16–17 inches. They're about as big as an eggplant. Baby is quickly running out of legroom and is now in the fetal position. There's fat accumulation under baby's skin now so they're no longer translucent. Baby is hard at work and continue to hone their skills in breathing and sucking.

Chapter 9: Month Nine

Finally! Baby could come any day now. You're probably hoping it's sooner rather than later. By now, you've probably got a birth plan in place, but it's time to start considering what could happen if you can't wait for nature to take its course.

It's also a good time to give more thought to how you'd like to look after your baby once they're here.

Planned Induction

It's always best to let nature take its course, but there are instances where nature could use a push. If healthcare providers are under the impression that delivering sooner is the best course of action, they'll suggest an induction.

Possible Reasons for Induction

- When the due date has come and gone and there are no signs of labor (post-term pregnancy).

- When your water breaks and labor doesn't start (premature rupture of membranes).

- Getting a uterine infection.

- Fetal growth restriction.

- When there is insufficient amniotic fluid surrounding the baby (oligohydramnios).

- Having diabetes, type 2 or gestational.

- Elevated blood pressure.

- Placental abruption.

- Medical conditions like obesity or kidney disease.

Elective Labor Induction

Elective labor induction is usually for convenience—there's no medical emergency attached to it.

To lower the baby's risk of health issues, a medical professional will verify that the gestational age of the baby is at least 39 weeks or older before inducing labor.

Recent studies have led to the provision of labor induction for women with low-risk pregnancies at 39 to 40 weeks. Starting labor early minimizes a number of risks, including those related to stillbirth, macrosomia (refers to growth beyond 8 pounds 13 ounces, regardless of gestational age), and the development of high blood pressure if the pregnancy progresses. The decision to induce labor should be a joint one between the expectant mother and her healthcare practitioners.

Risks

There are instances in which a woman shouldn't undergo labor induction. If you've had a C-section, or significant uterine surgery, placenta previa, or if your baby is breech or transverse, it might not be an option for you.

Other dangers associated with inducing labor include:

- **Bleeding after delivery**: The likelihood that the uterine muscles won't adequately contract after giving birth (uterine atony) increases when labor is induced. This can cause substantial bleeding after birth.

- **Failed induction**: If the proper induction techniques don't result in a vaginal delivery after 24 or more hours, the induction is deemed unsuccessful and might result in a C-section.

- **Infection**: Certain labor induction techniques, like rupturing the membranes may raise the danger of infection for both mom and baby.

- **Low fetal heart rate**: Oxytocin and prostaglandin (the medications used to induce labor) cause irregular or excessive contractions, which might reduce the baby's oxygen supply and drop its heart rate.

- **Uterine rupture**: These occur when the uterus tears along the scar line from a prior significant uterine surgery. The complications can be life-threatening, so in order to avoid that, an emergency C-section will be performed and the uterus removed if necessary.

What to Expect

Induction involves a number of steps, but depending on how you respond to each one, your doctor may not have to follow through with the next ones.

Cervical Ripening

Your doctor will need to start the ripening process if your cervix doesn't show any signs of softening, opening, or thinning to allow your baby to exit the uterus and enter the birth canal. The doctor will usually do this by applying topical prostaglandin to your cervix. It can come in the form of a gel or a vaginal suppository. A few hours after that, your cervix will be checked. Ripening is usually enough to initiate labor and contractions.

Sometimes the prostaglandin does ripen the cervix, but contractions still don't start. In that case, your doctor will move on to the subsequent steps.

If you've had any previous uterine surgery, you won't be given prostaglandin in an attempt to avoid uterine rupture. Your doctor might opt for a graduated dilator or catheter with an inflating balloon.

Membrane Stripping

Your doctor may be able to get labor started by swiping their finger across the delicate membranes connecting the amniotic sac if it's still intact. This is supposed to encourage the uterus to release prostaglandin, which should soften the cervix and allow contractions to start.

Although it isn't intended to break your water, it can happen, and it does tend to be painful.

Membrane Rupturing

Your doctor may artificially rupture the membranes to kick-start your contractions if your cervix has already started to dilate and efface but your water hasn't broken.

This involves manually bursting the amniotic sac with a device that resembles a long, sharp crochet hook. It can be uncomfortable, but it shouldn't hurt.

Pitocin

If none of the previous steps took effect and labor hasn't started, your doctor will progressively administer the drug Pitocin via an IV to trigger or intensify contractions. Pitocin is a synthetic version of the hormone oxytocin. Although you won't have anything to compare it to if this is your first child, Pitocin-induced contractions are stronger, more regular, and more frequent than natural ones. They start as quickly as 30 minutes after the Pitocin is administered. If you know you'd like an epidural, talk to your doctor about starting it while you receive Pitocin so that it will be ready when labor actually begins.

Breast vs. Bottle

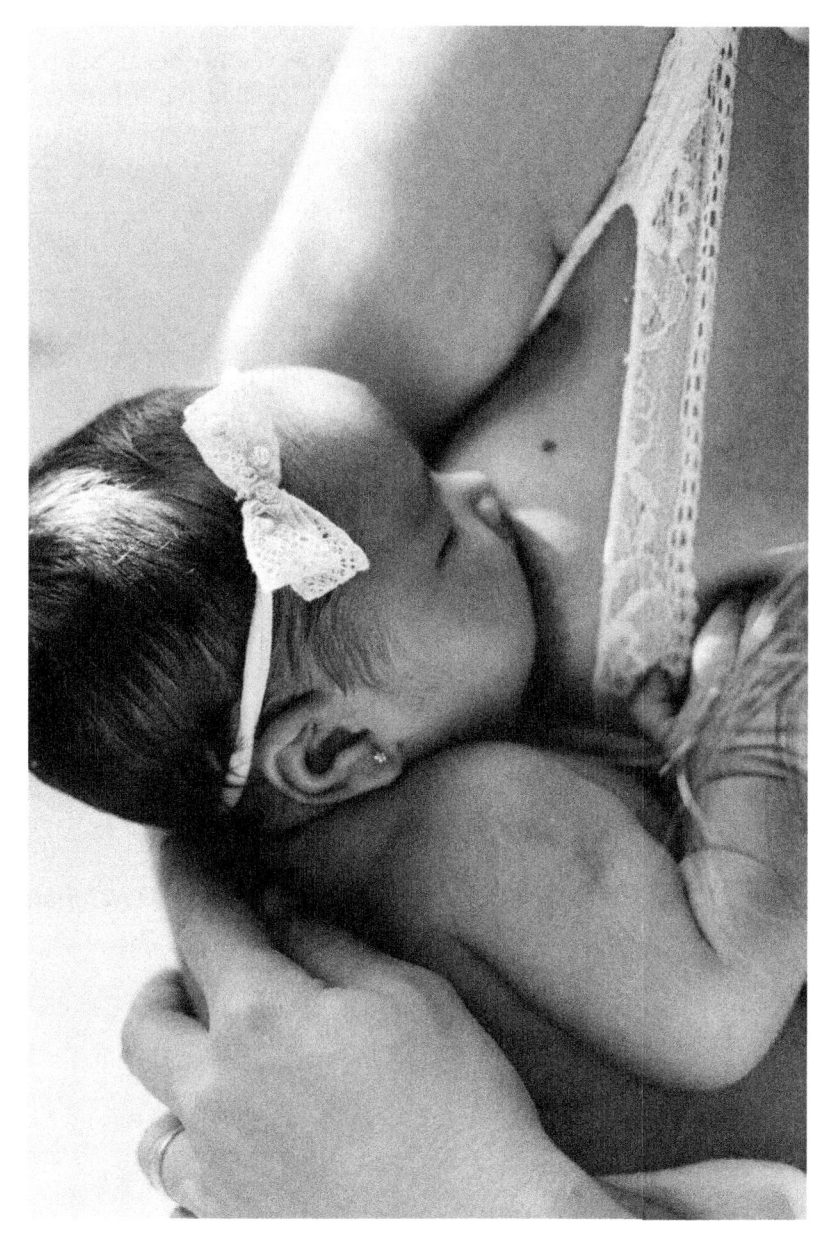

The feeding method that has the most benefits for both mother and child is breastfeeding. Health experts advise that babies should consume only breast milk for the first four to six months of their lives and then stick with it as a major source of nutrition until they are at least one to two years old.

Baby formula is designed to provide newborns with a nutritious supply of sustenance. There are several different formulas available for infants from the day they're born. The nutrients, calories, taste, digestibility, and price of infant formulas vary. There are options for almost every situation. Whether your baby is lactose intolerant, has a milk protein allergy, or has a metabolic condition, you will be able to find a formula for them.

At the end of the day, how and what you choose to feed your baby is your decision. All babies need to be fed.

Here are some of the benefits and drawbacks of both breastfeeding and formula feeding.

Breastfeeding vs. Formula Feeding Pros and Cons

Breastfeeding Pros

- All the nutrients that newborns need to grow and develop are in breast milk.

- The antibodies in breast milk help keep your baby healthy.

- Babies who are breastfed have a lower risk of developing respiratory illnesses.

- Breastfeeding can help your infant avoid health issues like allergies, eczema, ear infections, and gastrointestinal issues.

- It's easier for breastfeeding mothers to shed weight after giving birth.

- Breastfeeding possibly lowers the risk of diabetes and various cancers.

Breastfeeding Cons

- Discomfort in the nipples and breasts. Very common in the first week. Also, learning how to nurse can take a couple of weeks.

- Breast heaviness or engorgement.

- Obstructed milk ducts

- Insufficient milk to meet the baby's needs.

Formula Pros

- There's more freedom of movement because anyone can feed your baby.

- You can get away with longer intervals between feeds, because babies take longer to digest formula.

- You can actually measure and be sure of how much your baby consumes.

- Your baby will be able to bond with more family members during feeds.

Formula Cons

- Babies are not as well protected against Infections, illnesses, and disorders on formula.

- You have to properly mix and prepare the formula, while ensuring the temperature is right.

- All the accessories that come with bottle-feeding can be pricey.

- Babies may experience constipation and gas as a result of the formula.

Breastfeeding Myths

Baby won't consume enough milk

Virtually all women can produce adequate milk for their babies, regardless of breast or nipple size or shape.

The best way to keep your supply going is through early and frequent feedings and ongoing skin-to-skin contact.

When you've got a good supply going, the amount of breast milk you produce will precisely correspond with your baby's needs. Your body generates more milk as you breastfeed.

Your partner may feel left out

There are so many ways for partners to get close to the baby, and many ways for them to support you too, for instance:

- They can bring you water or snacks while you're feeding.
- Have skin-to-skin contact with the baby.
- Cuddling the baby.
- Changing diapers.
- Burping.
- Bathing the baby.

It makes your breasts sag

Your breasts won't sag because of breastfeeding. The ligaments supporting your breasts can swell because of pregnancy hormones. They also just may appear to sag as you age.

You can prevent it by wearing bras that fit properly.

You have to stop at 6 months

There is no stipulation on when you should stop breastfeeding.

The World Health Organization suggests that you (*Breastfeeding - Common Myths*, 2022):

- Breastfeed exclusively for the first six months.
- Continue breastfeeding while feeding supplemental foods, until two years and even beyond.

Your Baby's Development

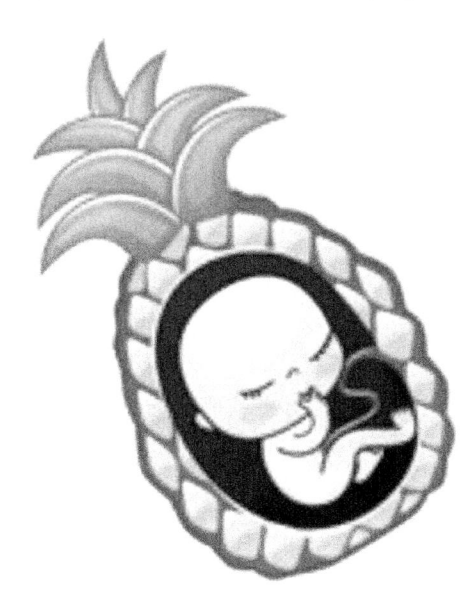

PINEAPPLE

As hormones that loosen and soften joints begin to take effect before labor, this last month may bring more joint flexibility and pelvic pain.

You'll also just be experiencing more and more of the same discomfort you've had for the past couple of months.

Baby is measuring in at 18–19 inches, and weighs in at roughly 6 pounds. They're about the size of a pineapple. They won't grow much more now; otherwise, you'd burst. Baby is pretty much fully developed and ready to go. They just need a couple more weeks inside so their digestive system can catch up with the rest of them.

Baby is probably eavesdropping on you because of their sharpened sense of hearing. They're also moving lower into your pelvis... Fun...

Trimester 4: The Stork Has Arrived

Chapter 10: Labor

Signs You're Going Into Labor Soon

Your back hurts

Most pregnant women experience back pain the entire time. But, if the pain intensifies or is central to your lower back, it may indicate that you are going through *back labor,* which happens when the baby is head down and facing forward. According to the Cleveland Clinic (n.d.), up to 32% of newborns are in this position in the beginning stages of labor.

Your baby's face is usually pressed against your spine as they go down into the birth canal, but when a baby's skull is on your spine, it can hurt. You'll feel the pain in your abdomen, but it'll mostly be localized in your back.

Some pregnant women may also have back pain-like contractions or back pain that radiates to or from their back. This may not be back labor, but any severe back pain may be an indication that labor is about to start.

You see a bloody show

For the entirety of your pregnancy, your cervix stays closed. It's clogged up with mucus that works to protect your baby from infection.

Once you go into labor, it's not needed anymore, so as labor progresses, the cervix starts to soften, dilate, and efface in anticipation of delivery, which causes the plug to make its way out. The mucus is expelled as a blob or like discharge, and it can weigh up to 1–2 tablespoons and measure as much as 2 inches.

As your cervix continues to dilate and efface, microscopic blood vessels rupture along its surface, tainting the mucus and giving it a brown (from old blood) or pink hue. Labor could start hours, days, or even weeks after you see it.

Losing your mucus plug is usually a sign that labor is starting, but keep in mind that it can be displaced gradually over time, so you won't always notice it. If you've still got it, or even trace amounts of it, it can indicate that delivery could happen soon.

Your water breaks

The amniotic sac doesn't always rupture prior to the onset of contractions. In reality, many women start their labor well before their water breaks. Also, the experience looks and feels different for everyone. For some, it's more of a little leak than a large gush.

But, if your sac does rupture on its own, it usually indicates that labor is about to start, if it hasn't already. About 90% of full-term pregnancies, 37 weeks or more along, experience spontaneous labor within 24 hours of the water breaking. Those that don't are likely to undergo an induction because after the amniotic sac has ruptured, the risk of infection increases (*Water Breaking: Understand This Sign of Labor*, 2019).

Timing Contractions

What Do They Feel Like?

Your womb thickens during a contraction before relaxing. A lot of women describe them as a feeling like severe period pains.

They will likely get longer, intensify, and become more frequent as labor progresses. Muscles constrict, and discomfort rises with a contraction; your belly actually becomes harder while it's happening. The hardness will subside as the muscles relax and the pain eases.

The contractions are lowering your baby and widening your cervix so they can go through the birth canal.

When to Start Timing

You can determine whether you are in actual labor by timing your contractions.

When your contractions start to happen closer together, and get stronger, start timing them. The best way to get an indication of their frequency is to start by timing three in a row. You can use your phone or a stopwatch.

Once they're happening at least every five minutes, and lasting a minute at a time, you should start making your way to where you're going to deliver.

What if I Don't Make It Out of the House in Time?

In the unlikely event that you are unable to reach the hospital in time, commit this piece of advice to memory so that you are ready.

If you're genetically predisposed to giving birth faster and you're aware of it, time your contractions from the beginning and go to the hospital just in case. If you spontaneously feel the urge to push after a short labor period, and you aren't at home, don't panic. Many babies have been born in moving vehicles. Even though it's unlikely, being ready for an emergency delivery at home could curb your worry and make you feel comfortable knowing that you can manage the situation.

A few years ago, the American College of Nurse-Midwives (ACNM) started a program called "Giving Birth in Place" to inform individuals on how to prepare for emergency deliveries at home.

They say it's best to stay where you are if you've got a strong feeling you won't make it to the hospital. It's recommended that you assemble a delivery-ready supply kit for emergency situations. The items should be stored out of reach of kids and animals in a waterproof bag. The following should be packed in:
- A bag of extra-large underpads with a plastic back to shield sheets from bodily fluids.

- Bulb syringe in a baby-safe size. It must be made of soft plastic, and be an ear syringe so it can fit in baby's nose.

- A chemical cold pack.

- A small isopropyl alcohol bottle.

- 12 maternity pads.

- One pack of large cotton balls.

- Sharp, clean scissors (to cut the cord).

- A box of single-use latex or plastic gloves.

- White shoelaces (to tie the cord).

- A hot water bottle (for the baby).

- Ibuprofen or acetaminophen.

- An antibacterial liquid hand sanitizer or a little bar of soap

- Six diapers.

Stages of Labor

Stage one

Your contractions intensify, and your cervix dilates to a diameter of 10 cm.

Stage two

You'll experience painful contractions, and eventually, the need to push. You'll receive instructions from your midwife on how to control your breathing during contractions. It is at this point that your baby will be delivered.

Stage three

After giving birth to your child, you push the placenta out. Stage three is also called "the afterbirth." Your midwife or doctor may offer you a shot to help you along.

Should I Shave?

The times have definitely changed. People are less worried about the little things. So a bit of hair down there isn't going to shock or worry your doctor.

The medical staff's role is to ensure that both you and the baby have a safe birth. They have no concerns or worries regarding the appearance of your perineum.

Hospitals used to shave women in preparation for delivery, but that's changed, and it's now recommended that you don't shave at all. At least not past 36 weeks gestation.

The belief was that shaving would prevent infection, but as time goes on and medicine advances, there's been evidence of a slight increase in infection after shaving.

Try not to worry about judgment; the chances of you facing any are slim to none. If you really must groom, opt for a wax or any other method that doesn't involve a razor.

Breath Techniques

Learn and practice regulated breathing techniques for labor pain management before you go into labor. By focusing on your breathing, you can keep your oxygen levels high, relax your muscles and mind, and get some relief from the discomfort.

Before giving birth, practice the breathing exercises below if you haven't already studied specialized breathing methods at a birthing class:

- **Belly breathing**

Try belly breathing when labor is still early. When you breathe in, let your belly expand outward; when you exhale, let your belly relax downward.

Place one hand right below your ribs on your abdomen, and the other on your chest.

Inhale deeply through your nose, allowing your abdomen to push your hand away. Your chest should remain still.

Put your lips together and exhale like you're whistling. Use the hand that is placed on your tummy to force all the air out.

During or in between contractions, do this exercise. Breathe slowly each time.

- **Pant-pant-blow breathing**

Belly breathing will be harder as labor progresses, so exhale six times per minute in a "pant-pant-blow" sequence as your contractions get stronger.

At the beginning of your contraction, inhale deeply through your nose.

Exhale by doing two brief blows followed by one longer blow. It sounds like "hee-hee-hooooo." You see it in movies.

It should take about 10 seconds to breathe in and out like this.

Keep breathing like this until the contraction stops.

Fetal and Internal Monitoring

Your doctor will want to examine your baby's health both during pregnancy and labor. They monitor baby by checking the heart rate and other vital signs.

There are two ways doctors monitor babies. On the outside of your tummy (external monitoring) and on the inside (internal monitoring):

- **External monitoring**: A fetoscope is a specialized instrument used to monitor the baby's heartbeat. It's a stethoscope with a distinct shape. The baby can also be monitored using a doppler.

- **Internal monitoring**: The medical staff attach an electrode onto the baby's head while in utero.

Your midwife keeps an eye on your baby's heartbeat during labor so they can identify any indication of trouble as soon as possible. The range of a healthy heart rate is 110 to 160 beats per minute.

The healthcare team might also make use of:

Intermittent Monitoring

Being monitored at regular intervals throughout labor.

The midwife may use a fetoscope or a doppler. She'll place one of the instruments on your belly to hear baby's heartbeat. She'll do so every 15 minutes in the first stage of labor and every five minutes in the second.

Should there be any concerns about you or your baby, they will start electronic monitoring.

Electronic Fetal Monitoring (EFM)

Continuously keep an eye on the two of you...

Medical staff will put electrodes on your belly. The electrodes are attached to a large machine that continually prints waves that signify your contractions and the baby's heartbeat. Instead of paper, some machines display everything on a screen.

Or, with your permission, they might place the electrodes directly on to baby's head so they can monitor the heartbeat.

EFM is usually used when you're past 42 weeks gestation, or when you ask for an epidural. It also gets recommended if:

- Your temperature or blood pressure are high.

- There are concerns about your baby's growth or heartbeat.

- Your waters are sparse, your waters break more than 24 hours before labor, or they are stained with meconium or blood.

- You're being induced, you're on oxytocin, or your labor's lasting longer than 8 hours.

Fetal Blood Sampling

A small blood sample is taken by an obstetrician to determine baby's heart rate.

If they're worried about your baby's heartbeat, your healthcare team will ask an obstetrician to check, and the doctor might advise you to get a blood sample. They will need your permission before they can do anything.

You tilt or sleep on your left side with your right leg lifted, and then your doctor will put a speculum in your vagina, make a little cut on your infant's scalp, and then get a drop or two of blood.

They're looking at the acid and oxygen levels in the blood sample. These results can indicate how well your baby is responding to labor.

If it's normal, you get to stay in labor. If it's not and your baby's in distress, your obstetrician could advise that they deliver your child right away.

What Positions Are Best for Labor?

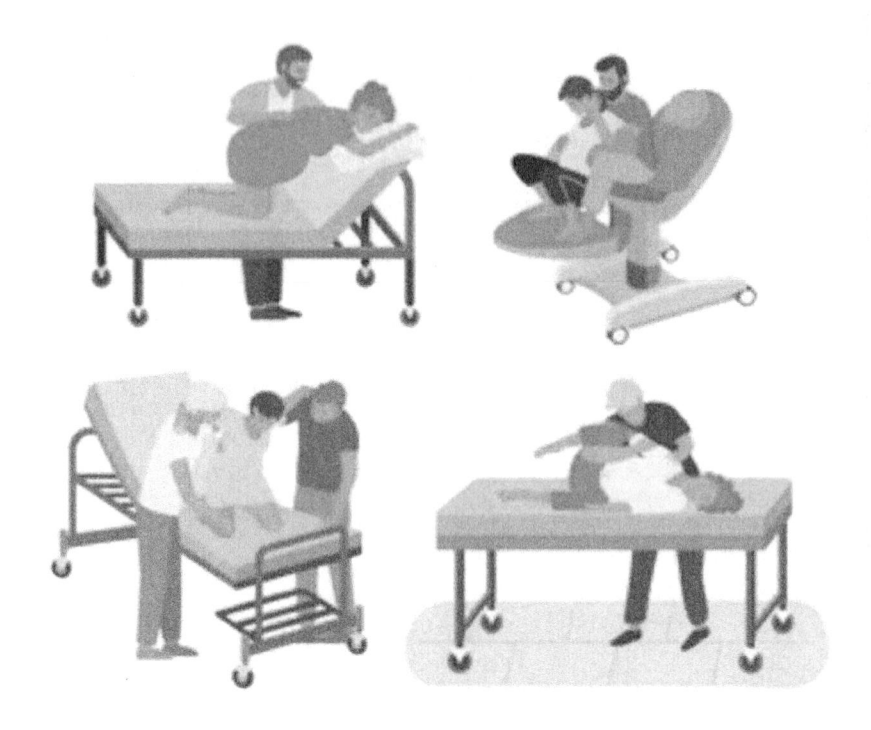

The immediate picture you have in your mind of a woman giving birth is her reclining in a hospital bed. In reality, women move about a lot during labor and change positions as their labor develops and the baby shifts positions.

Moving, maintaining balance, and shifting positions can:

- Help you determine your ideal birthing position.//
- Help the baby move down.
- Shorten labor time.
- Reduce discomfort.
- Help you to cope.
- Give you a sense of control over your labor.

Good Positions to Try

- Straddling a chair.
- Standing and leaning against something.
- Seated and leaning against a table.
- Standing and leaning on a birth ball that is perched on a bed.
- Hugging a birth ball while in a squatting position.
- Getting on all fours and kneeling.
- Sitting and bouncing softly on a birth ball.
- Kneeling over the back of your bed, or kneeling and leaning against your birth partner for support.

If you can, try to walk around as much as you can. You can try to maintain motion by shifting your weight from one foot to the other or by rolling your pelvis if you start to feel fatigued or your contractions become more intense.

Your birth partner will be able to give you massages or stroke your back in some of the positions listed above. It will help you release some endorphins, which might help a little with the pain.

Don't forget to take breaks when necessary, and don't give a second thought to how you look or sound during any of this. Medical staff have seen it all before and then some.

What Can Your Birthing Partner Do?

Birth partners can enhance the experience and make a woman feel supported while in labor. Here are some pointers on how to be a fantastic one:

- **Be prepared and ready**

Birth partners need to be fully prepared and on standby.

If a birth plan is in place, it should be discussed at length and in advance with the mom-to-be. A partner can learn about what to anticipate by taking birth classes together with the mom.

Ask mom if there's anything in particular that can be done to help her during labor and delivery. Ask about the things you shouldn't involve yourself with, as well. Know your boundaries; if there are aspects of the delivery you would prefer not to participate in directly, let it be known in advance.

If there's anything you're not confident with yet, make sure you learn and practice it in time for the birth.

- **Provide good company**

    During the early stages of labor, especially, keep mom company, ensure she's happy, and try to pass the time together.

    You might be able to spend time together walking, watching TV, listening to music, or reading. Literally, anything to get her mind off the discomfort.

    Do anything and everything you can to help her feel more at ease. She might want help taking a bath or shower. You can get her things to help soothe her, or help her maneuver that.

    Look after yourself too, and take breaks when you need to. Choose comfortable clothes and pack snacks for yourself so you can stay in peak shape.

- **Provide practical support**

    You can help in so many little ways. Driving mom to the hospital, carrying the bags, and getting her checked into the birthing suite or hospital.

    Once you're in the labor and delivery ward you can help her get comfortable in the bed, help her turn around if need be. A refreshment and a back rub would also go down really nicely.

If you've opted for a home birth, you can help set everything up. Then on the day, you can offer refreshments and keep the family updated with how things are going.

This step hinges on you, knowing well in advance how everything needs to happen.

- **Advocate for her**

You might need to let the midwife or doctor know what mom needs because you know her best. Help her communicate her wishes to them. Also, you might need to keep her updated on all new information that comes from the medical staff.

Even if she chooses something completely off from her birth plan, you should still support her choices.

- **Be flexible**

You can do all the preparation in the world, but you'll need to adapt to whatever's working or not working throughout labor because no two labors are the same. It's possible that everything can go as planned, but it's also possible that an urgent medical issue could occur and change how the labor progresses.

Whatever happens, try to let mom know and keep encouraging and reassuring her. She will feel less powerless and a bit more in control of the situation.

You might have to make very important decisions at the drop of a hat, or you might have to wait really long for her labor to progress. Be ready to be flexible and ride the wave of the day.

Chapter 11: Delivery

The hope for all deliveries is that they're straightforward. In the event that things don't go exactly according to plan, you should have some knowledge of the types of interventions that are used and how they affect you. That way you'll always be making informed decisions.

What's an Episiotomy?

Your vagina and perineum are incredibly elastic; they're able to expand to accommodate the birth of your child.

On occasion, a member of your healthcare team may need to make a cut in your perineum to widen the opening at your vagina. This is an episiotomy. It gets sewn up once the baby is born.

Episiotomies are only performed when necessary, so they don't happen for every labor.

They're done mostly to stop tearing or in situations where moms just need a bit of help. They're most likely in vaginal births.

Other Reasons for Episiotomies

- Baby's in distress. Their heart rate is either too fast or too slow; this could mean that they aren't getting enough oxygen.
- Your baby's breech.
- Your baby's bigger than average.
- Your doctor plans on using forceps or a ventouse.
- Your doctor advises that you have a quick labor because you have medical issues, like a heart condition.
- You've been exerting yourself for a while and are worn out.

- It's required to stop a third-degree tear from happening (a third-degree tear is a perineum muscular tear that also impacts the anus muscles).

Recovery

Keeping It Clean

To clean your perineum, use only warm water. Avoid rubbing it when cleaning. Witch hazel and salt are assumed to support the acceleration of wound healing, but there isn't any scientific proof of this. However, if you want to use them, there's no harm in doing so.

Wear underwear that's made of breathable materials, like cotton. Put on comfy, loose clothing while you're healing, because tight clothing may hurt you.

Clean your hands

- both before and after using the restroom.
- before and after cleaning your wound.
- when swapping out your pad.

If you live with young children, washing up and being clean are extremely important because they could be carrying an illness like Group A strep that could spread to your wound. Once it enters the bloodstream, things can become quite serious.

Going to the Loo

Wash your perineum each and every time you're done in the restroom. Put warm water around your vaginal area as well. Pouring warm water on your outer vagina while you urinate might also lessen the stinging sensation from the urine.

Lean forward toward your knees while urinating. This will assist in diverting urine away from the wound.

Your First Bowel Movement

After giving birth, your back passage and bottom may feel a little sore.

When you're ready to poop, your first instinct might be to worry about your stitches. You don't have to; pooping won't make you lose your stitches or open your incision. You can take steps to make pooping more bearable.

As you poop, place a clean pad at the side of your incision and gently push. This may relieve some of the pressure you'll feel on the wound.

Wipe gently from front to back. This lessens the chance of bacteria infecting the wound.

Do your best to avoid constipation. Drink plenty of water and consume foods high in fiber.

Pain Management

Paracetamol is safe to take, and it works well in relieving pain. If you're breastfeeding, you can take two 500-milligram pills every six hours.

Diclofenac pills or suppositories are also really good. Suppositories offer pain relief for a longer time and can be inserted once every 18 hours. If you're unsure about how to put them in, you can ask your midwife.

Aspirin can't be taken if you're breastfeeding.

If paracetamol and diclofenac don't work, call your doctor so they can check and see if it's infected.

Infection indicators:

- redness
- a yellow or green discharge

- extreme pain

Let the medical team know if you're breastfeeding so they can prescribe pain medication that's not harmful to your breastfed baby.

Forceps and Vacuum Births

Forceps and vacuum births are also called "assisted births." Your healthcare team only makes use of them when labor has stalled, or when delivery is about to end but is not progressing, and the health of you or your baby is at risk from an extended labor.

Forceps look like metal salad utensils that the doctor can use to guide your baby out of the birth canal by grasping them while they're still inside. A ventouse is a suction cup used to get your baby out of the birth canal. They don't happen too often, but they can be a helpful alternative to a cesarean.

What Happens?

Before anything happens, your healthcare team will need your permission.

If you haven't already had an epidural, you'll get a local anesthetic to numb your vagina and perineum. If your doctor has concerns, you might be taken to an operating room so that, if necessary, you can get a C-section.

To widen the vaginal orifice, your doctor might do an episiotomy. Your birth partner might still be able to cut the cord if they want to, because once your baby's out, they are placed on your tummy.

Forceps

Forceps are curved so they can fit around a baby's head. Doctors gently wrap the baby's head in the forceps, which are joined together at the handle. The doctor then carefully pulls while you push during a contraction.

There are lots of different types. Some are made specifically to turn the baby into the proper position for birth. For example, if the baby's lying to one side (occipito-lateral position) or facing up (occipito-posterior position).

Ventouse

The suction cup is attached to a tube that connects to a suction device. The baby's head is firmly supported by the cup, and then the doctor gently pulls the baby while you push during a contraction.

Forceps are usually suggested over a suction cup, especially if you're giving birth before 36 weeks. It's because forceps are less likely to harm the baby's head while it's still soft.

Why Would I Need One?

- You've got an underlying health condition like hypertension, so you're advised not to push.

- Your baby's heart rate is worrying.

- Your baby's in an awkward position.

- Your baby's energy is dwindling, and might be in distress.

- When you deliver a premature baby vaginally, forceps can assist in shielding your baby's head from your perineum.

Potential Risks

For you:

- **Anal incontinence**: After delivery, anal incontinence can occur, especially if there is a third- or fourth-degree tear. These tears are very common with assisted deliveries.

- **Urinary incontinence**: Urinary incontinence after delivery is quite common. It happens a lot after a forceps or ventouse delivery. You can prevent it with physiotherapy and pelvic floor exercises.

- **Higher risk of blood clots**: Blood clots in the pelvic or leg veins are more likely to occur after an assisted birth. You can avoid them by being physically active after birth. You can also wear anti-clot stockings, or your doctor might give you heparin injections.

- **Third and fourth-degree tears**: These kinds of tears affect:
    - 3 out of every 100 women giving birth naturally
    - 4 out of every 100 women in a ventouse delivery
    - 8–12 out of every 100 women in forceps delivery

For baby:

- A ventouse cup mark is left on a baby's head. It's called a "chignon," and it normally fades away within 48 hours.

- A bruise on a baby's head is called a "cephalohematoma." It affects 1 to 12 out of every 100 babies delivered with a ventouse. There's no cause for concern, and the bruise goes away with time.

- Marks on a baby's face from forceps. They disappear within a day or two.

- One in ten babies born via assisted delivery experience minor cuts on their face or scalp; they heal fast.

- Jaundice, which causes your baby's skin and eyes to turn yellow, should subside in a few days.

After an assisted delivery, you may stay in the hospital a little longer, but your recuperation time will be about the same as it would be for a natural birth. It takes around six weeks, but it can take longer if you're recovering from third- or fourth-degree tears. After about a month, the stitches dissolve. You should be able to control any lingering pain with over-the-counter drugs. Consult your healthcare practitioner if the pain is more serious.

The Placenta

Delivery after vaginal birth

Your uterus will continue to contract after the baby is born, so the placenta can advance. These contractions lack the intensity of labor contractions.

Sometimes you may be advised to push harder or have pressure applied to your tummy to get it out. Normally, it's out within 5 minutes, but some people may need more time.

Once you've given birth, you could be so preoccupied with meeting your baby that you don't even feel the placenta delivery. But, some women have reported having seen a second rush of blood that's typically followed by the placenta.

The umbilical cord is connected to the placenta. It doesn't hurt when it's severed because it doesn't have any nerves.

Delivery after cesarean

Your doctor will manually remove the placenta from your uterus during a cesarean delivery before stitching up the incisions.

The fundus (the top portion of your uterus) is then likely to be massaged after birth to help it contract and begin to shrink. They might prescribe medicine, like pitocin, to make your uterus contract if it's unable to do so naturally.

Your placenta will then be carefully checked to ensure it's fully intact after delivery. If it's found to have portions missing, your doctor can advise a uterine ultrasound to confirm. Excessive bleeding after delivery can be a sign that some placenta remains in the uterus. This is called "retained placenta."

Retained Placenta

The following factors could prevent the placenta from delivering fully:
- The cervix closes, leaving a very small gap through which the placenta can't pass.
- The placenta is too firmly fused to the uterine wall.
- During delivery, a piece of the placenta broke off and stayed behind.

The uterus must contract after delivery, so retaining the placenta is a serious risk. Once the uterus is tightened, the blood vessels inside it can stop bleeding. So having portions of the placenta left inside may cause bleeding or infection.

Your doctor will advise surgical removal as soon as possible.

In rare cases, the placenta is so closely bound to the uterus that the only way to remove it is a full hysterectomy.

If you have any of the following, you're at risk of having a retained placenta, for example:
- Prior instances of placenta retention.
- Prior to cesarean delivery.

- Having had uterine fibroids.

Should you be concerned about retaining your placenta, speak with your doctor so they can come up with a strategy to avoid it.

Once the mammoth task of delivering your baby is done, the doctors and nurses have to shift their attention a little bit to make sure your little one is okay. Shortly after giving you a bit of time with baby, they will start running routine tests and monitoring the both of you.

What Is an Apgar Score?

At one and five minutes after birth, babies are given the Apgar test. How well they tolerated labor is measured by the one-minute score. The five-minute score informs the medical professional of the baby's health outside the womb.

In some cases, the test gets carried out ten minutes after delivery.

The Apgar score was first created in 1952 by Virginia Apgar, MD (1909–1974).

A doctor, midwife, or nurse can perform the test. They look at the baby's:

- Heartbeat
- Skin color
- respiratory effort
- Muscle tone
- Reflexes

Each category receives a score of zero, one, or two depending on the baby's condition.

Heart rate

- Babies with no heartbeat receive a score of 0.

- Babies with a heart rate of less than 100 beats per minute receive a score of 1.

- Babies with heart rates over 100 beats per minute receive a score of 2.

Skin color

- If the baby's skin is pale blue, they receive a score of 0.

- If the baby's skin is pink, but their extremities are blue, they receive a score of 1.

- If the baby's skin is pink all over, they receive a score of 2.

Respiratory effort

- If the baby isn't breathing, they receive a score of 0.

- If the baby's breathing is slow and erratic, they receive a score of 1.

- If the baby cries straight after birth, they receive a score of 2.

Muscle tone

- Babies with loose, flaccid muscles receive a score of 0.

- Babies with a bit of muscle tone receive a score of 1.

- Babies that make vigorous movements receive a score of 2.

Reflexes

- If the baby doesn't respond to mild stimulation, they receive a score of 0.

- If the baby grimaces, they receive a score of 1.

- If the baby grimaces, coughs, sneezes, or cries loudly, they receive a score of 2.

Newborn Screening Tests

Your baby will undergo newborn screening when they are one to two days old. At birth, they are screened for dangerous but uncommon and usually treatable medical conditions. It involves tests for the heart, hearing, and blood.

Some babies are born with health conditions and don't show any signs, so screening can help find the ailment early so it can be treated. Early intervention is crucial since it could protect your baby from more serious health issues.

In the United States, newborn screening is provided for every baby. Every year, almost 4 million newborns are screened.

How's It Done?

1. **Hearing test**

    Used to test for hearing loss. Babies wear tiny headphones, and a sophisticated computer is used to monitor how they react to sound.

2. **Heart screening**

    Used to check for a class of heart diseases known as critical congenital heart defects (also called "critical CHDs" or "CCHDs"). It makes use of a quick test known as pulse oximetry. Using a pulse oximeter device and sensors applied to your baby's skin, pulse oximetry measures the amount of oxygen in your baby's blood.

3. **Blood test**

The blood test is administered to look for uncommon but dangerous medical disorders. Your baby's heel is pricked by a medical professional to obtain a few droplets of blood. They draw the blood onto a piece of paper and send it to a laboratory for analysis. By the time baby is five to seven days old, the results are ready. Ask your baby's doctor or the hospital staff for further information about the timelines for shipping blood samples to the lab and receiving test results back.

What if the Results Aren't Normal?

Most of these tests come back normal. If your baby's results are abnormal, they may just require additional testing. A diagnostic test is the next step to determine whether the baby has a health issue. Further testing is not required if the diagnostic test findings are normal. Your provider can advise you on what to do for your baby if the results are not normal.

One of the most common conditions we see in newborn babies is:

Jaundice

Bilirubin accumulation in the blood is the primary cause of jaundice. The breakdown of red blood cells results in the production of the yellow substance bilirubin.

Jaundice is common among newborns because they have a large amount of red blood cells that are constantly being broken down and replenished. Also, because a newborn baby's liver is still developing, it is less efficient at clearing bilirubin from the blood. The liver becomes more adept at processing bilirubin by the time they are about 2 weeks old, so jaundice resolves by this time without any negative effects on baby.

Jaundice can be hard to see on darker skin tones, so in those cases, you'd look at the palms and the soles of the feet.

Other signs of neonatal jaundice:

- Urine that is dark yellow (newborn babies' pee should be colorless).

- Light-colored poop (it should be yellow or orange)

These symptoms often manifest two days after birth and tend to subside on their own by the time the infant is about two weeks old.

Chapter 12: Postpartum

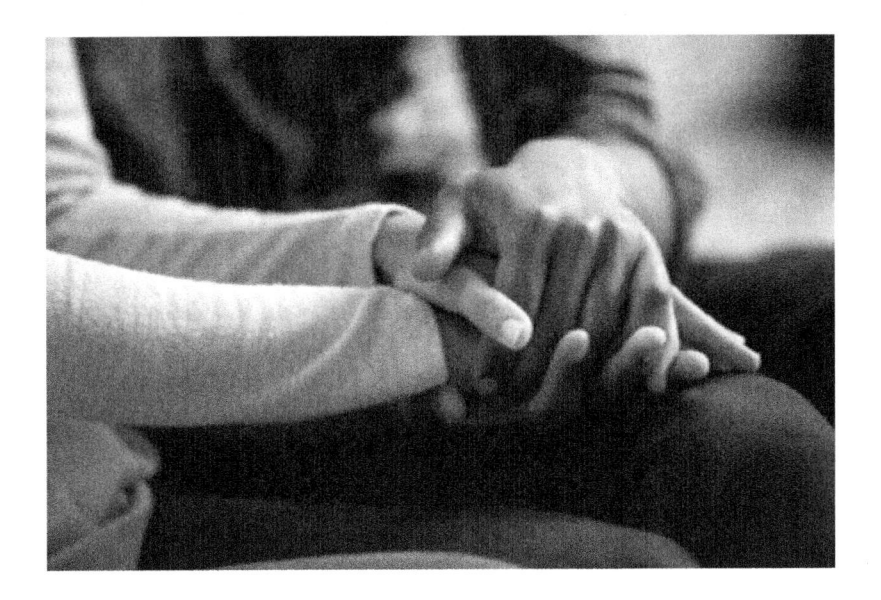

Emotions After Delivery

After you give birth, you go through a range of emotions that words can't describe. Your baby's here, your body still sort of feels pregnant, and your hormones are all over the place. It takes time for everything to balance out and go back to normal, so sometimes, as your body is adjusting, you can experience feelings of dread and anxiety.

In some cases, it manifests as full-on depression.

A lot of new moms go through the *baby blues*, which include unbalanced moods, bouts of crying throughout the day, anxiety, and trouble sleeping. It usually starts a couple of days after delivery and can last up to two weeks. Anything longer than that is most likely postpartum depression.

Postpartum depression is a more severe and pervasive type of depression that new moms endure. If it starts during pregnancy and persists after childbirth, it's called "peripartum depression." In very rare cases, some moms develop postpartum psychosis, which is a severe mood illness.

Postpartum depression is neither a weakness nor a deficiency in a person's character. A lot of the time, it's just a side effect of childbirth. Treating it as soon as possible will help you control your symptoms and strengthen your relationship with your baby.

Signs to Look Out For: Baby Blues

- Anxiety
- Weepiness
- Despair
- Moodiness
- Mood swings
- Trouble concentrating
- Increase or decrease in appetite
- Insomnia

Signs to Look Out For: Postpartum Depression

Postpartum depression can start off feeling like the baby blues, but the symptoms are more severe and persistent. So much so that they could eventually make it difficult for you to take care of your child and do other everyday tasks. Symptoms typically start to appear within the first few weeks of you being a mom, but they can start sooner—during pregnancy—or later—up to a year after delivery.

Symptoms include:
- All the symptoms mentioned above
- Excessive crying

- Withdrawing from those around you
- Having a hard time bonding with your baby
- Sleeping too often
- Fatigue
- Loss of interest and enjoyment in previously enjoyable activities
- Feelings of inadequacy
- Thoughts of self-harm and harming your baby
- Recurring suicidal thoughts

Signs to Look Out For: Postpartum Psychosis

Postpartum psychosis often appears within the first week following delivery. The symptoms are severe. Symptoms include:

- Paranoia
- Being very energized and unhappy
- Trouble sleeping
- Delusions and hallucination
- Feelings of obsession around your baby
- Feeling lost and confused
- Attempting to hurt yourself or your child

Postpartum psychosis needs to be treated right away because it might cause life-threatening ideas or actions.

Can My Partner Have Postpartum Depression?

According to studies, new dads can also experience postpartum depression. They can exhibit symptoms that mimic those of mothers with postpartum depression. They might experience changes in their regular eating and sleeping schedules, or they can feel depressed, exhausted, overwhelmed, or anxious.

The fathers who are most susceptible to postpartum depression are those who are young, have a history of depression, have issues in their relationship, or are financially strapped. PPD in your partner can have the same detrimental effects on your relationship and the development of your child as it would if you had it.

When to Seek Help

It sounds unrealistic, but it can be very hard to even realize, let alone acknowledge, that you've got the baby blues or PPD. If you show any signs, make an appointment with your obstetrician, gynecologist, or primary care physician. Get help as quickly as you can if you exhibit symptoms that point to postpartum psychosis.

Postpartum Body

Your hormones change during pregnancy to promote the development of your unborn child and get your body ready for labor. Once you give birth, they work to help your body recover, foster a bond with your newborn, and help you breastfeed.

The initial hormonal changes following delivery are:

- A decrease in estrogen and progesterone.

- The bonding hormone, oxytocin, increases and plays a part in the powerful maternal instinct you'll experience.

- To signal the production of milk, prolactin levels rise.

Your First Postpartum Period

The restarting of your period following delivery depends on a number of factors. The biggest being whether you've decided to exclusively nurse your baby.

Those who choose not to breastfeed usually get their period between four weeks and three months after giving birth, which is a lot sooner than those who do. Some breastfeeding moms get their period during that time period too, but most don't until they've started to wean or have completely stopped breastfeeding.

Postpartum Hair Loss

In the six months following childbirth, your hair may start to shed or even come out in clumps.

Most people lose around 100 hairs daily, but they don't fall out all at once, so you don't notice. When you're pregnant, your hormones prevent your hair from falling out, making it appear thicker.

Once you've delivered and your hormone levels return to normal, the hair you retained in pregnancy starts to fall out, so it can seem like you're losing hair.

Don't panic though, because you're not losing anything; just going back to normal. If you're breastfeeding, you may retain a bit of that hair, until such time as you decide to wean.

In about a year, everything should have stabilized, and you should start to see your hair going back to the way it was pre-pregnancy.

How You Can Deal With It

- **Get the proper nutrients**: Eat clean and continue taking your prenatal vitamins.

- **Be gentle with your hair**: Use a good conditioner, a wide-toothed comb, and only shampoo when absolutely necessary. This will help reduce tangling.

- **Choose the appropriate accessories**: Instead of using elastic bands to hold hair up, use scrunchies or barrettes, and avoid pulling hair into tight ponytails.

- **Use less heat**: Try to avoid using flat irons, curling irons, and blow dryers.

- **Less chemical treatments**: Postpone getting your hair straightened, permed, or highlighted until the shedding stops.

Postpartum Preeclampsia

Postpartum Preeclampsia is a dangerous disorder associated with high blood pressure. Any new mom who has just had a baby is susceptible. It's the same as preeclampsia in pregnancy but doesn't harm the baby.

Risks include:
- Death
- Organ failure
- Stroke
- Seizures

Warning signs:
- Abdominal pain (upper right quadrant)
- Swelling of the face and hands
- Nausea or vomiting
- Terrible headache

- Seeing spots (or other changes in vision)
- Respiratory issues or shortness of breath

Precautionary measures:
- Rely on your instincts
- Monitor your blood pressure
- Look out for warning signs and tell your doctor
- Determine whether a one-week follow-up appointment is required.
- Don't miss any follow-up appointments

Settling to Breastfeeding

For roughly the first month, new babies should be breastfed 8–12 times each day. Breastmilk is very easily digestible, so babies feel hungry all the time. Regular feedings in the first few weeks also help to promote your milk supply.

By the second month, baby will probably only be nursing seven to nine times a day.

Breastfeeding should be an on-demand thing in the first few weeks. That's roughly every 1.5 to 3 hours. The older babies get, the less they nurse. They also start to develop a more regular eating pattern. For some, it's every 90 minutes, while others wait two to three hours between feeds.

The span of time between feeds should never exceed four hours, even at night.

How do I measure the time between feeds?

The best way to measure the intervals between feeds is to count from the time baby starts feeding as opposed to when they finish. So if baby's first feed was at 5 a.m., and the subsequent feedings began at 7 a.m. and 9 a.m., respectively, you can safely say they're feeding every two hours.

In the beginning, it can definitely feel like all you're doing is nursing, but as the weeks pass, the time between feeds will start to increase.

How long should my baby nurse?

In the beginning, babies can take up to 20 minutes to nurse on both breasts. As they get older and become used to feeding, this may decrease and become five to ten minutes on each side.

The length of time your baby feeds depends on your baby's needs and whether or not:

- Your breast milk has come in (usually two to five days after birth).
- Your let-down reflex happens immediately into a feed. Let-down reflex is the thing that allows milk to flow from the nipple.
- Your flow is fast.
- Baby has a strong latch and can fit as much of your areola as possible in their mouth.
- Baby starts swallowing right away.
- Baby is sleepy or preoccupied.

When to alternate

Try your best to give each breast an equal amount of time to nurse throughout the day by switching while feeding. This helps maintain your milk production in both breasts and helps you avoid uncomfortable engorgement.

If you start with your left breast at a particular feeding time, then try to start with the right one the next time. If you know you struggle to remember things like this, you can do something to help yourself remember. Like putting a ribbon or safety pin on the side of the breast you started the feed with. If you've got the time and energy, you can use a notebook or an app to keep track.

Some babies do favor one breast over the other, so if you can't alternate during a feed, you can just switch between breasts at every feed. Don't put too much pressure on yourself to switch in the middle of a feed. Do what's comfortable for you and baby.

How often to burp

Try burping before switching. Sometimes just the motion of switching can be enough to make a baby burp.

Some babies need a lot of burping, some need less. It depends on the baby, and it can be a different story at every feed.

Burping frequently could help if your baby spits up a lot. Spitting up is normal, but a baby shouldn't vomit after eating. If you notice your baby spitting up all or most of a feed, you may need to seek medical care.

When should I stop?

Do whatever works best for you and your baby. The recommendation is exclusively for 4 to 6 months before introducing solids. Breastfeeding can continue with solids for up to a year or longer as a matter of choice. Try and do it for as long as you can because there are so many benefits for both you and baby.

According to studies, it can reduce a baby's risk of developing diarrhea, ear infections, and bacterial meningitis, or at least minimize the severity of the symptoms. Children who breastfeed are also less susceptible to asthma, diabetes, obesity, and SIDS.

Breastfeeding reduces uterine size and burns calories for mothers. In fact, moms who do might regain their pre-pregnancy weight and shape faster. Moreover, it lowers a woman's risk of developing:

- breast cancer
- hypertension
- heart disease and diabetes

It also could shield moms from ovarian and uterine cancer.

Breastfeeding Twins: Positions and Tips

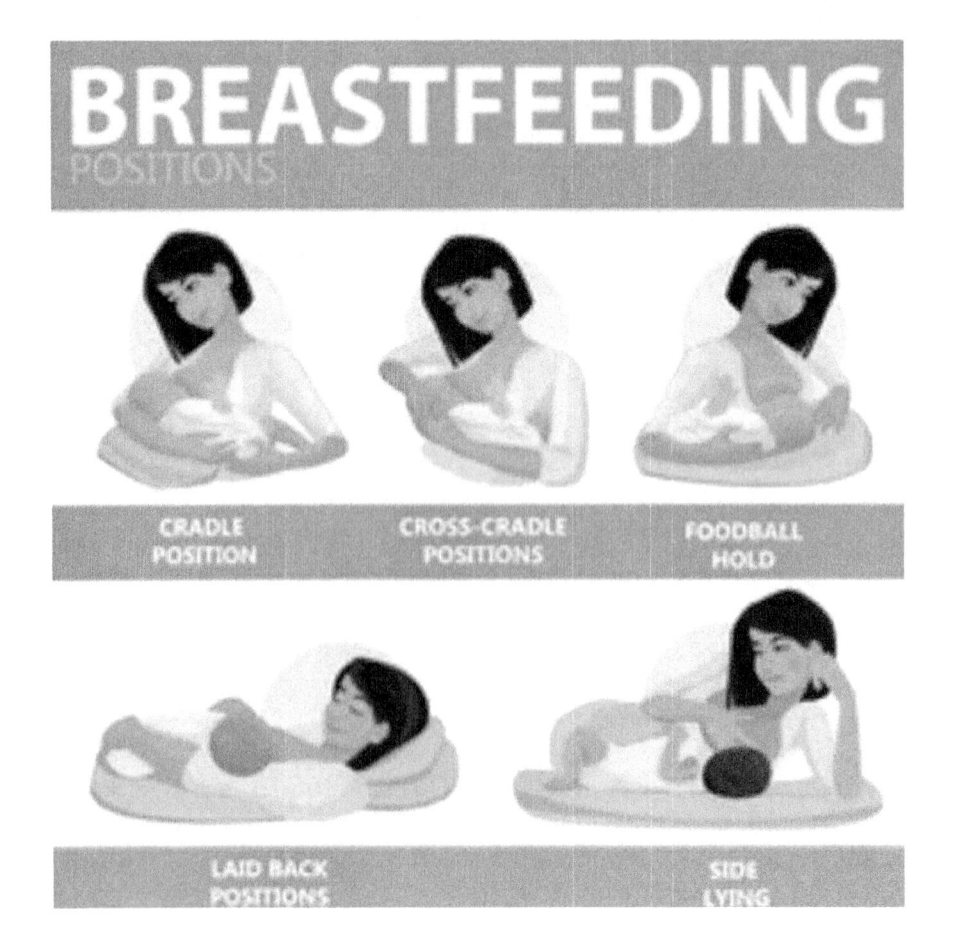

BREASTFEEDING POSITIONS

| CRADLE POSITION | CROSS-CRADLE POSITIONS | FOODBALL HOLD |

| LAID BACK POSITIONS | SIDE LYING |

BREASTFEEDING TWINS

Front Cross

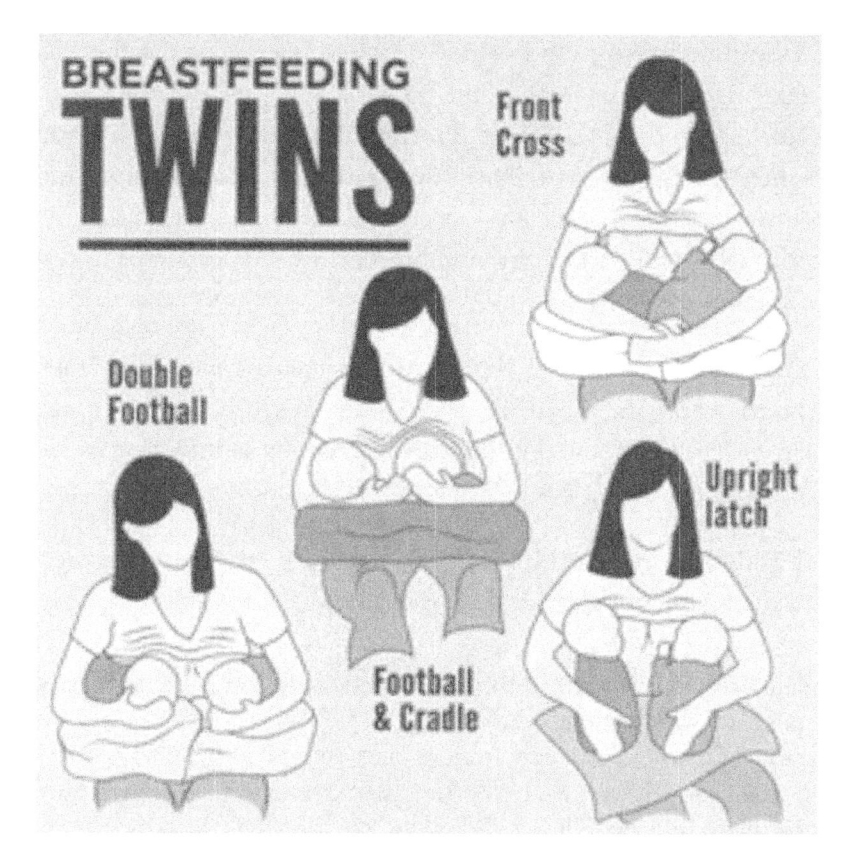

Double Football

Upright latch

Football & Cradle

Conceptualizing how to breastfeed twins is quite daunting. You might wrestle with the idea of feeding them one-at-a-time vs at the same time. You should do your best to have them on the same schedule and nursing at the same time. Keeping one hungry baby fed every couple of hours is a big undertaking; imagine that with two.

Here are some tips for nursing twins simultaneously:

Positioning

Nursing while sitting up can be hard, especially when it's nighttime feeding, but that's the safest and most efficient way to get both babies fed.

Find your position by process of elimination. Try out various positions until you find the most effective and pleasant one (Fierro, 2020):

- **Double or cross cradle hold**: A combination of the football and cradle holds. Both babies' torsos and legs are pointed to the side and in the same direction as they lay across mom. Their heads and upper backs are cradled by mom's hands and arms. One baby's legs are tucked under mom's arm (like in the football hold). And baby number two's head can actually rest on their sibling's body.

- **Criss-cross or front-V Hold**: Mom's hands cradle the babies' bodies from below while their heads rest on her forearms. Their legs are pointed in different directions as their bodies are crossed on Mom's lap.

- **Parallel or Saddle Hold**: Both babies are facing mom's chest while seated upright. Ideal for older babies who can sit.

Twins can breastfeed comfortably on a bed, sofa, or large armchair. Choose a space where there's enough room for everyone to spread out comfortably and where you can arrange everything you need so that it's close enough for you to reach. Before you start the feed, make sure you've got everything you'll need close by so you don't have to get up and interrupt the session. Make sure the babies are easy to reach before taking position. Try to alternate the babies so that both have access to each breast.

Breast engorgement

Breast engorgement is painful. It feels like they could pop at any time—it also feels warm, sensitive, heavy, and hard to the touch. Besides being uncomfortable, it can also lead to problems breastfeeding, so if you're able to recognize it early enough, you can get it treated.

A good number of moms experience it in the first few weeks. Hormone levels are changing, and milk production is high, so they swell. It's more than just the milk that makes them swell. Your breasts are on the receiving end of extra blood and fluids for milk production, so they swell and become congested. As time goes on and your body starts to go back to normal, it stops.

Causes

- **A feeding schedule**: The amount of milk a moms' breasts can hold without feeling uncomfortable varies. Moms who don't feed on demand regularly experience engorgement, mastitis, and insufficient milk production because their breasts aren't drained frequently enough.

- **Expressing**: Some moms like to kick their milk production into high gear by expressing and making more milk than their babies require. But if you find yourself going hours without expressing or nursing, your breasts can become engorged.

- **A baby that isn't latching**: You can maintain production and prevent clogged ducts or mastitis by routinely expressing milk until your baby is able to nurse comfortably.

- **Weaning too quickly**: Weaning can't happen all at once. It has to be gradual, so that your breasts can get used to producing less and less milk with time. Try hand- or pump-expressing just enough milk to relieve the feeling of fullness, being sure never to fully empty your breasts.

Treatment

- Try to nurse every 1.5 to 2 hours during the day and every 2–3 hours at night, starting at the same time each time. Try to make sure the first breast is empty before moving on to the second.

- To minimize swelling in between feeds, apply ice for 15 to 20 minutes at a time. You can use ice in any form as long as you're protecting your skin with some sort of cloth.

- Apply moist warmth to your breasts just before feeding for up to two minutes to encourage flow. Try a warm shower, a warm cloth, or submerging your breasts in warm water.

Clogged Ducts

Your breasts host a network of mammary ducts that transport milk from the breast to the nipple. If something like inflammation in the surrounding blood vessels and soft tissues obstructs the duct, milk may back up in them.

When a milk duct becomes blocked or obstructed, breast milk can't flow to the nipple.

It manifests as a red, tender, and an uncomfortable lump in your breast. It's crucial to understand the symptoms and how to treat it at home because it can result in infection.

Other symptoms include:

- Swelling or discomfort around the lump.
- Letdown causes pain.
- The disappearance of a lump after a feed or a pump.
- The disappearance of pain and discomfort after a feed.

Some moms get a blister on the nipple. It's called a "bleb." It's a tiny white dot on the nipple made up of debris from inflammation.

The causes of clogged ducts are the same as the ones for engorgement.

Treatment

The abbreviation BAIT can help you recall some of the best methods for unclogging a blocked duct:

- Breast rest: Avoid overstimulation or overfeed. If you are producing too much, reduce your output.
- Advil: Take 800 milligrams every eight hours for two days.
- Ice: Lay on your back and apply ice for ten minutes at a time every 30 minutes.
- Tylenol: Take 1,000 milligrams of Tylenol every eight hours for two days.

Mastitis (an infection) can develop as a result of not treating a blocked milk duct.

Mastitis

Mastitis symptoms develop fairly quickly. They include:
- Chills and body aches.
- Fever
- Red, swollen, pain-filled breasts
- Severe pain while breastfeeding or pumping

If you experience any symptoms, call your obstetrician right away because it needs to be treated with antibiotics.

Bottle-Feeding

How to Prepare Utensils

Everything you need for a bottle-feed must be sterilized and properly prepared. Poor cleanliness or improper preparation could make a baby gravely ill.

These are the steps to follow:

1. Sanitize your hands.

2. In warm, soapy water, clean the bottles, discs, lids, teats, and tongs.

3. Follow the manufacturer's recommendations while sterilizing. Everything can be sterilized using boiling water, a steam kit, or a chemical sterilizer. The best sterilizer is a steam one. Microwaveable or plug-in sterilizers are good too.

4. Before removing the bottles from the sterilizer with the tongs, wash and dry your hands.

5. After sterilization, do not rinse the utensils.

If your bottles are closed properly after sterilization, they will be clean and ready to use for up to 24 hours.

How to Prepare Formula

You'll need the following:

- a sterile prep area
- a minimum of six bottles, lids, discs, and teats
- formula
- a reliable source of water
- A kettle
- a little teat brush and a bottle brush

Use wide-necked bottles if you have vision problems, as they are easier to work with and fill.

These are the steps to follow:

1. Boil water in a kettle, then leave to cool for no longer than 30 minutes. This is so that the water is at least 150 °F.

2. Clean your prep space thoroughly. Use soap and warm water to wash your hands and a fresh towel to dry them.

3. To determine how much water and powder you need, carefully read the directions on the label of the formula.

4. Pour the stipulated amount of boiled water into a sterilized bottle. Be careful, it's still hot.

5. Add the stipulated number of scoops to the bottle. Too much or too little can make baby ill. Properly reseal the container to keep out moisture and germs.

6. To mix, gently swirl the bottle around until well mixed, or use a sterilized spoon to stir. Avoid shaking the bottle to avoid air bubbles.

7. Set the bottle in a big bowl of cold water if you need to cool it down quickly. Just make sure the cold water doesn't go over the bottle's neck or touch the neck.

8. Pour a tiny bit of milk on the inside of your wrist to make sure it's not hot. It should be lukewarm.

9. Feed baby and dispose of any milk the baby didn't drink in two hours.

10. Wash and rinse the bottle after every feed.

How to Give a Bottle

Sit so that you and baby are comfortable.

Always keep the bottle in your hand and baby in your arms.

Never let your child feed on their own. While feeding, your baby maintains eye contact with you, and this helps with bonding and can give you a bit of time to relax.

Never rest the bottle on or lean it against:

- a regular pillow
- a self-feeding pillow
- any other support structure

Your baby might choke if you do this.

Paced Feeding

Pacing is so important. Your baby will be able to regulate how quickly and how much milk they consume.

The best way for you and baby to get used to bottle-feeding is through paced feeding. It's comfortable for baby, and you can avoid overfeeding.

These are the steps to follow:

1. Hold the bottle horizontally while holding baby in an upright position on your lap.
2. Play around baby's top lip with the teat until they open their mouth.
3. Let baby suckle on the teat.
4. Tilt the bottle ever so slightly so that the teat fills with milk.

5. When baby stops for a break, lower the bottle so there's no milk in the teat.

6. Look to your baby for cues on when to feed and when to pause. Stop when they appear satisfied.

When your baby has had enough, they'll show it, so don't feed them beyond what they're willing to handle.

You can use a cup with handles if your child is older than six months and prefers not to drink from a bottle.

Until baby learns how to feed themselves, only pour a small amount of liquid into the cup at a time. This will save you from lots of spillage and waste.

To avoid excessive spitting up or vomiting, keep baby upright for at least 30 minutes after feeding. Use a smaller teat if you are experiencing issues with vomiting. If a teat is too big for your baby, it probably has a much faster flow and that may be triggering your baby's gag reflex.

Bonding With Your Baby

The universal idea of mothers bonding with their babies, is that they are immediately connected to their babies the second they're born. That's true for some, and not for others.

You carried your baby, so you've loved them from the beginning, that's a given. But the truth is that once the baby's out, they're essentially a stranger. It's normal for you to need some time to get to know them.

Many new parents require a bit of time to connect. When you bond with your baby, you start to feel an unwavering love for them. It's something that develops gradually, sometimes over the course of a year. So it's perfectly okay if you don't experience these intense feelings in the first few days or weeks following delivery.

There are things you can do to foster a close relationship with your baby, but there are also things that can impede the bonding process. It will eventually happen with time and with constant, close contact with your baby.

Why is it important?

Bonding is essential for development.

Your baby will believe the world is a safe place to play, learn, and explore when they get what they need from you. It could be as small as a smile, touch, or snuggle. These things establish the framework for your child's growth and welfare throughout childhood.

The act of bonding promotes your baby's physical and mental development. Frequent human interaction causes the baby's brain to release hormones. These hormones promote brain development. And, as your baby's brain develops, memory, cognition, and language develop too.

How to bond with your baby

Try the following:

- Speak to your baby in calming, reassuring tones. You could talk about the weather, or tell tales. Your baby will learn to recognize the sound of your voice and have a good foundation on which to learn language as they get older.

- Sing. Your baby will probably enjoy the rhythm and tones of songs and music.

- Look your baby in the eye when you talk and sing. Express yourself with your face too; that way, your baby will learn the relationship between words and feelings.

- Touch and cuddle your baby often. They can sense even the slightest touch. Gently stroke your baby when you're doing mundane things like changing a diaper or giving a bath.

- Always respond when your baby cries. Even if you haven't the slightest clue why they're crying, your responsiveness indicates to them that you'll always be there for them.

- Hold your baby close. Set some time aside to rock or cuddle your baby skin-to-skin.

- Make your baby feel secure physically. When holding your child, support their head and neck well. You can also swaddle them to mimic the safe environment of the womb.

Even after taking these steps, you might not feel the bond with your child that you believe you should, but there's no need to feel bad or embarrassed. The bond will develop the more time you spend together. More so if you've got support and time for self-care.

Here are some things to look out for that might slow the process of you bonding with your baby:

- The baby blues
- Postpartum depression
- A lack of support and time for self-care

Baby's First Bath

For a lot of parents, bath time is their favorite time to spend with their new babies. It's a great opportunity to connect without any interruptions. But these days, there's a lot of debate (mostly online) about how and when to bathe your newborn. Something that was a standard practice for centuries is now a source of uncertainty and even fear.

Most hospitals have typically washed babies within the first hour of their birth, but that's changing.

The World Health Organization advises waiting at least 24 hours after birth—or at least 6 hours if a full day is impractical for cultural reasons—before giving a newborn its first bath.

Reasons why it's recommended to delay the first bath include:

Breastfeeding and bonding: Premature bathing of the infant can interfere with early breastfeeding, skin-to-skin contact, and bonding. One study found that delaying the baby's initial bath by 12 hours led to a 166% increase in nursing success compared to babies who were bathed right away.

Dry skin: The vernix is a white waxy substance that covers babies' skin prior to birth. It's like a natural moisturizer and may have antibacterial properties. It should be left on the skin for a while to prevent the drying out of their sensitive skin. Preemies would greatly benefit from this because of how easily their skin can be damaged.

Blood sugar levels and body temperature: Babies who get bathed immediately could be more susceptible to hypothermia. Also, for some babies, that first bath can feel slightly stressful, which can increase their risk of experiencing a decrease in blood sugar (hypoglycemia).

Babies don't require baths every day because they don't perspire or become unclean enough to need them.

For the first year, three baths a week are enough. Anything more than that can cause your baby's skin to become dry.

Stick to sponge baths for the first couple of weeks or until the cord falls off.

Safety tips for a sponge bath:
- Ensure you've got everything ready before you start.
- Place baby on a flat surface that's comfortable for them, and convenient for you.
- Wash baby's face first.

- Keep baby warm.

You can start immersing your baby in water once the belly button area is healed. It's best to be gentle and quick with his first few baths. If baby seems at all uncomfortable, you can go back to giving sponge baths for a week or so, then try a normal bath again. Your baby will let you know when they're ready to make the switch.

Safety tips for a regular bath:

- Use a baby bath or sink.
- Don't use bath seats.
- Use touch supervision.
- Never leave a baby alone in the bath, even for an instant.
- Check the water temperature.
- Keep baby warm.
- Use soap sparingly as it dries the skin.
- Clean gently.
- Have fun.
- Get out, dry off, and moisturize.

Once you've got the fundamentals down, bath time becomes so easy. Just make sure baby is safe and comfortable, and don't forget to enjoy every moment.

Looking After the Cord

It can take up to three weeks for the umbilical cord stump to dry out and fall off. Here's how you can gently treat the belly button area in the interim:

- **Keep it dry**: Once upon a time, parents were told to swab the stump with rubbing alcohol following each diaper change. It's been discovered that this may destroy bacteria that dries the cord so it can fall off. It's best to just let it breathe. To avoid suffocating it, keep the front of your baby's diaper folded down.

- **Only do sponge baths**: Although getting the stump wet is harmless, sponge baths make it easier to keep it dry.

- **Let it fall off naturally**: Avoid the urge to remove the stump yourself.

Things to lookout for:

It's common to notice a little blood close to the stump as it heals. The cord stump may bleed a little when it comes off, similar to a scab.

But, if the umbilical area oozes pus, the surrounding skin turns red and inflamed, or the area forms a pink, moist bump, call your baby's healthcare practitioner. These might be indicators of an infection in the umbilical cord. To prevent the illness from spreading, quick treatment is required.

Moreover, if the stump hasn't detached after three weeks, consult your baby's doctor. This could be a symptom of a deeper issue, like an infection or immune system dysfunction.

Six Weeks Postpartum

Sex After Delivery

A lot of women swear off sex once they've given birth, but it's just talk. It's bound to happen at some point. Chances are you won't be in the mood, and it may be a bit uncomfortable at first, but here's all you need to know:

How Soon After Delivery Can I Do It?

The medically approved time frame, regardless of delivery method, is four to six weeks. If you're going to experience any post-birth complications, it's likely to happen in the first two weeks following delivery. So waiting will allow your body more time to recover.

You may also have a reduced sex drive, exhaustion, vaginal dryness, pain, postpartum discharge, and vaginal tears. You might have to wait longer if your vaginal tear needs surgical repair.

Will It Hurt and What Can I Do?

Your vagina may become dry and sore due to hormonal changes, especially if you breastfeed. If you are recovering from an episiotomy or perineal tears, you could feel some discomfort during sex as well.

To make it more comfortable:

- **Pain management**: Try to prepare by taking pain-relieving measures like emptying your bladder, having a warm bath, or taking an over-the-counter (OTC) painkiller. Use ice wrapped in a cloth towel on the area if you feel a burning sensation.

- **Employ lubricant**: If you feel vaginal dryness.

- **Experiment**: Talk about alternatives to penetrative sex, like reciprocal masturbation, massages, and oral sex. Be honest about what feels good and what doesn't.

- **Set aside time**: Schedule sex if you need to. Preferably when you're not too tired or nervous.

What Can I Do if I'm Just Not Interested?

When adjusting to life after delivery, there is more to intimacy than just sex. Be open with your spouse. If you're not feeling sexy or if you're worried that it will hurt, communicate that. Keep up your intimacy in other ways until you're ready to engage in sex. Even if it's just a few minutes when you get a break, or after the baby goes to sleep, spend time alone together. Find different ways to show your love.

If you're still having trouble, keep an eye out for postpartum depression's telltale signs and symptoms. Contact your doctor if you suspect postpartum depression. Early intervention means early healing.

Always remember that maintaining good health and making time for self-care might help you keep the passion alive.

What Are the Positives?

Quickies are here to save the day: Fun tidbit about sex after birth: It doesn't have to last for hours on end. Have your spouse stimulate you, and then you do everything in your power to maintain your interest in the present. To stay present, concentrate on the feeling of what's being done to you and what you're doing in return.

Sex doesn't only have to happen at night: Weekends, during baby's nap, is the ideal time to connect. It can relieve some of the pressure you might feel at night and become something to look forward to.

It could get better after birth: It sounds strange, but many moms find that they enjoy sex more now than they did before becoming parents. Delivering a baby exposes us to a variety of feelings, and as a result, our bodies—particularly our genitalia—become more sensitive, enhancing our capacity for pleasure.

Our internal organs can also be precisely repositioned during childbirth, increasing their receptivity to stimulation.

Your sex drive will eventually come back: You'll want to have sex again after giving birth, the same way you'll want to sleep again, go on outings, and even give birth again. Give yourself time to heal and get used to your new lifestyle.

Contrary to popular belief, having more children does not mean having less sex. You will eventually come to the realization that life with kids will always be hectic, but you simply have to soldier on and have fun whenever and wherever you can.

Common Partnership Issues After Baby and How to Solve Them

The transition from coupledom to parenthood is thrilling, exhilarating, and amazing. It's also taxing, frustrating, and worrying—a combination that could be harmful to the romantic bond that originally led to you becoming parents.

Sustaining a marriage after having a child requires a lot of time and effort, which is ironic because those are probably the two things you don't have. Making efforts to maintain your relationship pays off in the long run. You'll have more time to spend appreciating one another because you won't spend much time feeling resentful of one another.

Here's why it's so hard, and how you can make things go more smoothly:

- **Chores**: Before having a baby, it was easier to get chores done. But the chores don't disappear once baby's home. If chores pile up, it can lead to frustration on both sides. So the best thing to do is have a visual aid in place that states which chores need to be done and by whom. Alternate if you need to, and always be clear about what you need. Nobody can read your mind, so be direct. Make it a standard practice to thank your partner after they finish a task. They might be more responsive to requests in the future if you express gratitude. Niceties also foster a more healthy environment.

- **Difference of opinion**: Not many people have parenting plans in place, and the conversations about how things should be done don't happen as often as you'd think. It's usually once the baby arrives that parents start to notice how different their opinions on raising babies are. If parent A chooses to do things their way, they should be willing to deal with whatever happens as a result of the method they employ. For instance, the parent who lets the baby take a nap too close to bedtime should be willing to stay up with the baby when they won't sleep.

Compromises should be made on issues like feeding and sleep training. There is enough information out there to allow parents to come to an agreement.

- **Less quality time**: Before baby, there was probably a nice balance between your personal lives and your life as a couple. After baby, you probably spend more time together, but it's not in a way you're used to. You're together all the time, but because it's not quality time, there becomes a disconnect. The solution is to carve out alone time for yourselves as individuals, time to enjoy each other's company as a couple, and family time. Balance is key.

- **No alone time**: A baby is a round-the-clock commitment, so it's no wonder you don't get time to yourself. The first three months are likely to be all about baby, but after that, you should start considering ways to pop out and do something for yourself.

- **Potentially overbearing family**: Grandparents love grandchildren, aunts, and uncles love niblings. It's good for your baby to be surrounded by and showered with love, but you have to put boundaries in place before extended family overwhelms you. Try and think of the rules you'd like to enforce for your family before you give birth. Communicate them, so that everybody's on the same page and nobody gets hurt.

- **Money worries**: Money is a big deal. It's a contributing factor to the breakdown of a lot of relationships. If you feel stressed about money, you're not going to take it out on your baby, you'll take it out on dad and vice versa. The solution to this is preemptive planning, a lot of talking, and a lot of compromising.

Your First Checkup: What to Expect

A postpartum checkup is a medical exam you have soon after giving birth to make sure you're healing properly. Even if you feel well, you should go. Postpartum care is crucial because new mothers run the risk of developing serious, even fatal health issues in the days and weeks following delivery. Postpartum care reduces the number of new moms who suffer from health issues that could prove fatal.

What's a Postpartum Care Plan?

Together with your healthcare practitioner, you can create a postpartum care plan. It makes it easier to get ready for your postpartum medical treatment. Don't wait to develop your plan until after you deliver. Set it up while you're still pregnant.

Chat with your provider about:

- Their contact details.
- Your postpartum checkups.
- Your reproductive plan and birth control.
- Health issues or post-pregnancy complications that need treatment.
- The normal emotional and physical changes following pregnancy.
- PPD and other mental health issues following pregnancy.
- Feeding baby.

What Happens at a Checkup?

Your healthcare professional checks to make sure you're recuperating after delivery and adjusting to life as a mom. You can expect a full physical that includes:

- Blood pressure, weight, breasts, and belly check
- A pelvic exam
- Checks on any health conditions you had during pregnancy, i.e., diabetes and hypertension
- Check to see if your immunizations are up to date.
- Birth control.

There will also be conversations about any problems you faced while pregnant and your feelings about being a mother.

Baby's First Checkup: What to Expect

Your baby's first checkup will actually be by a pediatrician at the hospital right after the birth. The doctor will perform a physical exam of baby's overall health, assess their reflexes, and offer advice if there are any issues with weight or feeding.

Sometimes, the doctor might need to see your baby a few times a day for the first couple of days in the hospital. This would only happen if your baby has jaundice, or issues with weight or feeding.

The subsequent checkup will normally take place at your preferred clinic three to five days after delivery. Your baby's first week on earth is really important to their health. They are completely new to the world and are learning how to live, and adapt to new surroundings. Everything's new to you too, so doctors want you to know they're there for you.

How Far in Advance Should I Book the Checkup?

How to pick your baby's first doctor? The decision is ultimately up to you, but here's what to take into account:

- Choose a clinic close to home.
- Find a doctor you connect with by reading up on them online.
- Find a practice that lets you easily access baby's medical and immunization records online.
- Choose a medical professional who is well-trained and experienced. Board certification is something you can seek out.

What Happens at the Checkup?

Before the checkup, some clinics require you to fill out online documents pertaining to your baby's health and development and how you're adjusting to motherhood.

Once you arrive, a nurse will gather any additional paperwork you have completed and ask you a few routine questions. They'll also measure your baby's head circumference, length, and weight.

The doctor will then come in and review the growth chart with you to make sure your baby is gaining weight and developing normally. They will also ask about baby's feeding schedule, sleeping habits, and bowel movement.

Finally, the doctor will perform a thorough head-to-toe check to assess baby's general health and look for signs of abnormalities or developmental delays. They'll perform:

- A head check
- A hip check
- A reflex check
- An umbilical cord check

There will be a time in your appointment for you to speak with the doctor and ask any questions. Some clinics have a nurse line that you can call whenever a question comes up or if you feel like you need some guidance.

What Should I Take With Me?

As a new parent, it's natural to feel stressed out, especially when you're sleep deprived. Hence, getting ready for the baby's medical appointment beforehand is a smart method to maintain composure and efficiency.

Here are a few items to bring:

- A bottle
- A blanket
- An extra outfit
- Your insurance card
- Paperwork from the hospital if you have any
- A feeding journal if you keep one
- Diapers and wipes

Conclusion

Dear First-Time Mother,

I want to take a moment to commend you on your incredible journey through pregnancy. The moment you learned you were expecting, your journey of joy, excitement, and anticipation began. And through it all, despite the difficulties and uncertainty of bringing new life into the world, you have exhibited incredible courage, tenacity, and grace.

You have dealt with morning sickness, exhaustion, and a plethora of other physical side effects associated with conceiving a child. You have given your body proper care, fed your child, and made countless other sacrifices. You have balanced the emotional ups and downs that pregnancy can bring while managing your job, household duties, and the never-ending stream of doctor's appointments and testing.

You have shown your unwavering love and dedication to your unborn child throughout it all. You have built a relationship with your infant that will last a lifetime by talking, reading, and singing to them. For the sake of your child's health and welfare, you have made several sacrifices and set aside your own demands.

You could have started this journey as a first-time mother feeling unsure and unprepared. To finish this chapter, keep in mind that you have grown into a strong and capable caretaker, equipped with the force of unwavering love and a fresh appreciation for the wondrous experience of motherhood.

I want to remind you that you are a true warrior and an inspiration to everyone you know as you get ready for the next stage of your adventure. You will remain led by your fortitude, tenacity, and love in the coming years. As you continue on your path, please know that you have our love and support as you reach this incredible milestone.

Sincerely yours, Elizabeth Benson

If you have enjoyed this book, please leave a helpful review on Amazon.

Glossary

Albumin: A protein that may show up in your urine during pregnancy. It might be a symptom of preeclampsia or another illness. At your prenatal visits, your midwife will examine your urine for albumin.

Antenatal: It pertains to the entire pregnancy, from conception to delivery, and literally means "before birth."

Birth canal: The pathway that a baby passes through during delivery. It's made up of the cervix, vagina, and vulva.

Catheter: A flexible, thin tube made of plastic that can be used for a variety of therapeutic or diagnostic operations. Catheters can be used for drainage, such as from a surgical site or the bladder, as well as for the injection of fluids or medications into specific bodily parts.

Colostrum: The milk that your breasts produce around the end of your pregnancy and in the early days following the birth of your child. It is highly concentrated and packed with antibodies to guard your infant from infections. Colostrum seems rich and creamy and can occasionally be quite golden in color.

Cot death: The unexpected passing away of a seemingly healthy infant in their sleep. Also known as SIDS.

Down's syndrome: A genetic disorder characterized by an excessive number of chromosomes. People who have Down's syndrome are more likely to experience some health issues and have some degree of learning difficulty. Their facial features and physical development are also impacted.

Dystocia: A labor that stagnates. Shoulder dystocia is when a baby's shoulders become stuck after the head has been delivered; labor dystocia is when contractions do not strengthen and cervical change stops.

Embryo: Refers to the growing baby during the first eight weeks of pregnancy.

Fetus: Refers to the growing baby from eight weeks onwards.

Fundus: The upper part of the womb.

Gingivitis: Red, sensitive, and bleeding gums that can progress into periodontitis, if neglected.

Hemoglobin: Red blood cells contain hemoglobin, which transports oxygen from the lungs to every area of the body. Because they create more blood during pregnancy, pregnant women need to produce more hemoglobin. Insufficient production can cause anemia, which will make you feel extremely exhausted. During prenatal visits, your hemoglobin levels are checked.

Hypotension: Low blood pressure. While in childbirth, some women who receive an epidural experience hypotension.

Hypoxia: When the mother's blood pressure is too low, or the cord is compressed, the baby does not receive enough oxygen.

Lanugo: Fine, soft hair that covers baby at around 22 weeks. At full gestation, the lanugo fades, but it could still be there on premature babies.

Meconium: Your baby's first stools, or bowel movements. Meconium is made up of mucus and bile that babies consumed when they were in the uterus. It has a tar-like consistency, is green or black in color, and is odorless.

Neonatal care: The treatment provided to preterm or ill newborns. It occurs in a neonatal unit, which is especially created and furnished to take care of them.

Oedema: Swelling, most frequently of the hands and feet. Although it is typically nothing to worry about, if your high blood pressure suddenly worsens, it may indicate preeclampsia.

Perinatal: The period just before and following a birth.

Pica: The urge some pregnant women have to eat things like dirt, chalk, or clay. It is believed to be related to anemia caused by iron deficiency.

Postnatal: The window of time from the moment a baby is born until they are roughly six weeks old.

Precipitous birth: One that occurs very quickly, usually in less than three hours.

Rubella: A virus that, if contracted by the mother in the first few weeks of pregnancy, can have a significant impact on unborn children. Since the majority of women have received their rubella vaccinations, they are not in danger. If you are considering becoming pregnant and doubt your immunity to rubella, request a blood test from your doctor.

Steroids: Synthetic hormones that could be administered to a pregnant woman experiencing preterm labor in an effort to hasten the fetus's lung development.

Zygote: The fertilized egg just prior to its first division and development into an embryo.

References

Abedin, S. (2022, September 11). *Water Birth Information: Benefits and Risks of Water Birth*. WebMD. https://www.webmd.com/baby/water-birth

Advantages of bottle-feeding. (n.d.) BIBS. https://bibsworld.com/blogs/guides/advantages-of-bottle-feeding

Aggarwal, N. (2021, November 18). *Postpartum Checkups: When They Occur and What to Expect*. Thebump. https://www.thebump.com/a/postpartum-checkup

Apgar score. (2016). Medlineplus. https://medlineplus.gov/ency/article/003402.htm

Baby movements in pregnancy. (n.d.). Tommys https://www.tommys.org/pregnancy-information/pregnancy-symptom-checker/baby-fetal-movements

Baby's first doctor appointment. (2021, February 18). HealthPartners Blog. https://www.healthpartners.com/blog/what-to-expect-at-babys-first-doctor-appointment/

Back pain during pregnancy: 7 tips for relief. (2019). Mayo Clinic. https://www.mayoclinic.org/healthy-lifestyle/pregnancy-week-by-week/in-depth/pregnancy/art-20046080

Balonwu, V. (2015, December 1). *Miscarriage Causes And Treatment - Health And Medical Information*. Viviennebalonwu. https://www.viviennebalonwu.com/2015/05/miscarriage-causes-and-treatment.html

Bleeding during pregnancy Causes. (2022, January 20). Mayo Clinic. https://www.mayoclinic.org/symptoms/bleeding-during-pregnancy/basics/causes/sym-20050636#:~:text=Normal%20vaginal%20bleeding%20near%20the

Bonding and attachment: newborns. (2020, November 8). Raising Children Network. https://raisingchildren.net.au/newborns/connecting-communicating/bonding/bonding-newborns#when-bonding-and-attachment-arent-easy-nav-title

Braxton Hicks contractions. (n.d.). HSE.ie. https://www2.hse.ie/conditions/braxton-hicks/#:~:text=Braxton%20Hicks%20contractions%20happen%20when

Breast Milk Is Best. (2021b, December 8). Johns Hopkins Medicine. https://www.hopkinsmedicine.org/health/conditions-and-diseases/breastfeeding-your-baby/breast-milk-is-the-best-milk#:~:text=Compared%20with%20formula%2C%20the%20nutrients

Breastfeeding - Common myths. (2022, May 25). HSE.ie. https://www2.hse.ie/babies-children/breastfeeding/a-good-start/common-myths/

Breastfeeding vs. Formula Feeding Information. (2021, May 24). Mount Sinai Health System. https://www.mountsinai.org/health-library/special-topic/breastfeeding-vs-formula-feeding

C-Section (Cesarean Birth): Procedure & Risks. (2022, August 14). Cleveland Clinic. https://my.clevelandclinic.org/health/treatments/7246-cesarean-birth-c-section

C-Section (Cesarean Section): Procedure, Risks & Recovery. (2022, August 14). Cleveland Clinic. https://my.clevelandclinic.org/health/treatments/7246-cesarean-birth-c-section#recovery-and-outlook

Carlson, J. (2020, February 27). *8 Dangers of Smoking While Pregnant.* Healthline. https://www.healthline.com/health/smoking-and-pregnancy

Causes of second trimester loss. (n.d.). The Miscarriage Association. https://www.miscarriageassociation.org.uk/information/misca

rriage/second-trimester-loss-late-miscarriage/causes-of-second-trimester-loss/

Charles, A. (2021, June 14). *10 Foods and Drinks with Caffeine.* Healthline. https://www.healthline.com/nutrition/foods-with-caffeine

Choosing your birth partners | Labour & birth articles & support. (2022, August 18). National Childbirth Trust. https://www.nct.org.uk/labour-birth/dads-and-partners/choosing-your-birth-partners#:~:text=Whoever%20you%20choose%20as%20your

Clogged Milk Duct: Causes, Symptoms & Treatment. (2022, March 10). Cleveland Clinic. https://my.clevelandclinic.org/health/diseases/24239-clogged-milk-duct

Collier, S. (2021, June 25). *How can you manage anxiety during pregnancy?* Harvard Health. https://www.health.harvard.edu/blog/how-can-you-manage-anxiety-during-pregnancy-202106252512

Common Foods to Avoid. (n.d.). Community Care Midwives. https://communitycaremidwives.com/common-foods-to-avoid.html

Cottrell, S. (2022, April 21). *Is It Safe To Take a Bath While Pregnant?* Parents. https://www.parents.com/pregnancy/my-body/is-taking-a-warm-bath-in-the-last-trimester-safe/

Danielsson, K. (2022, December 6). *Find out When It's Time to Call a Doctor If Your Baby Isn't Kicking.* Verywell Family. https://www.verywellfamily.com/what-to-do-if-your-baby-is-not-kicking-2371400

De Bellefonds, C. (2023, February 24). *Are Changes in Fetal Movement and Baby Kicks Normal?* What to Expect. https://www.whattoexpect.com/pregnancy/fetal-development/changes-in-fetal-movement/#worry

Diehl, W. (2018, May 21). *Do I Have Postpartum Depression or Just the Baby Blues?* Right as Rain by UW Medicine.

https://rightasrain.uwmedicine.org/mind/mental-health/do-i-have-postpartum-depression-or-just-baby-blues-0

Doctor, M. (2022, March 15). *Postpartum Check Up: All You Need To Know | theAsianparent Philippines*. Ph.theasianparent.com. https://ph.theasianparent.com/all-you-need-to-know-about-postpartum-check-up

Does a Hot Bath Induce Labor? (2021, March 2). WebMD. https://www.webmd.com/baby/does-a-hot-bath-induce-labor

Donaldson-Evans, C. (2005, April 25). *Watch Your Baby's Growth at Week 4*. WhattoExpect. https://www.whattoexpect.com/pregnancy/week-by-week/week-4.aspx

Donaldson-Evans, C. (2021, June 1). *Why Might Your Practitioner Decide to Induce Labor?* What to Expect. https://www.whattoexpect.com/pregnancy/labor-induction/#definition

Donaldson-Evans, C., & Murkoff, H. (2021a, June 24). *Week 20 of Pregnancy*. What to Expect. https://www.whattoexpect.com/pregnancy/week-by-week/week-20.aspx

Donaldson-Evans, C., & Murkoff, H. (2021b, June 24). *Week 32 of Pregnancy*. What to Expect. https://www.whattoexpect.com/pregnancy/week-by-week/week-32.aspx

Donaldson-Evans, C., & Murkoff, H. (2022a, June 24). *16 Weeks Pregnant*. What to Expect. https://www.whattoexpect.com/pregnancy/week-by-week/week-16.aspx

Donaldson-Evans, C., & Murkoff, H. (2022b, June 24). *Week 8 of Pregnancy*. What to Expect. https://www.whattoexpect.com/pregnancy/week-by-week/week-8.aspx

Donaldson-Evans, C., & Murkoff, H. (2022c, June 24). *Week 12 of Pregnancy*. What to Expect. https://www.whattoexpect.com/pregnancy/week-by-week/week-12.aspx

Donaldson-Evans, C., & Murkoff, H. (2022d, June 24). *Week 24 of Pregnancy*. What to Expect. https://www.whattoexpect.com/pregnancy/week-by-week/week-24.aspx

Donaldson-Evans, C., & Murkoff, H. (2022e, June 24). *Week 28 of Pregnancy*. What to Expect. https://www.whattoexpect.com/pregnancy/week-by-week/week-28.aspx

Donaldson-Evans, C., & Murkoff, H. (2022f, June 24). *Week 36 of Pregnancy*. What to Expect. https://www.whattoexpect.com/pregnancy/week-by-week/week-36.aspx

Drug use and pregnancy. (2019, April 1). Stanford Medicine. https://www.stanfordchildrens.org/en/topic/default?id=illegal-drug-use-and-pregnancy-85-P01208

Dunkin, M. A. (2022, August 8). *Childbirth Classes: Lamaze, Bradley, Alexander, and Other Types*. WebMD. https://www.webmd.com/baby/childbirth-class-options

Ectopic pregnancy - Symptoms and causes. (2018, September 8). Mayo Clinic. https://www.mayoclinic.org/diseases-conditions/ectopic-pregnancy/symptoms-causes/syc-20372088

Engorged Breasts - avoiding and treating. (2016, January 28). La Leche League GB. https://www.laleche.org.uk/engorged-breasts-avoiding-and-treating/

Episiotomy why you might need one. (2019, June 19). HSE.ie. https://www2.hse.ie/pregnancy-birth/birth/episiotomy/why-you-might-need-one/

Equipment for bottle-feeding. (2022, September 14). HSE.ie. https://www2.hse.ie/babies-children/bottle-feeding/equipment/

Exercise in Pregnancy. (2020, December 2). NHS https://www.nhs.uk/pregnancy/keeping-well/exercise/

Family Health History and Planning for Pregnancy. (2019). Centers for Disease Control and Prevention. https://www.cdc.gov/genomics/famhistory/famhist_plan_pregnancy.htm

Fierro, P. P. (2020, October 27). *Correctly Positioning Your Twins for Breastfeeding.* Verywell Family. https://www.verywellfamily.com/how-to-breastfeed-twins-together-4114638

Forceps Delivery: What to Expect, Risks & Recovery. (2022, June 12). Cleveland Clinic. https://my.clevelandclinic.org/health/treatments/23260-forceps-delivery

Forceps or vacuum delivery. (2020, December 2). NHS https://www.nhs.uk/pregnancy/labour-and-birth/what-happens/forceps-or-vacuum-delivery/

Freeborn, D., Trevino, H. M., & Burd, I. (2022, January 4). *Fetal Monitoring.* Nationwidechildrens.org. https://www.nationwidechildrens.org/conditions/health-library/fetal-monitoring

Gestational diabetes - Symptoms and causes. (2017, April 24). Mayo Clinic. https://www.mayoclinic.org/diseases-conditions/gestational-diabetes/symptoms-causes/syc-20355339

Gibran, K. (2018). *On Children by Kahlil Gibran - Poems.* Academy of American Poets. https://poets.org/poem/children-1

Glossary of useful terms. (2009). Hscni.net. https://www.publichealth.hscni.net/

Goodenough, G. (2021, January 18). *The Pros and Cons of Formula Feeding.* Ready, Set, Food! https://readysetfood.com/blogs/community/the-pros-and-cons-of-formula-feeding

Graves, G. (2022, December 4). *A Simple Birth Plan Template for First-Time Parents.* Parents. https://www.parents.com/pregnancy/giving-birth/labor-and-delivery/how-to-write-a-short-simple-birth-plan/

Greenspan, Y. (2016, January 21). *The Importance of Reading While Pregnant.* Literary Hub. https://lithub.com/the-importance-of-reading-while-pregnant/

Group B strep (strep B) and pregnancy. (2020, July 1). Tommy's. https://www.tommys.org/pregnancy-information/pregnancy-complications/group-b-strep-strep-b-and-pregnancy

Group B strep disease - Symptoms and causes. (2019). Mayo Clinic. https://www.mayoclinic.org/diseases-conditions/group-b-strep/symptoms-causes/syc-20351729

Group B Streptococcus (GBS) in pregnancy and newborn babies. (2017, May 1). Royal College of Obstetricians and Gynaecologists. https://www.rcog.org.uk/for-the-public/browse-all-patient-information-leaflets/group-b-streptococcus-gbs-in-pregnancy-and-newborn-babies/

Gurevich, R. (2022, September 16). *Why You Have Mood Swings During Pregnancy and How to Cope.* Verywell Family. https://www.verywellfamily.com/mood-swings-during-pregnancy-4159590

Healthy diet during pregnancy. (2022, June 22). Healthdirect Australia. https://www.pregnancybirthbaby.org.au/healthy-diet-during-pregnancy#balanced-diet

Hecht, A. (2006, December). *Exercise During Pregnancy.* WebMD. https://www.webmd.com/baby/guide/exercise-during-pregnancy

Hepatitis B. (2012, April 25). American Pregnancy Association. https://americanpregnancy.org/womens-health/hepatitis-b/

High Blood Pressure During Pregnancy. (2021, May 6). Centers for Disease Control and Prevention. https://www.cdc.gov/bloodpressure/pregnancy.htm#:~:text=Gestational%20Hypertension&text=It%20is%20typically%20diagnosed%20after

How To Deal With Emotions After Giving Birth. (2017, November 13). Parenthood Times. https://parenthoodtimes.com/emotions-after-giving-birth/

How to give a baby a bottle. (2022, December 14). HSE.ie. https://www2.hse.ie/babies-children/bottle-feeding/how-to-give-baby-bottle/

How your baby is monitored during labour. (2021, November 4). HSE.ie. https://www2.hse.ie/pregnancy-birth/labour/preparing/monitoring/

Howland, G. (2021, October 12). *Mama Natural Birth Course vs. Lamaze Childbirth Classes.* Mama Natural. https://www.mamanatural.com/mama-natural-vs-lamaze-birthing-classes/#:~:text=Lamaze%20focuses%20on%20healthy%20childbirth

I can't stop crying after the birth of my baby. (2019, August 4). National Childbirth Trust. https://www.nct.org.uk/baby-toddler/crying/i-cant-stop-crying-after-birth-my-baby

Iftikhar, N. (2020a, June 27). *How to Know When to Go to the Hospital for Labor.* Healthline. https://www.healthline.com/health/pregnancy/when-to-go-to-the-hospital-for-labor

Iftikhar, N. (2020b, August 31). *Understanding Fetal Position.* Healthline. https://www.healthline.com/health/baby/fetal-position#possible-positions

Inducing labor: When to wait, when to induce. (2022, May 4). Mayo Clinic. https://www.mayoclinic.org/healthy-lifestyle/labor-and-delivery/in-depth/inducing-labor/art-20047557#:~:text=Can%20I%20request%20an%20elective

Kegel Exercises: How to and & Benefits. (2023, January 2). Cleveland Clinic. https://my.clevelandclinic.org/health/articles/14611-kegel-exercises

Larson, J. (2020, April 22). *When to Worry About Fetal Movement: Decreases and Increases*. Healthline. https://www.healthline.com/health/pregnancy/when-to-worry-about-fetal-movement#decreased-movement

Lauretta, A. (2021, August 4). *When To Announce Your Pregnancy*. Forbes Health. https://www.forbes.com/health/family/when-to-announce-pregnancy/

Lessing, D., & Indeed editorial team. (2022, October 1). *55 Inspiring Quotes About Learning (Why They Are Helpful)*. Indeed.com. https://ca.indeed.com/career-advice/career-development/quotes-about-learning

Lukasik, E. (2016, February 3). *Emergency birth: What to do when you can't get to the hospital*. Pregnancy Magazine. https://www.pregnancymagazine.com/pregnancy/emergency-birth-cant-get-to-hospital

Marcin, A. (2019, October 2). *What Is Hypnobirthing? Technique, How-To, Pros and Cons*. Healthline. https://www.healthline.com/health/pregnancy/hypnobirthing

Masters, M. (2021, June 22). *Can You Take Baths While Pregnant?* What to Expect. https://www.whattoexpect.com/pregnancy/looking-good/pampered-parts/bathing.aspx#bath

Masters, M. (2022, February 22). *Is Your Hair Falling Out?* What to Expect. https://www.whattoexpect.com/first-year/postpartum-health-and-care/postpartum-hair-loss/

Matta, C. (2022, October 30). *Can I Get Botox While Pregnant?* Verywell Family. https://www.verywellfamily.com/can-i-get-botox-when-pregnant-5198014#:~:text=Risks%20of%20Using%20Botox%20While%20Pregnant

May I break your waters? Information on Artificial Rupture of Membranes. (2014, June 12). Aimsireland. http://aimsireland.ie/may-i-break-your-waters-information-on-artificial-rupture-of-membranes-2/

McTigue, S. (2020, March 26). *What Are the Earliest Signs of Being Pregnant with Twins?* Healthline. https://www.healthline.com/health/pregnancy/signs-of-twins#chances-of-twins

Medications for Pain Relief During Labor and Delivery. (2022, December 4). ACOG. https://www.acog.org/womens-health/faqs/medications-for-pain-relief-during-labor-and-delivery#:~:text=An%20epidural%20block%20(also%20called

Medicines During Pregnancy. (2022, February 23). Myhealth https://myhealth.alberta.ca/Health/Pages/conditions.aspx?hwid=uf9707#:~:text=Deciding%20about%20medicines%20during%20pregnancy

Miles, K. (2021, February 4). *Forceps delivery and vacuum delivery.* BabyCenter. https://www.babycenter.com/pregnancy/your-body/forceps-and-vacuum-deliveries_1451360

Moderate Amounts of Caffeine Not Linked to Maternal Health Risks. (2021, November 11). Pennmedicine.org. https://www.pennmedicine.org/news/news-releases/2021/november/moderate-amounts-of-caffeine-not-linked-to-maternal-health-risks

Moldenhauer, J. S. (2022, September 3). *Prelabor Rupture of the Membranes (PROM).* Women's Health Issues: MSD Manual Consumer Version. https://www.msdmanuals.com/home/women-s-health-issues/complications-of-labor-and-delivery/prelabor-rupture-of-the-membranes-prom

Movement and positions during labour. (n.d.). Tommys https://www.tommys.org/pregnancy-information/giving-birth/movement-and-positions-during-labour

Myths: Smoking and Pregnancy | Smokefree Women. (2019, June 1). Smokefree.gov. https://women.smokefree.gov/pregnancy-motherhood/quitting-while-pregnant/myths-about-smoking-pregnancy

Nair, A. (2020, October 27). *Postnatal Examination: Purpose, Check Ups, Questions to Ask.* Parenting.firstcry.com. https://parenting.firstcry.com/articles/your-postnatal-examination-what-to-expect/

Nall, R. (2016, November 28). *Placenta Delivery: What to Expect.* Healthline Media. https://www.healthline.com/health/pregnancy/placenta-delivery

Navsaria, D. (2020, March 3). *Bathing Your Baby.* HealthyChildren.org. https://www.healthychildren.org/English/ages-stages/baby/bathing-skin-care/Pages/Bathing-Your-Newborn.aspx#:~:text=The%20World%20Health%20Organization%20(WHO

Newborn screening tests for your baby. (2020, July). March of Dimes. https://www.marchofdimes.org/find-support/topics/parenthood/newborn-screening-tests-your-baby

Nguyen, H. (2021, September 29). *Postpartum recovery: What to expect.* HealthPartners Blog. https://www.healthpartners.com/blog/what-to-expect-after-giving-birth/

Ogunyemi, D. (2022, January). *Bonding With Your Newborn: What to Know If You Don't Feel Connected Right Away.* Acog.org.

https://www.acog.org/womens-health/experts-and-stories/the-latest/bonding-with-your-newborn-heres-what-to-know-if-you-dont-feel-connected-right-away#:~:text=Many%20new%0parents%20need%20more

Opt-Out| Pregnant Women, Infants, and Children. (2019). Centers for Disease Control and Prevention. https://www.cdc.gov/hiv/group/gender/pregnantwomen/opt-out.html

Overview - Newborn jaundice. (2019). NHS. https://www.nhs.uk/conditions/Jaundice-newborn/

Pacheko, D. (2020, October 30). *Pregnancy & Sleep: Tips, Sleep Positions, & Issues.* Sleep Foundation. https://www.sleepfoundation.org/pregnancy#:~:text=Common%20Sleep%20Disorders%20and%20Problems%20During%20Pregnancy.%20The

Pain relief in labour. (2020, December 2). NHS https://www.nhs.uk/pregnancy/labour-and-birth/what-happens/pain-relief-in-labour/

Patient Information Induction of Labour. (2017). NHS https://www.hdft.nhs.uk/content/uploads/2018/07/Birth-Induction-of-Labour-leaflet.pdf

Pearl, E., & Joseph, B. (2022, March 5). *Can I Still Drink Coffee While I'm Pregnant? (for Parents).* Nemours KidsHealth. https://kidshealth.org/en/parents/preg-caffeine.html

Perineal massage during pregnancy. (2021, November 22). HSE.ie. https://www2.hse.ie/pregnancy-birth/labour/preparing/perineal-massage-during-pregnancy/

Placenta praevia (low-lying placenta). (2021, February 26). HSE.ie. https://www2.hse.ie/conditions/placenta-praevia/#:~:text=Placenta%20praevia%20happens%20when%20the

Placental abruption - Symptoms and causes. (2022, February 25). Mayo Clinic. https://www.mayoclinic.org/diseases-conditions/placental-abruption/symptoms-causes/syc-20376458#:~:text=Placental%20abruption%20occurs%20when%20the%20placenta%20partly%20or%20completely%20separates

Pollack, S. (2021, September 9). *HR Headaches: When and How Should I Tell My Employer That I'm Pregnant?* Workest. https://www.zenefits.com/workest/hr-headaches-when-and-how-should-i-tell-my-employer-that-im-pregnant/#:~:text=baby

Postpartum Depression - Symptoms and Causes. (2018b, September 1). Mayo Clinic. https://www.mayoclinic.org/diseases-conditions/postpartum-depression/symptoms-causes/syc-20376617

Postpartum Emotional Deluge. (n.d.). Bodily. https://itsbodily.com/blogs/birth-recovery-postpartum/postpartum-emotions-changes-after-giving-birth

Postpartum Preeclampsia: Risk after Delivery Remains. (2019, May 29). DONA International. https://www.dona.org/postpartum-preeclampsia-risk-after-delivery-remains/#:~:text=Unfortunately%2C%2075%25%20of%20maternal%20deaths

Pregnancy 101. (2019). National Geographic [Video]. YouTube. https://www.youtube.com/watch?v=XEfnq4Q4bfk+B5:B29

Pregnancy and Bladder Control. (2020, November 6). Cleveland Clinic. https://my.clevelandclinic.org/health/articles/16094-pregnancy-and-bladder-control

Pregnancy and Heartburn. (2015, May 3). Cleveland Clinic. https://my.clevelandclinic.org/health/diseases/12011-heartburn-during-pregnancy

Pregnancy Emotions & Mood Swings: Challenges Every New Parent Faces. (2018, June 16). ForWhen. https://forwhenhelpline.org.au/parent-resources/pregnancy-emotions-mood-swings/#:~:text=The%20third%20trimester%20can%20be

Pregnancy Glossary: Your A to Z Guide to Pregnancy Terminology. (n.d.). What to Expect. https://www.whattoexpect.com/pregnancy/glossary

Pregnancy nutrition: Foods to avoid. (2017, March 31). Mayo Clinic. https://www.mayoclinic.org/healthy-lifestyle/pregnancy-week-by-week/in-depth/pregnancy-nutrition/art-20043844

Pregnancy Stretch Marks: Prevention & Treatment. (2022, July 11). Web-Pampers-US-EN. https://www.pampers.com/en-us/pregnancy/pregnancy-symptoms/article/pregnancy-stretch-marks

Pregnancy Weight Gain Calculator. (2009, March 8). Calculator.net. https://www.calculator.net/pregnancy-weight-gain-calculator.html

Pregnancy. (2021, May 4). ADA. https://www.ada.org/resources/research/science-and-research-institute/oral-health-topics/pregnancy

Prenatal care checkups. (2017, June 18). March of Dimes. https://www.marchofdimes.org/find-support/topics/planning-baby/prenatal-care-checkups

Prenatal care: 1st trimester visits. (2018, August 6). Mayo Clinic. https://www.mayoclinic.org/healthy-lifestyle/pregnancy-week-by-week/in-depth/prenatal-care/art-20044882

Prenatal care: 2nd trimester visits. (2022, August 4). Mayo Clinic. https://www.mayoclinic.org/healthy-lifestyle/pregnancy-week-by-week/in-depth/prenatal-care/art-20044581

Prenatal Care—The Full Guide. (n.d.). Pampers https://www.pampers.com/en-us/pregnancy/prenatal-health-and-wellness/article/prenatal-care

Prenatal screening for genetic conditions. (n.d.). Department of Health Australia. https://www.healthywa.wa.gov.au/Articles/N_R/Prenatal-screening-for-genetic-conditions

Prenatal testing: Is it right for you? (2020, August 25). Mayo Clinic. https://www.mayoclinic.org/healthy-lifestyle/pregnancy-week-by-week/in-depth/prenatal-testing/art-20045177

Preparing baby formula. (2022, November 10). HSE.ie. https://www2.hse.ie/babies-children/bottle-feeding/preparing-baby-formula/

PUPPP Rash: Symptoms, Causes, Treatment & Prevention. (2022, February 9). Cleveland Clinic. https://my.clevelandclinic.org/health/diseases/22374-puppp-rash#:~:text=PUPPP%20is%20an%20itchy%20rash

Recovering after an episiotomy. (2019, June 19). HSE.ie. https://www2.hse.ie/pregnancy-birth/birth/episiotomy/recovering/

Recovering from a perineal tear. (n.d.-c). Tommys. https://www.tommys.org/pregnancy-information/after-birth/recovering-perineal-tear

Rh Factor Blood Type and Pregnancy. (2020, April 27). American Pregnancy Association. https://americanpregnancy.org/healthy-pregnancy/pregnancy-complications/rh-factor

Richardson, J. H., & Littleton, K. (2015). *Breastfeeding FAQs: How Much and How Often (for Parents).* KidsHealth. https://kidshealth.org/en/parents/breastfeed-often.html

Ridgeon, E. (2021, May 7). *Spinal anaesthesia in labour and childbirth.* My BabyManual.

https://mybabymanual.co.uk/childbirth/delivery/spinal-anaesthesia-in-labour-and-childbirth/

Rigsby, K. (2019, December 13). *I'm Pregnant. When Should I Go to the Doctor?* Ntmconline.net. https://ntmconline.net/im-pregnant-when-should-i-go-to-the-doctor/

Riley, L. (2009, November 3). *Q&A: What Happens If I Can't Make it to the Hospital?* Parents. https://www.parents.com/pregnancy/my-life/emotions/qa-what-happens-if-i-cant-make-it-to-the-hospital/

Romito, K., Bailey, T. M., Husney, A., & Jones, K. (2022, February 23). *Breathing Techniques for Childbirth.* Myhealth.alberta.ca. https://myhealth.alberta.ca/Health/pages/conditions.aspx?hwid=tn7421

Rosenblum, N. (n.d.). *Breastfeeding 101: Q&A with Lactation Expert Nadine Rosenblum.* Hopkinsmedicine.org. https://www.hopkinsmedicine.org/health/wellness-and-prevention/breastfeeding-101-qanda-with-lactation-expert-nadine-rosenblum

Ruddy, E. Z. (2022, May 6). *9 Surprising Truths About Postpartum Sex After Birth.* Parents. https://www.parents.com/parenting/relationships/sex-and-marriage-after-baby/how-to-have-great-postpartum-sex/

Savchenko, M. (2019, July 9). *How to Prepare for Breastfeeding Before Your Baby Arrives.* Flo.health - #1 Mobile Product for Women's Health. https://flo.health/being-a-mom/your-baby/baby-care-and-feeding/how-to-prepare-for-breastfeeding#:~:text=Most%20obstetricians%20and%20lactation%20consultants

Sex after pregnancy: Set your own timeline. (2022, December 6). Mayo Clinic. https://www.mayoclinic.org/healthy-lifestyle/labor-and-delivery/in-depth/sex-after-pregnancy/art-20045669#:~:text=While%20there

Sex in trimester one, two and three of pregnancy | Pregnancy articles & support. (2022, August 18). National Childbirth Trust. https://www.nct.org.uk/pregnancy/relationships-sex/sex-trimester-one-two-and-three-pregnancy

Sickle Cell Disease. (n.d.). Johns Hopkins Medicine https://www.hopkinsmedicine.org/health/conditions-and-diseases/sickle-cell-disease#:~:text=Sickle%20cell%20disease%20is%20an%20inherited%20blood%20disorder%20marked%20by

Silver, E. (2019, January 16). *Why you shouldn't shave down there before labour.* Today's Parent. https://www.todaysparent.com/pregnancy/giving-birth/why-you-shouldnt-shave-down-there-before-labour/

Slaughter, E. (2019). *What are the Effects & Dangers of Alcohol During Pregnancy?* American Addiction Centers. https://americanaddictioncenters.org/alcoholism-treatment/dangers-pregnancy

Smyth, R., Markham, C., & Dowswell, T. (2013, June 18). *Amniotomy for shortening spontaneous labour.* Cochrane.org. https://www.cochrane.org/CD006167/PREG_amniotomy-for-shortening-spontaneous-labour

Stages of labour. (2023, January 4). HSE.ie. https://www2.hse.ie/pregnancy-birth/labour/preparing/stages-labour

Stein, E., Gordon, S., & Riley, L. (2022, December 19). *Signs of Approaching Labor: How to Tell Your Baby is Coming Soon.* Parents. https://www.parents.com/pregnancy/giving-birth/signs-of-labor/signs-of-approaching-labor/

Sumner, C. (2005, October 3). *8 Marriage Issues You'll Face After Baby and How to Solve Them.* Parents. https://www.parents.com/parenting/relationships/staying-close/marriage-after-baby/

Swollen ankles, feet and fingers in pregnancy. (2019, May 17). HSE.ie. https://www2.hse.ie/conditions/swollen-ankles-feet-fingers-pregnancy/

Ten tips for birth partners. (2020, December 2). National Childbirth Trust. https://www.nct.org.uk/labour-birth/dads-and-partners/ten-tips-for-birth-partners

Terreri, C. (2013, October 20). *How to Use Water for Comfort in Labor.* Lamaze International. https://www.lamaze.org/Giving-Birth-with-Confidence/GBWC-Post/how-to-use-water-for-comfort-in-labor

The Essential Hospital Bag Checklist. (2022, November). My Expert Midwife. https://myexpertmidwife.ie/blogs/my-expert-midwife/essential-items-for-your-hosp

Think You Can't Breastfeed After Implants? Think Again. (2021a, August 8). Johns Hopkins Medicine. https://www.hopkinsmedicine.org/health/wellness-and-prevention/think-you-cant-breastfeed-after-implants-think-again

Thomas, L. (2017, August 8). *Labor: what is the "show"?* News-Medical.net. https://www.news-medical.net/health/Labor-what-is-the-show.aspx

Timing your contractions - when to go to the hospital. (2023, January 4). HSE.ie. https://www2.hse.ie/pregnancy-birth/labour/signs-labour/timing-your-contractions/

Today's Parent. (2018). *What to expect in your First Trimester of pregnancy | Pregnancy Week-by-Week* [Video]. YouTube. https://www.youtube.com/watch?v=cfn04QUO4B8

Todd, N. (2017, February 13). *How Can I Handle My Labor Pain?* WebMD. https://www.webmd.com/baby/guide/pregnancy-pain-relief

Toxoplasma from Food Safety for Moms to Be. (2020). FDA. https://www.fda.gov/food/people-risk-foodborne-illness/toxoplasma-food-safety-moms-be

Traveling While Pregnant or Breastfeeding. (2020, February 11). Johns Hopkins Medicine. https://www.hopkinsmedicine.org/health/conditions-and-diseases/traveling-while-pregnant-or-breastfeeding

Umbilical cord care: Do's and don'ts for parents. (2022, February 24). Mayo Clinic. https://www.mayoclinic.org/healthy-lifestyle/infant-and-toddler-health/in-depth/umbilical-cord/art-20048250#:~:text=A%20baby

Understand how COVID-19 might affect your pregnancy. (2022, September 7). Mayo Clinic. https://www.mayoclinic.org/diseases-conditions/coronavirus/in-depth/pregnancy-and-covid-19/art-20482639

Understand the symptoms of depression during pregnancy. (2019, June 5). Mayo Clinic. https://www.mayoclinic.org/healthy-lifestyle/pregnancy-week-by-week/in-depth/depression-during-pregnancy/art-20237875

University of Michigan (2020). A randomized controlled trial of the hypnoBirthing program: Effects on labor, stress and pain. *BMC Pregnancy and Childbirth, 20*(1), 1-10. doi:10. 1186/s12884-020-27040-6

Vaccination Considerations for People who are Pregnant or Breastfeeding. (2020, February 11). Centers for Disease Control and Prevention. https://www.cdc.gov/coronavirus/2019-ncov/vaccines/recommendations/pregnancy.html

Vaginal Birth After Cesarean (VBAC): Facts, Safety & Risks. (2021, August 23). Cleveland Clinic. https://my.clevelandclinic.org/health/articles/21687-vaginal-birth-after-cesarean-vbac#:~:text=If%20you

Varicose Veins During Pregnancy: Types, Causes & Treatment. (2022c, May 25). Cleveland Clinic. https://my.clevelandclinic.org/health/diseases/23331-varicose-veins-in-pregnancy

Vitamins and supplements during pregnancy. (2022b, October 17). Healthdirect Australia. https://www.pregnancybirthbaby.org.au/vitamins-and-supplements-during-pregnancy#vitamins-and-minerals

Water Births (2017, April 26). American Pregnancy Association. https://americanpregnancy.org/healthy-pregnancy/labor-and-birth/water-births/#:~:text=Benefits%20for%20Mother%3A&text=Buoyancy%20promotes%20more%20efficient%20uterine,blood%20pressure%20caused%20by%20anxiety.

Watson, S. (2021, December 2). *Coping with pregnancy loss.* BabyCenter. https://www.babycenter.com/pregnancy/your-life/coping-with-pregnancy-loss_4006

Weiss, R. E. (2021, September 13). *How to Combat Boredom During a Long Labor.* Verywell Family. https://www.verywellfamily.com/things-to-do-during-labor-to-prevent-boredom-4111058

When breastfeeding or feeding expressed milk is not recommended. (2019c, December 14). Centers for Disease Control and Prevention. https://www.cdc.gov/breastfeeding/breastfeeding-special-circumstances/contraindications-to-breastfeeding.html

When Is It Safe to Deliver Your Baby? (2020). University of Utah. https://healthcare.utah.edu/womenshealth/pregnancy-birth/preterm-birth/when-is-it-safe-to-deliver.php

Wild, S., & Nierenberg, C. (2018, March 27). *Vaginal Birth vs. C-Section: Pros & Cons.* Live Science. https://www.livescience.com/45681-vaginal-birth-vs-c-section.html

Your antenatal appointment schedule. (n.d.). Tommy's. https://www.tommys.org/pregnancy-information/im-pregnant/antenatal-care/your-antenatal-appointment-schedule

Your body after the birth (the first 6 weeks). (n.d.). Tommy's. https://www.tommys.org/pregnancy-information/after-birth/your-body-after-birth

Your postpartum checkups. (2018, July). March of Dimes. https://www.marchofdimes.org/find-support/topics/postpartum/your-postpartum-checkup

Image References

Mendes, L. (2021). *Breastfeeding baby* [Image]. Unsplash. https://unsplash.com/photos/L0cDMFldZgg

The First-Time Dad's Roadmap to Pregnancy and Parenthood

A Guide to the Emotional and Psychological Challenges of Fatherhood

Book 2

Introduction

A lot has changed in recent years. The world as we know it has shifted from what it once was. During the course of this change, many aspects and practices of everyday life similarly transitioned from what they were before. One of these things was parenting. Over the last few years, if not decades, we have come to recognize parenting for the collaborative effort it truly is. In the process, we discovered that fatherhood, in particular, is a much more nuanced and nebulous endeavor than we gave it credit for.

Raising children has never been easy, and finding your footing as a father becomes increasingly difficult the more this practice shifts and evolves. Right about now, you might be wondering why you can't just turn to your parents' methods and replicate them for your own children. After all, they were adults when you were born, and you are an adult now, waiting on your own bundle of joy. The trouble is, you're not exactly in the same place they were back then. Khandwala et al. (2017) report that the average age of fathers in the United States has been raised by approximately 3.5 years since 1975. Modern-day dads are getting introduced to child-rearing at increasingly older ages. This same study demonstrated that US dads are, on average, 31 years old when they welcome their first child. Along with that, we must consider that 9% of newborn infants have fathers who are at least 40. The average age of a first-time mother has followed a similar pattern.

A dad's age isn't the only thing that contributes to the shifting face of fatherhood. The context in which fatherhood takes place has also shifted over time. Today, fathers are more involved with their families than ever. Dads are no longer faceless, breadwinning entities. In the 21st century, child-rearing and domestic responsibilities are more equally dispersed, and fathers contribute to more areas of life than in previous decades. While many modern fathers still work and contribute to household income, a greater effort is made to spend time with their children and to be active participants in the child-rearing process. In fact, according to the *Changing face of fatherhood - more family time* (2021), there are many dads out there who seek out more flexible work arrangements and hours so that they are more readily available to their families.

Additionally, we must consider the fact that fatherhood hasn't developed in isolation. In recent decades, the family structure itself has undergone significant change. In addition to households with same-sex parents, there has been an uptick in single fatherhood, stay-at-home dads, and familial structures where childcare is expanded beyond those in one particular house. Now more than ever, children of divorced parents are likely to have a more expansive support network, particularly if both parents remarry. The face of fatherhood has never been more different or more diverse. This is a good thing, as it opens up the wonders of parenthood to a whole new group of people who previously viewed it only from the sidelines, even in their own families.

If I were to take a wild guess, I'd say that you and I are meeting one another in the pages of this book because you yourself are about to become a father for the first time. Most likely, the euphoria has worn off somewhat, and you've come to realize what parenthood actually is. It can be a daunting task to tackle, especially the first time around. The only thing you can be sure of is the numerous twists and turns that will characterize the process of child-rearing.

It's possible that your worry about your impending parental status comes from your own childhood experience. Perhaps you are determined to be the antithesis of your own father and support your wife and child through every step of this journey. If that's the case, then let me reassure you that you've completed the first step of parenthood: Looking at what your parents did and choosing to do the opposite. As a teenager, this was rebellion. As an adult, it's just good parenting sense.

If you are worried that you don't have all the skills and knowledge you need to be a good first-time father, rest assured that the purpose of this book is to teach those very same things. More importantly, by the time you reach the final page, you will not only be fully equipped to tackle parenting head-on, but you will have gained a holistic picture of what fatherhood is. This includes not only supporting your child and partner but also knowing when to take a step back and look after yourself.

After all, your well-being is connected to that of each of the people in your life, and the better you are doing, the more your family will flourish.

Admittedly, these are quite big promises, especially if we consider how far-reaching the change is that we hope to affect. However, as a parent of four kids myself, I've been through that introductory gauntlet myself. Moreover, with a background in psychology, I understand that the theory underlying the tactics outlined in this book is sound and will prove effective in making a change. Most important of all, the techniques, skills, and knowledge we will explore have all been applied in my own life. It is because of this experience that I ask you to trust me now. I have seen firsthand how drastically we can change our parenting abilities if we have even a little more knowledge. It may be daunting, and it won't happen overnight, but rest assured that you won't be walking this road alone.

Chapter 1:

Facing Your Fatherhood Fears

From the time you first learn that your title is about to change to "Dad," you may find that an ever-increasing number of worries are creeping into your mind. These concerns can range from anxiety about your parenting style to spiraling about all the ways in which you can make a mess of child-rearing. The good news is that nothing is set in stone and that you can make the changes needed to be an excellent father. The bad news is that these worries won't ever quite go away. Once the little one arrives, your stress will shift towards all the external influences they will encounter and will remain there for the rest of your days. It's a raw deal, but that's parenthood for you.

The very first step you can take towards quelling your fears is by becoming an involved father. The impact of an involved father stretches far beyond dividing up duties and doing the pajama drill. Children whose fathers actively played a role in their raising experience had heightened levels of security and more easily developed the desire as well as the ability to explore the world around them. This, in turn, helps keep the developmental process moving. Additionally, fathers who are involved during the years of early childhood development (ECD) are able to contribute to their children's self-esteem, as well as contribute to the strengthening of their cognitive functioning, and may even shape the way they view risk-taking. This extends into adolescence when teens of involved fathers demonstrate a higher likelihood for academic success as well as a lower risk for substance use and teenage pregnancy. This comes full-circle during young adulthood, when the positive nature of a father-child bond directly contributes to important life events such as healthy romantic relationships, positive parent-child bonds with their own children, career success and stability, and even economic prosperity.

These benefits were outlined by the South Carolina Center for Fathers and Families (2019), which has similarly collected the following statistics: In households where fathers were actively involved, children were

- twice as likely to pursue tertiary education.
- at a lowered risk for teenage pregnancy by as much as 75%.
- approximately 80% less likely to be incarcerated at any point during their lives.

Conversely, households in which fathers are more distant, uninvolved, or absent have delivered the following statistics:

- Children from these homes constitute approximately 71% of all high school dropouts.
- 90% of children who run away from home or experience homelessness have uninvolved fathers.
- 63% of suicides among youth can be traced to households with absent fathers.

Responses to Pregnancy News

Your journey to fatherhood starts the moment you hear the news about the pregnancy. Reactions to this news vary and can fall anywhere along a spectrum ranging from euphoria to dumbfounded shock. The important thing to note is that, whatever your emotional experience, there is no right way to react to hearing that you'll be having a baby. Some prospective fathers will jump for joy, elated that they are finally getting the family they've planned and worked for. Others may need more time to process the news and may have difficulty wrapping their heads around the abstraction of having a baby (if this is you, don't worry; once the baby arrives, the abstract becomes real very quickly). Still, there are others who may feel a mixture of happiness, shock, and confusion. The point is, as long as you don't run for the hills, there is no specific or perfect way to react to this news.

Tapp (2017) chronicles the responses from various men elicited by pregnancy news. These reactions covered just about the full spectrum of human emotion and included the following:

- "I cried. Not ashamed to admit it, either. We had been trying to conceive for a long time. I was ecstatic!"

- "I kept repeating, 'Are you sure?' It upset her because she thought it meant I wasn't happy, but I just wanted to be sure before I got my hopes up."

- "I think I was in shock. I didn't say anything for a few minutes, and then I kept repeating, 'I am going to be a dad.' It took a long time for it to sink in."

- "I can't remember exactly what I said because it's all jumbled up, but it was a mix of, 'You're so beautiful, I am so happy, and this is wonderful.' I was on a high for days."

- "I think I said, 'Are you happy?' My wife was up for a big promotion at work, and I realized this could affect her career negatively. It wasn't an immediate happy reaction because it was complicated."

- "I screamed, 'YES!" for about ten minutes. Then I called everyone I knew; I was so excited."

There is no such thing as a perfect reaction, largely because there is no such thing as a perfect parent. News of a pregnancy may be particularly complicated, and that's perfectly normal. Some people try to become parents intentionally, and for others, it may be a complete surprise. Don't shy away from these feelings. The time ahead will be full of twists and turns, and the clearer your head is, the better you will be able to navigate this road.

The Common Worries of New Dads

The unknown territory that lies ahead may scare you in any number of ways. But as always, we have to remember that these are problems we can deal with. For instance, you may be worried about all the changes the baby will bring, that it will overshadow all other parts of your life and that it will force you into adult roles you aren't ready for. The fact of the matter is that, yes, having a child will change a great many things in your life. However, what will not change is the fact that you still have needs and desires. There's no reason why you shouldn't be able to do the things you love; you just have to make it work. Talk to your partner, determine what she needs or wants, and find a way for both of you to be happy without neglecting the baby. Consider giving one another a night off from baby duty or leaning on your support network for some time away from home.

Your concerns might be more heavy, specifically regarding miscarriages or the well-being of your partner. Different mothers will require different types of care, vitamins, and prenatal preparation. From your side, do what you can to ensure that your partner experiences as little stress as possible during the pregnancy. If there are things that may pose a danger to her or the baby, limit their exposure to these things or remove them entirely.

Many dads-to-be may become concerned with their lifestyle choices or those of their partner, specifically as they relate to the use of alcohol, drugs, and other negative lifestyle choices. With regards to the former, you can remove all alcohol from your home to avoid slip-ups during pregnancy. As a show of solidarity, you can stop drinking during pregnancy as well. If drugs are being used (meaning anything from nicotine to more illicit substances), your best bet would be to quit as soon as possible. Should addiction be a factor, get your partner the help she needs. If it's something more manageable, like smoking, you can quit alongside her or otherwise find some means of incentivization to help her kick the habit. Later on, we'll be exploring diet during pregnancy, and you can use that information to craft healthier food habits for the both of you.

Next, we come to a worry we've already touched on: anxieties surrounding your capabilities as a father. If you're worried that you won't be a good father, remember that it's a learning process. You don't need to know parenting from A to Z the moment your baby arrives. Over time, you will pick up more and more knowledge and learn what it takes to be a good dad. Additionally, remember that you won't be doing this alone. Talk to your partner about your fears or consult other dads in your life to get some help and advice.

If your worries about fatherhood center around inadequacy or concerns that you will replicate your own father's absence or mistakes, it is essential that you open up and share these feelings with the people in your life. Even if your dad was hands-on, you may still have similar concerns. Whatever your experience, remember that you possess the capacity to be an amazing father; all you have to do is unlock it and harness its power to protect and nurture your child. As for those worries tied to your own father's approach, the fact that you have identified them as problematic is already a step in the right direction. The next step is discussing this with your partner and collaboratively forming a parenting strategy.

Moving over to something a bit more pragmatic is the worry surrounding household finances after the baby has arrived. Despite the fact that news of impending fatherhood may trigger the compulsion to switch into provider mode, modern parenting conventions mean that you probably won't be shouldering the financial burden alone. However, even in double-income households, child-rearing is an expensive endeavor. As such, draw up a baby budget before the little one's arrival. By having a good idea of what to expect from parenting, monetarily speaking, you will be able to start putting money aside or finding new avenues of income well ahead of time.

Other common worries you may come across in anticipation of becoming a father for the first time include stress originating from strained relationships with your family and friends. If these connections are unhealthy or unmaintained, you may find yourself without a much-needed support network. The same goes for a strained relationship with your partner. If things are bad between the two of you, you may be concerned about how you are meant to co-parent. In both situations, the best course of action is to talk through and attempt to resolve your issues. If you and your partner's issues have been present for a while and you find yourself unable to resolve things by yourself, consider calling in professional help.

You might also find yourself preemptively worried about your child's well-being after birth. This may result from there being some distance between you and your family after birth or because your family structure may not be as "traditional" as others. If you are worried about this, it's important that you make an effort to establish rules and rituals before your child is born. Make a point to communicate with them or spend time with them, even if it means doing so virtually.

Finally, many first-time dads worry about their baby's genetic abnormalities and what effect they will have on the child's life. Put simply, there is very little you can do to prevent these abnormalities from making their presence known. What you can do, however, is consult a doctor to find out what the extent of their effects will be. More often than not, your doctor will also be able to advise you on how you can help lessen these effects or how you can make your child's environment more accessible. Minimize your worry by preparing ahead of time. In this manner, you will be well-prepared to assist your child in meeting their unique needs if they have genetic abnormalities.

Stress: The Consequence of a New Dad's Worries

If you have worries about first-time parenting, then there's an excellent chance that you are experiencing stress. Just as your worries may take a number of forms, so can your stress also result from a number of different things. It's important to identify your stress triggers before finding a way to deal with them. Common triggers for first-time fathers include:

- The sudden pressure of becoming responsible for another human being's welfare.

- Feeling a lack of control over your current situation and the future that lies ahead.

- The prospect of facing major life changes.
- Being overwhelmed by the responsibilities that come with being a parent.
- Uncertainty of the way forward.
- Health-, pregnancy-, and finance-related worries.

Luckily, there are some things you can do to reduce the stress these triggers cause. Remember that the lower your stress levels are, the greater your paternal impact will be. This counts for the time before birth as well as the weeks and months afterwards.

Be Prepared

You don't have to know everything about parenting right away, but having some knowledge won't do any harm. This learning includes accompanying your partner to prenatal and birthing classes and providing support during doctor's appointments. If you'd like something more hands-on, offer to babysit for a friend or observe as they go about their parenting activities.

Make Use of Your Time

Preparing to be a father is a stressful thing, and engaging in some self-care will help you lower those stress levels and remain functional. However, you also have to plan ahead for the time after your little one is here. If it is available to you, arrange with your company for paternity leave. If not, save up your vacation days and cash them in at the time of birth. Though the ideal would be that you stay with your partner and child for the first few weeks after birth, even a few days will be helpful.

Make Time for Your Partner

Once your child gets here, nearly the entirety of your focus will be centered around nurturing and keeping them safe. As such, use the time before they arrive to carve out some quality time for you and your partner. It doesn't have to be elaborate, but it must be unrelated to parenting. Take the time to strengthen your bond and remind one another that you are there to provide support. In doing so, you enter the world of parenthood with somebody by your side on whom you can depend.

Get Some Help

Talk to other parents in your life to gain insight into what the process of child-rearing is really like. Additionally, make sure that you and your partner have people whom you can call or lean when you are in need of some help. If a conversation with friends isn't enough to ease your worries, you can also seek out professional assistance. Talk to your general practitioner or even a therapist and ask for all the information you feel you need.

Lend a Helping Hand

Lending a hand where and when you can will help make the pregnancy easier. In addition to helping in this way, you can also take the time before the birth to do as much preparation as you can. Practice things like changing a diaper or drawing a bath so that you have some proficiency at this when the time comes.

You can employ these tactics before your baby arrives. However, there's no guarantee that your stress will just disappear if you are well prepared. If your worries persist after birth, there are a number of tactics that may help bring your blood pressure down.

Don't Be Afraid to Ask for Help

Your support network exists for a reason. If you and your partner are struggling, reach out and ask for some support. If your issues are something more severe, consider making an appointment with a doctor, therapist, or counselor to help you solve the problem before it worsens.

The Common Worries of New Moms

For every concern you have as a first-time dad, there are ten more worries plaguing your partner (a first-time mom), and chances are they are ten times more intense. When you are worried that your partner is experiencing this type of stress, or if she confides in you about her experience, there are measures you can take to help her get through those moments of difficulty.

Pregnancy Complications

Worries about the pregnancy process are common, especially for first-time parents. Ensure that your partner maintains a regular schedule of appointments with the obstetrician gynecologist (OB/GYN). In doing so, you will catch any complications, abnormalities, or issues early and be able to make informed, proactive decisions.

Miscarriage

You and your partner may share this particular concern and with good reason. It's estimated that between 10% and 20% of pregnancies end in miscarriage (Mayo Clinic Staff, 2021). Losing your unborn child is rough in and of itself, and unfortunately, the blow can't always be cushioned by determining the cause. There are many instances in which the reason for the miscarriage cannot be determined, though chromosomal aberrations are thought to be a leading cause. If the miscarriage results from something else, it's important to know that it's no one's fault. As the pregnancy goes on, the risk of miscarriage decreases, and you should largely be out of the woods once your partner finishes her first trimester.

Worries About Doing Parenting Wrong

Parenting is a complex task to perform, and mistakes are a natural part of the experience. However, slipping up doesn't mean that you'll fail entirely, and the more you try, the better you'll get. Ensure that you practice what you can before the baby arrives and do this side-by-side with your partner. The two of you can help each other improve your technique and can support one another in moments of panic. Reassure her that by simply being there, loving, nurturing, and protecting her baby, she's already hitting it out of the park.

Fatherhood and Masculinity

As you make your way along the journey to, and eventually through, fatherhood, you may increasingly find yourself engaging in introspection and self-reflection. Many prospective fathers do this with the express purpose of determining how their sense of self will shift as they become parents. More specifically, many first-time fathers will start asking these questions in order to figure out how to navigate and combine their masculinity with the expectations levied by fatherhood.

The first thing to note is that there is no right or wrong way to be a man. You are who you are, and that's perfectly alright. Secondly, we must remember that gender roles have become increasingly fluid over the last four decades, evolving from the 1980s when women more regularly started entering—and remaining in—the workforce (Hylton-Schaub & Bryant, 2021). Because of these changes, modern man takes on many forms, none of which is wrong. Positive portrayals of masculinity across the spectrum of its existence aren't wrong. However, expressions that tend toward the discriminatory, prejudiced, and offensive must naturally be avoided and recognized for their toxicity.

Once you have determined what it means to you to be a man in the 21st century, it's time to move on to another equally pertinent question: What does it mean to be a father in the modern age? While gender roles have certainly become more malleable, there are still many stereotypes that blight the concept and practice of parenthood. Too often, women are placed in the role of primary caregiver, tasked with being responsible for the baby's emotional and physical well-being. Conversely, men are still often expected to appear as the distant, barely-present breadwinner. Not only are these ideas antiquated and tinged with feelings of sexism, but this dichotomization of the traditional mother/father roles in a family fails to match the reality of modern parenting.

Despite the fact that modern fathers actively wish to be more involved in the child-rearing process, they face significant obstacles, primarily the fact that many companies do not provide paid paternity leave. Moreover, due to outdated gender norms, many fathers worry about how they will be perceived if they choose their family or child over their career. And yet, the effects of an actively involved father far outweigh any backwards views anyone else may hold. By having paid paternity leave at your disposal, you are able to establish a healthy bond between you and your child. By bonding with them and establishing a secure attachment style, you can positively impact their neural, social, and emotional development. Being with your family can also improve your health, lower your death risk, and steer you away from health-damaging behaviors. These benefits extend to your partner as well, as extended, paid leave is known to mitigate the effects of postpartum depression, reduce the rate of infant mortality, and even increase the duration of breastfeeding in the first six months after birth (de Souza et al., 2022). Really, it's a win-win situation all around.

At the end of the day, being a modern father means making the decision to be involved with your family and doing what you can to facilitate this. You alone cannot change the systems in place, but you can find a way to make them work for you. Understanding this is an example of what we can describe as healthy masculinity. Hylton-Schaub and Bryant (2021) define healthy masculinity as the understanding of a man's responsibilities and assignments. Consequently, "when we know our assignment as men, we also understand that if we love our family, we need to be around as long as possible to be the best that we can be." Healthy masculinity sees you move away from those old ideals in which you repress or ignore your emotions. A healthily masculine man understands that, in order to care for and love those around him, he must face his own trauma and do the work to resolve his own emotional issues.

This feeds into what we consider today to be a good man. We can describe a good man, first and foremost, as someone who takes accountability for his actions and who does not attempt to distance himself from responsibility or blame. Additionally, traits denoting a good man include having an open, receptive heart and putting his influence and skills to use for the betterment of all those in his life.

Similar to our examination of healthy masculinity, we turn to Hylton-Schaub and Bryant (2021) for their definition of its opposite, toxic masculinity, which they describe as "traits or characteristics that are poisonous to the idea of what a man should be." They further describe men who are toxically masculine as those who objectify and needlessly sexualize women, who make excessive use of alcohol and drugs, and who continue to uphold antiquated, harmful beliefs regarding the roles of men and women in family structures. The actions and attitudes of these men are damaging to the progress we hope to make towards equality, as well as the ever-evolving perception of what a man and a father may be.

It's essential to understand that these definitions of healthy and toxic masculinity and the paternal traits that are associated with each are not limited to fathers in the West. Rather, these attitudes are found across cultural and racial lines. Toxic masculinity proves harmful wherever it presents itself across the globe. Conversely, healthy masculinity improves the fatherhood experience for all dads. We can attribute this to the fact that, despite certain cultural customs and specifications, children require the same things from their fathers across the board. Kids need their fathers to teach them, to model appropriate behavior, and to help them grow and develop so that they may become well-adjusted adults. Most important of all is the fact that children all over the world need their father's love and support, regardless of their racial, cultural, or ethnic background.

If we examine what children need from their fathers as they grow up, it's worth taking a look at how fathers contribute differently than mothers to the child-rearing process. The greatest contribution a father makes lies in his approach. Traditionally speaking, mothers tend to be gentler and more watchful of their children. By contrast, fathers encourage exploration and allow their kids to learn about the realities of life. This means that they don't shelter them, and if their kids fall, they will help them get back up but will also use it as a teachable moment. Crucially, we mustn't pit the two approaches against one another. Instead, consider that the mother's approach is meant to supplement the father's and vice versa.

We close out this section by taking a more serious look at how we enable the perpetuation of antiquated gender norms within the realms of parenting. What it essentially comes down to is that many young boys today are being given limited access to the world. They aren't presented with a holistic picture of what a man (and, by extension, a father) can and should be. Instead, outdated ideals and behaviors are promoted in a push for conformity. In doing so, we are failing our boys. We need to teach them to embrace all the different aspects of their personhood, to lean into emotions instead of away from them, and to view themselves as more than just a set of traditionally masculine traits.

This type of change is essential, but unfortunately, it cannot happen on an individual level alone. We need true systemic change in order to shift the conversation around and perspective on fatherhood. This means that we must all engage in self-reflection to identify and unpack our views on fatherhood and masculinity and to rectify those aspects that are no longer viable. On an institutional level, corporations must make it easier for fathers to access paid paternity leave. Governmental departments must ensure that medical professionals, educators, and all those involved with the process of parenting are making an active effort to involve fathers in the process and to acknowledge the importance of their role in the lives of their children (Promundo, 2019).

Are You Ready to Be a Dad?

When preparing to be a father, there is perhaps nothing more difficult than truthfully gauging how prepared you are for the time ahead. In order to help you understand the state of mind you occupy in anticipation of fatherhood, answer the questions listed below. Be honest with yourself, and if any of your answers give you cause for concern, read on to see which steps you can take to remedy the situation.

1. Am I ready for the changes that will come with fatherhood, both in terms of my own life as well as my relationship with my partner?

2. Do I need to have kids so I can feel loved, or will I be able to fulfill their emotional needs without expectations?

3. Is becoming a father a rite of passage or something I genuinely want to do?

4. Even though my partner and I will co-parent, will I be able to handle taking care of my kids by myself?

5. Am I emotionally equipped to be a father?

6. When I think of having and raising kids, what are the first emotions that appear?

7. In terms of finances and resources, will I be able to provide for my family, at least in part?

8. Are my partner and I compatible enough to handle coparenting?

9. Will I be able to handle it if something goes wrong during pregnancy or childbirth?

10. Do I have what it takes to be a good father?

If your answers to the above questions have you doubting your readiness, take a look at the following tips for help along your first-time dad journey:

- Sit down with your partner and discuss your approach to discipline and the strategies you would use to deal with misbehavior.

- Do your research. Watch videos, read books, and listen to podcasts to help you prepare for the little one's arrival.

- Become invested in your partner's pregnancy. Be curious, and engage with her to find out about her experience. Ask questions and help out whenever you can.

- Envision the type of father you hope to be, and make a list of things you will do in order to achieve this goal.

- Figure out the household finances and budget for the time after the baby has arrived.

- Find other dad-friends who can help you with questions and concerns.

- Construct a self-care routine you can continue after the baby has arrived.

- Don't compare yourself to your friends, family, agemates, or even your own partner when it comes to parenting aptitude and skills.

- Go easy on yourself, and remember that it is a learning process.

What Type of Dad Do You Want to Be?

An essential part of learning to be a father is determining who you'd like to be when stepping into the role of dad. The first step in this discovery is examining your own childhood and unpacking the way in which you were raised. Though you can use both your parents as references, reevaluating your father's parenting style might be more relevant to your goals here.

Think back to the way in which your father taught you skills across all areas of life, covering emotional, social, physical, and even academic competencies. Next, identify the approaches and techniques he used that you would like to replicate with your own children. It may be helpful to talk to your dad and ask him why he made certain parenting choices. In doing so, you will gain deeper insight into the logic behind his child-rearing style and be able to make an informed decision about your own. Regardless of how much of his style you intend to utilize, you have to remember that you aren't your dad and that your child isn't you. Things have changed a lot since you were a kid, and your use of older techniques will have to adapt to the times.

Once you have determined how much of your parents' approach you want to keep, it's time to decide what type of father you'd like to set out to be on your own. Ask yourself what you hope your child will learn from you and how you would go about teaching these lessons. Moreover, practice some self-reflection and ask yourself what you believe the role of a man and father to be when it comes to raising their children. Which values do you hope to impart to your children? What type of relationship do you want with them? Finally, what type of father will you be?

Relationships Australia Victoria (2019) has identified seven different types of fathers. Keep in mind that a good dad possesses a few characteristics and traits from each different type. The seven different types of dad are:

1. The responsible father: Excellent at organization, this father arranges for their children's appointments, medical and otherwise, and helps them stay on top of academics and extracurricular activities.

2. The thoughtful father: Actively using their memory, this father constantly considers their children's needs and desires. They know their children well, understanding where their strengths and weaknesses lie. Moreover, this father plans ahead to ensure that their child's needs are met.

3. The nurturing father: Experts in childcare, this father ensures that their children are nurtured, protected, and healthy.

4. The affectionate father: This dad's love language is, well, love. Affirmations of affection are regularly conveyed through hugs, kisses, and verbalizations of love.

5. The interactive father: Collaboration is the name of the game for this dad. This type of father helps their child to communicate and develop their ideas, as well as helping them to learn emotional and creative competencies through play. The interactive dad encourages decision-making and expression and wants to be involved in learning the rationale behind it all.

6. The sharing father: Teamwork is the way for the sixth type of father's dream to work. A collaborative approach is employed when it comes to parenting, and these fathers recognize their co-parent's skills, weaknesses, and values and help build a parenting model that combines the best of both caregivers.

7. The providing dad: Falling slightly more under traditional perceptions of fatherhood, the final type of father is the breadwinner. He provides in a financial sense, but he also takes charge and provides a sense of security for his loved ones.

As the first chapter of your fatherhood story comes to an end, you should have a good idea of what to expect in the time leading up to becoming a parent. For all the different intricacies and details, it all boils down to one word: preparation. Do your best to support your partner and be as well-equipped for parenthood as you can be. Once you've mastered that, you can steel yourself and turn the page to discover the many, many changes that becoming a first-time father brings—other than having a child in your home.

Chapter 2:

The Fatherhood Effect

When you and your partner welcome your first child, you can expect just about everything in your lives to change. Suddenly, all your attention is focused on this one tiny person, and you schedule your entire life around this very same small being. However, if we hope to gain a truly comprehensive understanding of what fatherhood entails, we will need to examine those changes that occur before the baby has even arrived.

The first of these changes is perhaps one of the most famous: baby brain. Also known as pregnancy brain, this phenomenon is characterized by psychological and neurobiological changes within the brain of an expectant mother. These changes trigger a brain fog and may result in difficulty performing certain cognitive functions. Along with this, "momnesia" is also often accompanied by symptoms such as forgetfulness, issues with retaining information, clumsiness, absentmindedness, weakened or shortened concentration, disorientation, and difficulty reading and remembering the names of people or things (de Bellefonds, 2022).

While it may seem disconcerting if your ordinarily sharp-minded partner is suddenly confused or cognitively distant, pregnancy brain is a natural occurrence and shouldn't be cause for worry. Furthermore, while many people only focus on this phenomenon in the time leading up to birth, your partner may experience symptoms of baby brain up until six months after your baby has arrived. Some mothers have even reported traces of pregnancy brains lasting well into the time their infants have become toddlers (Barth, 2020).

With the definition of pregnancy brain locked down, we can turn to a very important question: What causes this phenomenon? Simply put, we don't know. There are many variables that are present during pregnancy, and no two experiences are exactly alike. That being said, while we can't definitively point to one single cause, there are certain factors that have been identified as contributors to the experience of a baby brain.

The first thing is the significant change happening within your partner's endocrine system. Hormone changes are a well-known hallmark of the pregnancy experience, and secretions of estrogen and progesterone skyrocket during those nine months. These increases are compounded by changes in sleeping patterns. Many pregnancies are impacted by bouts of insomnia. If this problem persists, the constant lack of sleep may impact your partner's cognitive reasoning abilities.

For first-time parents, the pregnancy brain may be especially prominent in the time leading up to the baby's arrival, as stress is reported as a leading cause of the phenomenon. The anxiety caused by the prospect of becoming a parent can be overwhelming, as I'm sure you've noticed, and the effects of this worry can impair your partner's ability to concentrate and may even affect their memory. Finally, we may be able to trace the experience of a baby's brain to actual changes in your partner's brain structure. This is the result of her brain streamlining itself, eliminating surplus neural networks, and creating new ones that will help with the experience of motherhood (de Bellefonds, 2022).

So, your partner has a baby brain, and her mental faculties aren't what they used to be. What can you do to help? You can start by planning out a daily routine. This will combat forgetfulness, and the longer your partner maintains her routine, the better her memory will be able to function. Be sure to include smaller tasks such as hydrating and physical exercise in this routine.

You can also lighten her load by taking on some of the responsibilities she would usually cover. Free up more of her time so that she can rest and get that much-needed sleep. While you can incorporate this into the daily routine to ensure she can sleep in a bit, it will also be helpful if you just encourage her to take 30 minutes of free time so she can take a nap. One of the things you can take over is grocery shopping if you don't normally do it. While you're down there, be sure to buy some "brain foods" that will help minimize the effects of pregnancy on the brain. These foods include the following:

- Leafy greens such as spinach or kale.

- Fruits rich in antioxidants, such as blueberries.
- Eggs help increase certain nutrients in the body.
- Food rich in omega-3 fatty acids. This includes fatty varieties of fish, such as salmon.

You can actively help your partner work on her baby brain by having a game night filled with brain-boosting activities. Play word games or games involving numbers. Making use of things such as Sudoku, crosswords, and puzzles will act as a sort of cognitive workout. By playing alongside your partner, you can demonstrate your support and work in some time for bonding and relaxation. On that same note, be sure to approach each of the methods, as well as your partner's entire experience with pregnancy brain, with love, kindness, and patience.

Dad Brain: Is It a Thing?

There is a possibility that your own cognitive functioning may suffer in the lead-up to becoming a parent. If you are dubious, rest assured that we will cover all the different causes and effects. The first thing you need to know going in is this: Yes, dad brain exists, like it or not. The second is that fathers-to-be tend to experience this phenomenon to a lesser extent, and as with pregnancy brain, its ultimate purpose is to prepare you better for fatherhood.

The Science Behind Dad Brain

The first and most commonly observed cause of the dad brain is changes in the cortical structure of the brain. Attributed to neuroplasticity, these changes occur in the brain region responsible for executive function, attention, planning, and empathy. The reason for this change is to improve the new dad's parenthood skills, as he will be able to anticipate, identify, and see to his new child's needs (Sun, 2022). While many of its effects and causes resemble those of the pregnant brain, this phenomenon doesn't properly set in until after the baby has arrived. Despite the fact that you may be taking steps to prepare for the task of being a father, it's only after you have become one that your brain shifts into this "dad mode."

As you learn to navigate these new parental waters, your brain undergoes the necessary changes to ensure that nothing (and no one) capsizes. In the process, your brain gains more gray and white matter in the aforementioned cortical regions, leading to the development of new neural pathways that stimulate the acquisition of new parenting skills. We can also observe hormonal shifts similar to those of an expectant first-time mother. The effects of hormones may already trigger some symptoms in dad brain before birth, as exposure to the mother's pregnancy hormones may impact the father's own endocrine system. This impact is seen most prominently in hormones such as estrogen, vasopressin, oxytocin, and prolactin, the levels of which may all increase in the months leading up to fatherhood. Estrogen and prolactin are perhaps the most effective in the time before birth. Estrogen promotes a shift in mindset, encouraging nurturing and attentiveness. This is achieved through the conversion of testosterone into estrogen. As the former's levels plummet, the latter's rise, and they may continue to do so for several months after the end of the pregnancy (Wu, 2018). This dip in testosterone may follow an initial decrease in the first weeks of pregnancy, which is also typically marked by a decrease in cortisol in the male body.

On the other hand, prolactin may affect the new dad during the pregnancy months by mimicking symptoms felt by the expectant mother (more on this later). The last two hormones, vasopressin, and oxytocin, are both linked to the strength of paternal-familial bonds. Wu (2018) reports that these biochemicals enhance paternal care instincts and a desire to establish a father-child bond. Moreover, elevated levels of vasopressin have been found to lead to an increase in fidelity, making for a stronger, more closely linked family unit.

All of the changes you experience with dad brain are linked to being a primary caregiver—the very thing you are preparing for. More importantly, dad brain isn't limited to specific types of parents. In terms of primary caregivers, both heterosexual mothers and homosexual fathers, the changes and fluctuations described above are experienced in those regions of the brain responsible for the understanding of social cues and the processing of emotions. Fathers who are secondary caregivers experience similar effects but to a far lesser extent.

The Positive Effects of Dad Brain

The hormonal fluctuations that come with dad brain are especially beneficial, as men with lower levels of testosterone tend to be more responsive to the cry of an infant and, as such, make better caregivers. These men similarly develop more intricate skills of empathy and sensitivity. Lower testosterone also allows for a freer flow of oxytocin and dopamine, neurochemicals famous for their role in bonding parents with their children.

Higher levels of these hormones are found in fathers, mothers, and children alike in the time after birth. Oxytocin is elevated, and as such, bonds are formed more easily, which may be particularly profound. Dads, in particular, have the chance to establish a strong parent-child connection, as their increased attentiveness means that they will spend more time with their newborn. Oxytocin works its magic through interaction, and the more present the dad, the higher the level of interaction. As the child matures, the relationship becomes more sophisticated and builds positively on the foundation laid in those early days.

It's worth noting that while the new neural pathways carved into the mind of a first-time dad all contribute to his parenting skills, this process isn't catalyzed naturally. In contrast with the natural occurrence of the baby brain in expecting moms, soon-to-be dads don't have a cerebral switch that gets flicked by external or internal factors. Instead, the greatest effects of dad brain are felt through learning. By making an intentional shift in mindset and behavior, new fathers become more adept at child-rearing. At the same time, the new skills they pick up allow them to form deeper, more profound bonds with their newborns.

What Remolds a New Father's Brain?

Though dad's brain is essentially gained through experience, it's important to understand that these changes happen over time and can only happen through parent-child interaction. The higher your level of interaction with your child, the more significantly you will experience the effects of dad brain. However, if you are a secondary caregiver or spend too little time with your baby, you will find that your brain structure and hormone levels will shift more subtly and possibly for a shorter period of time. However, before you panic about how much time you can spend with your newborn, it's worth noting that there are factors beyond your control that may influence the number of one-on-one hours you get with your baby. Social and cultural norms in your part of the world may dictate that you spend your time on pursuits other than childcare. Moreover, many first-time dads may encounter psychological obstacles when attempting to tap into the power of the dad brain. It's important to remember that while there is a measure of instinct involved, parenting is a learning process, and your dad brain will develop over time.

More on Paternal Instinct

Traditionally speaking, men have been cast in the role of protector when the family unit is put together. This forms part of the concept of paternal instinct, which is defined as "the instinctual bond which develops between a father and his child throughout pregnancy and the life of that child" (*Paternal Instinct: What is it [and why is it important]*, 2020). Though partially influenced by societal standards and norms, the father's role as protector does seem to be largely natural. Men are born with the instinctual drive and ability to function as a presence of safety and stability in the lives of those they care for.

Much emphasis has traditionally been placed on maternal instinct, but we are coming to understand that its paternal counterpart is equally as important. Though still often designated as providers and protectors, modern men understand that this extends beyond material wealth.

Leaning into paternal instinct means providing emotional support and generosity, as well as being compassionate. In all its forms, protection is an integral part of a father's masculinity. While this may sound slightly antiquated, we can see how far-ranging and malleable this sense of protectiveness is. Stenson (2023) identifies five distinct ways in which modern fathers seek to protect their loved ones:

1. Fathers protect the women in their lives, including their spouse, mother, and daughter. This form of protection is motivated both by instinct and by an observance of the prevalence of misogyny in the world.

2. Fathers step in to protect their spouse from external threats or aggressions, which sometimes include antagonistic behavior from their children.

3. Providing can also be seen as a form of protection in that it prevents the family from falling into poverty and illness.

4. Much of a father's protective instincts are focused on shielding their children from external and internal threats. In the case of the former, they offer protection against things such as bullies, and in the case of the latter, they protect them from the consequences of dangerous or impulsive behaviors.

5. A father's protection is delivered through education and character-building. This form of protection is intended to provide children with emotional and cognitive skills that will prove conducive to their development. Ultimately, the goal is to imbue them with knowledge, values, and attitudes they will be able to implement as means of protection in their own lives someday.

Stenson's fifth form of protection is regarded as the most important, partly because it overlaps the most extensively with the core tenets of paternal instinct, but largely due to the fact that it sets children up for long-term success.

In addition to acting as a safeguard against the evils of the world, paternal instinct also helps with the establishment and maintenance of a parent-child bond. Traditionally, we tend to view the mother-infant bonding process as more important, given that women are most often the primary caregivers. However, we now understand that modern parenting attitudes have shifted and that fathers are increasingly involved in the child-rearing process. By focusing on the paternal roleplayers, we can see that father-infant bonding is just as important. In fact, not only is this bond equally significant, but the time in which it forms closely resembles its maternal counterpart. Between eight and 10 months, infants form links with their mothers, and studies have demonstrated that the same connections are made with fathers during this time. Despite this similarity, we can also identify that father-infant bonding takes place differently, with the connection arising largely from stimulating interaction such as play (Hewlett, 1991).

Our understanding of paternal instinct isn't the only thing that has changed over the years. At the very start of this book, we looked at how the role of the modern father has evolved with time. A great portion of this evolution can be attributed to shifts in cultural and societal perspectives and ideas. However, as significant as the changed face of fatherhood is, it's important for us to understand that culture has played a role all along and that it didn't dictate the existence of distant fathers. At least not everywhere.

To understand the role of culture, we must look to the Aka people, who reside in the southern region of the Central African Republic, as well as the northernmost parts of Congo-Brazzaville. Within this culture, children are fiercely protected, nurtured, engaged with, and are the recipients of gentle discipline as opposed to outright punishment. More importantly, fathers play an immensely important role in the child-rearing process, contributing to the child's care and development just as much as their spouse. For more than 12 hours a day, Aka fathers are less than an arm's length away from their infant and hold their kids for an average of one hour during the day, switching to about a quarter of the nighttime. By contrast, fathers in the West average between 10 and 20 minutes a day in which they hold their children (Hewlett, 1991).

The reason for this extensive father-child interaction comes from the cultural ideals held by the Aka people. Within their society, egalitarianism is the order of the day. This means that men hold no position of superior authority over women, domestically or otherwise. Additionally, we see strong spousal bonds between parents as well. A sense of community permeates every aspect of Aka culture, and collaboration is found in everything they do. In the gathering of materials and resources, men and women work together to accumulate what they need to sustain their families and communities. Within the domicile, this translates to a more equal dispersal of power, a closer bond between the two, and more cooperative, positive parenting techniques. Finally, we must consider the importance of egalitarianism as a whole. In the Aka culture, everyone is capable of doing anything. There are no "masculine" or "feminine" activities or roles. Everyone pitches in and contributes to everything, from raising and harvesting crops to soothing a crying baby. Crucially, an Aka man's masculinity isn't diminished by his involvement with his kids. Instead, the stronger his presence, the more securely he will feel tied to his cultural values.

Hewlett's study began in 1984, nearly four decades ago. At the time, his comparisons between African and Western paternal behaviors demonstrated immense disparities across nearly every aspect of child-rearing. However, nearly a quarter of the way into the 21st century, we can see that fathers in the West are increasingly coming to adopt mindsets and habits similar to those of the Aka people and are picking up more of the slack when it comes to raising their own children. This is a good thing, as we are seeing a concerted effort to move from the individualist familial practices of the past towards a more collectivist family dynamic.

Pregnancy Symptoms in Fathers

We close out our exploration of the effect of fatherhood by taking a look at the physical influence of being a first-time dad. More popularly known as the gaining of "sympathy weight," the phenomenon is actually known as couvade syndrome. For an easier-to-understand name, we can also use the term "sympathetic pregnancy" (Dale, 2023). This syndrome arises in the non-pregnant partners of soon-to-be parents and involves the former experiencing symptoms of pregnancy that only the latter would typically experience.

Couvade syndrome is a nebulous part of the realm of parenting knowledge, as it isn't formally considered a physical or psychological affliction. Its occurrence is thought to be linked to our society's evolving ideas regarding fatherhood. Because soon-to-be dads are more involved in their partner's pregnancy, they are more exposed to the symptoms and changes that come along with the process. This may contribute to their developing a sympathetic pregnancy.

In addition to this, two causes of Couvade syndrome have been linked to emotionality in fathers. The first is a type of empathy called "compathy," which is described as the symbiotic sharing of another person's feelings. In this case, this sharing extends to physical experiences as well. Compassion is used to deal with the stress and fear that accompany the idea of impending fatherhood. The second emotional cause is termed "loading" and involves the assumption of another person's physical or psychological load. Couvade originating from this cause is seen most often in first-time fathers who have severe anxiety about becoming a father, as well as those who are bonded to their partner particularly closely. Other less common causes of the syndrome have been identified as envy and hormonal changes (Dale, 2023).

Sympathetic pregnancies usually manifest during the first or third trimester. Their effects usually end soon after childbirth. If you are concerned that you are developing this syndrome, be on the lookout for the following symptoms:

- Abdominal pain.
- Fluctuations in appetite.
- Nausea and vomiting.
- Flatulence.
- Problems related to digestion and the gastrointestinal system.
- Gaining or losing weight.

- Diarrhea.

- Constipation.

- Skin problems such as irritation or inflammation.

- Toothaches.

- Leg cramps.

- Depressive symptoms.

- Symptoms related to anxiety disorders.

Treating couvade syndrome has no real standard structure, but health care professionals should be consulted if you fear that you might have developed the condition. However, because many symptoms arise from feelings of anxiety or unpreparedness, there are steps you can take to minimize their effects. These steps include:

- Having an open and honest conversation with your partner about parenthood. Discuss your expectations, your fears, and your plans. Share what is troubling you and the parts of fatherhood you are looking forward to. Even if you don't find a solution to your problems, simply talking through your feelings can help lessen their weight on your mind.

- Plan ahead and prepare well in advance. Take prenatal classes, read parenting books, and babyproof your house. While you will never be 100% ready to be a dad, you can ensure that you take as many preparatory steps as you can. They will help ease your mind and, of course, come in handy when your baby arrives.

- Take care of yourself. Step out for some time alone or engage in self-care to manage your anxiety levels. You may want to consider consulting a mental health care professional to unpack the influence your mind's activities are having on your body.

If there is one thing we can take away from all this, it is that becoming a parent leaves no part of your life untouched. While baby and dad brain may not always elicit the best feelings or experiences, it's helpful to remember that there are ways to deal with them and that certain aspects of the phenomena serve a helpful purpose. More importantly, it's essential to recognize that things will change when you become a dad and that these changes will be both good and bad. That being said, you will feel much more in control (and much less sympathetically pregnant) if you have a plan in place for when you welcome your little bundle of joy into the world.

Chapter 3:

Navigating the Expectant Path—Preparing the Perfect Pregnancy Plan

One of the most potent weapons in your preparatory fatherhood arsenal is a well-structured pregnancy plan. This plan, which covers everything you need to do in anticipation of the birth as well as for the first year after, will be your most trusted guide as you approach fatherhood. A pregnancy plan can take many forms and will invariably differ from family to family, depending on needs, resources, and familial structure.

This plan includes everything from birthing classes to birthing techniques and more. It's crucial that you and your partner communicate honestly throughout the planning process, especially as you may differ on certain aspects thereof. For instance, while many of us may think of hospitals and stirrups as the traditional birthing setting, water births have enjoyed an uptick in popularity over the last few years. More specifically, hospital water births have become more popular, with approximately 10% of all American hospitals offering the option of water immersion for delivery (Chertoff, 2018).

Some other facts you might not know about water birth include the following:

- Maintaining a consistent water temperature is essential to the process, as it helps both mother and baby avoid experiencing excessive heat or chill.

- When the baby exits the birth canal, they are removed face down, allowing for the drainage of fluids from the mouth and nose.

- In the moments after birth, the baby is placed in the mother's arms, and their bodies can remain underwater. What's most important is that both of their heads remain above the surface.

- A water-birth baby's coloring may look distressing for a moment or two. They don't turn that shade of newborn pink right away and take a minute or so to oxygenate their systems properly. When this is done, the rosiness sets in.

- These births don't take place entirely in the water. After the baby is delivered, the mother is helped to a bed where she will deliver the placenta. This helps to more accurately estimate blood loss and intervene more appropriately if necessary.

- Even mothers who have tested positive for Group B Strep (GBS) can undertake water birth. Intravenous antibiotics will still be administered, and mother and baby alike will be kept as safe as possible.

This is the type of information you will need to consider when putting together your pregnancy plan. Ultimately, you and your partner should choose what works best for you and which will keep your baby the safest during the process.

Creating a Birth Plan

According to Healthdirect Australia (2022), a birth plan is a "written record of what you would like to happen when you are having your baby." This plan not only helps the expectant mother take control of the birthing process but can also make you, as the soon-to-be father, more involved in the process. Birth plans function as a useful referential framework you can use to guide you through the time leading up to the birth, the event itself, and the time after. These plans are customized to suit each family's specific situation. However, despite the differences in details, the contents of birth plans are largely the same. In general, they include:

- The location where the birth will take place.
- Who will be with the mother during the birth?
- Who will be the birth partner, and what will they do during the birth?
- How much mobility will there be during labor?
- Coping and supporting strategies, such as preferred birthing positions, massage techniques, and breathing exercises.
- Options for pain relief.
- What will happen if intervention is required?
- Who will hold the baby after the delivery, as well as who will cut the umbilical cord?
- What is the plan regarding breastfeeding and the maintenance of skin-to-skin contact.
- Whether you want to opt for the vitamin K injection for your newborn.

Given the comprehensiveness of the birth plan, you can already start compiling its contents during the second trimester. You can start putting together your birth plan as early as you'd like; however, it's recommended that you commit the final version (or a near-final version) to paper sometime between weeks 32 and 36.

Tips for Creating a Birth Plan

It's important that you start compiling your birth plan early. Later on in this chapter, you will see that part of this plan is the attendance of antenatal classes. Be sure to find classes in your area as soon as possible so that you can work their attendance into your schedule well in advance. This brings us to the second thing to consider: research. There's a lot of information that will be thrown at you as a first-time dad, all of which you will be able to cope with more easily if you do some reading up on your own.

Furthermore, communicate with your partner. Lay your cards on the table regarding what either of you envisions, not only for the time of the pregnancy and birth but also in the months that follow. Communicate openly and honestly, exploring the birth methods, preparations, and arrangements your partner feels comfortable with, as well as those that are within your means to facilitate. As you build your birth plan, remember to consult your healthcare provider regularly. Make use of the scheduled check-ups, as well as any additional consultations if necessary, to ask questions and discuss your options. You also have to prioritize. Certain measures will need to be in place well in advance (think antenatal classes, the contracting of a midwife's services, etc.), while others can be dealt with even after the baby has arrived. Make sure you have it all in order. Finally, draft a birth plan ahead of time. Seeing it all laid out in black and white will give you a chance to look at the entire picture and make the necessary adjustments.

Important Questions to Discuss With Your Partner

As you build your birth plan, there are a large number of things you have to take into consideration. With the sheer quantity of information you are meant to put down in this plan, it can be confusing to know where to start. Below is a list of questions you and your partner can work through to get the process started. Remember that flexibility exists. If you see that something you decided to use during the birth won't work out, you are free to come back to the plan and tweak it. Get your birth plan brainstorming started with the following questions:

- Where will the birth take place?

- Who will be in the room when the baby is delivered?

- Is there a particular birthing method you prefer over others?

- When labor sets in, who will be notified, and how will they receive the news?

- Will the birth be documented? If so, how?

- Will medication be used during the birth process?

- If medication will not be used from the outset, how will its necessity be communicated?

- If the birth takes place in a hospital, will the standard post-birth procedure, i.e., the first bath, as well as the administering of ointments and inoculations, be followed?

- If something should go wrong during the birth and your original plan cannot be followed, what will your backup be?

- After the birth, will visitors be allowed? If so, who is welcome to drop by?

- Where in the house will it be most comfortable for both mother and baby in the days after the birth?

- What does postpartum depression look and feel like?

- If symptoms of postpartum depression begin to arise, who will be contacted, and at what point?

- Will the baby be breastfed, or will you make exclusive use of a bottle?

- How will nighttime feedings be handled?

- Where will the baby sleep?

- Will co-sleeping be considered? If so, which precautions will be taken to ensure the baby's safety?

These questions cover only a portion of what you have to consider when compiling a birth plan, so don't be afraid to deepen your discussion. Bring up any relevant concerns or queries and work through them together.

Choosing a Birthing Method

The selection of a birthing method is, naturally, one of the most important components of any birth plan. This particular decision may be relatively difficult to make, especially as there are many factors to be considered. However, as you explore your options, remember to keep in mind that no birthing method is 100% foolproof. Nevertheless, the chosen method should work best for your partner and baby, keeping them safe during delivery. Keep in mind that, though your input is certainly valuable, this decision is ultimately your partner's to make. Though there are a number of different types of delivery, there are really only two main birthing methods.

The first birthing method is one of which many of you may feel wary: the cesarean section. Known more popularly as a C-section, this method can be selected ahead of the birth or alternatively used if complications present during the process of vaginal delivery. Having a C-section presents a number of advantages and disadvantages. In the category of the former, we find that this procedure has a standard means of execution. This means that decisions regarding the birthing location, use of pain management medications, and recovery after birth are already set. C-sections are performed in hospitals with the patient under regional anesthesia. Recovery typically lasts between two and four days, with the newborn and mother both remaining under the watchful eye of medical staff.

On the flip side of the coin, the pre-established aspects of this birthing method means that there is little to no possibility of personalization. While C-sections are largely safe procedures, the inability to select pain management strategies and the continuation of the birth process may be distressing to some prospective parents. Moreover, this operation is relatively invasive, as an incision is made along the abdomen, and the baby is delivered through this incision. Recovery may be more difficult than that following vaginal delivery.

With regards to vaginal delivery, we see pros and cons in equal measure. When the baby is delivered through the birth canal, which many consider the "traditional" way of giving birth, parents have more control over the birthing process. Not only is the mother present throughout, but variables such as pain management and changes caused by complications can be dealt with in a manner that works for the parents. Additionally, vaginal delivery has been demonstrated to reduce a number of health risks in newborns. Among these are the reduced probability of developing food allergies, lactose intolerance, and respiratory issues (Mustela USA, 2020).

That being said, no one birthing method is entirely without its disadvantages. Vaginal delivery, in particular, poses some relatively serious risks for mother and baby alike. This birthing method may sometimes cause the baby to suffer some physical injury or trauma as they move through the birth canal. Moreover, there are more uncontrolled factors present than during a C-section. As such, if there is no clear plan for the resolution of complications, further danger is posed to the mother and baby as a number of emergent medical conditions may arise. In terms of impact on the body, vaginal delivery is no less traumatizing than a C-section.

What this all comes down to is that there are two options when it comes to birthing methods. However, whether you opt for a C-section or choose a variation on vaginal delivery, it is important to understand what each process entails so that you may make an informed decision.

Vaginal Delivery

The most common type of delivery, often referred to as "natural childbirth," delivery through the birth canal is a relatively straightforward process (Rothstein, 2022). While many new parents would choose this option given its relative lack of complexity, we must understand that natural childbirth may not always be possible, even if it was the plan from the start.

We can identify two methods of intervention doctors may use during labor should complications arise. The first of these is known as an amniotomy, though you may be more familiar with its colloquial description of "breaking the water." Though not technically a means of induction, this procedure does create a rupture in the amniotic sac surrounding the baby, allowing for drainage of the amniotic fluid. The purpose of the amniotomy is twofold. Firstly, it can help speed up labor proceedings. Secondly, should the need arise, by removing the amniotic fluid, your healthcare provider can monitor your baby's well-being and track any changes that may take place. The second procedure is known as episiotomy and involves making an incision along the perineum so that the vaginal opening may be enlarged. This is usually done so that vaginal delivery is still a viable option and may help deal with complications that arise during labor.

Vaginal delivery has its advantages and disadvantages, much like any medical procedure. On the one hand, this type of delivery has demonstrated reduced risk of infection, shorter recovery periods, and hospital stays, as well as the opportunity to personalize the birthing experience. On the other hand, if no pain management medications are used, this type of delivery can be extremely painful. Additionally, physical injuries are a real possibility, and relying on natural childbirth may prove unpredictable, as some babies may arrive earlier or later than expected (Rothstein, 2022).

Assisted Vaginal Delivery: Vacuum or Forceps

Assisted vaginal delivery involves the use of medical instruments to help remove the baby from the birth canal. The reasons for this type of delivery vary and may include the labor lasting too long, the mother becoming too tired to continue the process, a delay in the progression of the process, or complications arising that place both mother and baby in distress (Cleveland Clinic, 2018). It's very unlikely that you will be able to plan for an assisted vaginal delivery in advance, as its execution is contingent on the fulfillment of several criteria. However, it will be helpful to indicate in your birth plan that this means of delivery is one you would like to employ as a backup.

Most commonly, the methods used during assisted deliveries are delivery using forceps and vacuum extraction delivery. The former involves the use of a surgical tool resembling tongs, which are placed on the baby's head. Once in the grasp of the forceps, the baby is guided out of the birth canal. Vacuum extraction involves the placement of a small suction cup on the baby's head. The attached pump is activated, pulling the baby out of the birth canal. This is done in tandem with the mother pushing the baby through the canal.

Given the fact that this type of delivery involves only a small deviation from the standard procedure for vaginal births, its advantages and disadvantages remain largely the same. Because the need for assistance is determined during the labor process, it's important to note that your obstetrician or birthing professional will use their judgment to select the tool for use, as different situations warrant different approaches.

Cesarean Birth

While C-sections can certainly be scheduled in advance as a matter of preference, there are a number of factors present at the time of birth that may also require you to opt for this type of delivery. Chief among them is the instance in which the baby turns from the traditional birthing position. This means that the baby is either in the breech position, meaning they have turned so that they come out bottom first, or in the transverse position, meaning they have turned sideways. Other reasons for a C-section include a birth involving multiple infants or a particularly large baby.

You may want to consider a cesarean birth in the case of high-risk pregnancies, as the control provided by the procedure protects the health of both mother and baby. If you schedule a C-section in advance, you also have more control over the birthing process and its timing and won't need to rush to your birth location when labor begins spontaneously. Though the positives are certainly legion, it's also worth noting that recovery from the operation may take as long as eight weeks. Undergoing this process while juggling the pressures of parenting a newborn can be especially arduous.

Vaginal Birth After Cesarean (VBAC)

If your partner has been pregnant before and delivered via C-section, she may be eligible for VBAC. This type of delivery is considered only when the pregnancy has been stable and free of complications. Moreover, your partner's candidacy is limited to giving birth after only one C-section. If she has had more than one cesarean, she becomes ineligible for this procedure, and you will have to schedule delivery via the procedure once more. In addition to this, you will only be considered for VBAC if the cause of the cesarean is not present in the current pregnancy. For instance, if your partner had to deliver that way because of high blood pressure and she still has this condition now, she would be unable to deliver via VBAC.

VBAC births have fewer complications, allow for increased participation during labor and birth, and have comparatively short recovery times. However, it must be noted that a VBAC birth does pose a risk, especially as uterine rupture is more likely if your partner has already delivered via C-section (Rothstein, 2022).

Scheduled Induction

Scheduled inductions are most commonly used for pregnancies that have extended beyond the typical 40-week period. Though rarely done before the 39th week, an induction may be done if it is medically necessary for the baby to arrive earlier. Typically, however, this type of delivery is done once your partner has passed her due date and the baby has developed enough to be fit for birth.

On induction day, your partner will be admitted to the hospital and will be given an intravenous medication known as Pitocin, which will catalyze the contractions that begin the labor process. Given the set of clinical procedures attached to this type of delivery, scheduled inductions are largely safe as medical help is constantly available. It also allows for more control on your part, and you can stick to your birth plan more closely. However, it isn't entirely perfect. Primary among the disadvantages of an induction is that it may be necessitated by complications related to your partner or your baby, which presents its own set of challenges. However, assuming that everything is fine on that front, the only real disadvantage that remains is the fact that your partner will be unable to perform unmedicated, natural childbirth.

Water Birth

Water births set the labor process in a hot tub-like bath filled with warm water. As with other forms of vaginal delivery, there is some variety to be found with water births, as the mother can choose to either give birth while half submerged or to move to another, more elevated position once the baby must exit the birth canal.

The increase in popularity enjoyed by water births is due in no small part to the fact that they may be performed in hospitals, birthing centers, or even in the comfort of your own home. Determining where the birth will take place can relieve some of the stress attached to the process. Additionally, water births are recommended for the freedom of movement they provide as well as for the reduction in blood pressure the calming water brings (Rothstein, 2022). Water births are also purported to be less painful and can help you safely and effectively manage your partner's pain.

As always, we must examine both sides of the coin. While advantageous in many ways, water births can also be a logistical nightmare, especially if you choose your home as your birthing location. Additionally, if complications arise, mother and baby will have to be taken to a medical facility, which may prove difficult if not dangerous. Less severe disadvantages include the inability to use medications for induction or epidural anesthesia. There are some concerns that water births may pose a greater risk for infection due to the mother spending the majority of the labor process in the same pool of warm water. The danger attached to this risk is negligible and should not dissuade you from considering a water birth as a viable means of delivery.

Choosing a Birth Location

Once you have settled on the type of delivery you would like to use, it's time to determine exactly where you will be welcoming your child into the world. Keep in mind that certain birthing methods, such as vaginal deliveries involving procedures and scheduled inductions, cannot take place at home and should only be performed by a qualified healthcare professional. If your desired type of delivery is more flexible in terms of locale, work through this section and weigh your options. Consider the fact that, at the end of the day, you should have the birth in the place that will be the safest for your partner and baby.

When selecting your location, there are a number of things to take into account beyond personal preference. You have to take into account the logistics surrounding the birth as well as the support you and your partner will need in the time after. As you consider where you want the birth to take place, make sure to factor in the following:

- The proximity of your birth location to a hospital (if you choose to use your home or a birthing center) and how you will get there in an emergency situation.

- Which methods of pain management are available during labor.

- The resources available for your baby should complications arise, for example, medications or a neonatal intensive care unit (NICU).

- How comfortable and private the delivery rooms are.

- The number of people who make up your support system that will be allowed in the room.

- The resources and support available for breastfeeding.

- Whether your baby will remain with your partner in the room or if they will be removed to a nursery.

Hospital

Given the location to which most parents default, delivering your child at the hospital is a safe option to consider, especially for first-time parents. The primary advantage of a hospital is the extensive support you will receive from a team of qualified doctors and nurses who will guide you through the process and who will know how to intervene if necessary. Moreover, the resources for these interventions are readily available, and you will receive the help you need before complications worsen. Another medicinal benefit is the availability of pain medication to help you through labor. If your newborn requires some additional medical care, most hospitals have a NICU where your baby will be treated. Other benefits of a hospital delivery include your ability to maintain a limited number of visitors after birth.

In terms of post-birth care, most hospitals will also furnish you with some supplies to help you start parenting once you are discharged. You may also find that your hospital has a lactation consultant to help you with any difficulties regarding breastfeeding. Finally, something we can chalk up in favor of a hospital birth is that insurance providers will cover more of the expenses than those incurred for a home or birthing center delivery.

However, for all the resources available, making use of a hospital as a birth location may make the process a bit more alienating and may make parents feel as though the birth proceedings are beyond their control. Hospitals are streamlined to function as effectively as possible according to previously established policies, many of which may not make you feel at your most comfortable during the birth process. If their way of doing things doesn't align with your birth plan, it will fall on you to make compromises. Additionally, because they follow a specific plan, hospitals may allow for less freedom of movement during labor and may advise your partner against giving birth in the position she prefers.

Though a perk in some instances, the cap on visitors may interfere with your plan of having your baby surrounded by loved ones at the moment of their birth and in the days after. You may also find yourself surrounded by unfamiliar faces as the hospital staff rotates. Doctors' routine of working on-call after hours may mean that the person delivering your baby isn't the one who has accompanied you through the pregnancy. Overall, the drawbacks tied to hospital births are more emotional in nature. Medically speaking, these birth locations are as safe as houses. However, having little control over the process can be disorienting, and having a negative emotional experience may translate into physical effects, so be sure to take into account what matters to you when making this decision.

Home

Home births have become increasingly viable options in the last few years. This is partly a result of the rise in water births, many of which hospitals are unable to support. Their popularity may also be due to modern parents' desire to have more control over the day of birth and to welcome their child in a comfortable, familiar space. This is the most prominent benefit of choosing a home birth, though the decision comes with a variety of other additional pros.

This birth location will all but ensure that your baby arrives via vaginal delivery and will give you as much time with them as you'd like without them being wheeled off to a nursery. If religious or cultural practices play a role in the birth process, you may have more freedom to enact them at home. You have more freedom in general, as you can determine who is there with you and for how long. Under the tutelage of a doula or midwife, your partner will also be able to try out a variety of birthing positions to find the one that fits her best. Also, given that the entire process is likely to take place in your living room, there are fewer costs attached to a home birth.

Despite how alluring these perks may seem, there are a number of things to consider before settling on a home birth. First among them is a financial factor, such as the fact that your insurance is less likely to cover the same portion of costs as it would for a hospital birth. However, depending on your plan, you may be able to claim a reimbursement. In addition to the potential financial implications, you may also have to consider other variables related to the birth itself. At-home births have been linked to increased danger for the baby to experience seizures, nervous system disorders, or even death (Mayo

Clinic Staff, 2018). That being said, remember that no birth location is entirely free of danger. Additionally, home births may be difficult to execute logistically, and you may have to buy a number of items in addition to typical baby supplies. You should also keep in mind that your home will have to be as close to sterile as possible, which may make housekeeping a pain in the days leading up to the birth.

It's important to note that home births, in spite of how much control they afford you, cannot be performed alone. Even though friends and family might be present, your partner needs to have a qualified healthcare professional lead and assist them through the process. In most cases, this will be a doula or midwife (more on them in a moment), though some obstetricians do participate in home births.

Finally, you have to keep in mind that a home birth may not always be possible to take place entirely at home. If complications arise, you may need to visit a hospital, so factor this into your preparation for the day. High-risk pregnancies are usually recommended for hospital births, as complications may not be resolved in time if the mother and baby have to be transported from another location. If you do decide on a home birth, you will have to keep a watchful eye out for anything that may require more serious medical attention. This includes the following:

- If your partner develops a fever.

- If your partner is in pain, and needs relief beyond what you can provide at home.

- If your partner experiences excessive bleeding.

- If your partner has high blood pressure.

- If the labor process has stalled, and isn't progressing as fast as it should.

- If your baby enters the breech or transverse positions.

- If your baby starts experiencing distress as they attempt to move out of the birth canal.

Birthing Center

If you and your partner would like the birth process to take place without the use of medication but don't want to rearrange your entire house, consider using a birthing center. These centers are "low-tech birthing [options] for moms-to-be who desire [an] unmedicated childbirth experience" (Brown, 2022). Though they can be freestanding facilities, many birthing centers are attached to or situated right next to a hospital. This makes it easier to find medical help should the need arise.

Similar to home births, birthing center deliveries are commonly performed by qualified midwives, though other healthcare professionals may also lend a hand, depending on the structure of the facility. Birthing centers can be thought of as a combination of a hospital and a home. Delivery rooms in these facilities are larger and more comfortable, and while healthcare professionals are involved in the process, little-to-no medication is involved. It's worth noting that this isn't limited to pain relief, which many birthing centers restrict to alternative options such as acupuncture or breathing exercises. Other common interventions associated with birth are also excluded from the birthing center procedure, and they are unlikely to do things such as labor induction, the administration of intravenous medication, and continuous fetal monitoring.

A birthing center may also appeal to you if you would like to have greater privacy and more freedom during the birth process. As with home births, the healthcare professional assisting your partner is likely to allow her to try out several different positions in which to deliver. These facilities have shorter periods of required stay, and you will be able to leave the birthing center between four and eight hours after your baby has arrived. Perhaps the greatest reason to consider a birthing center lies in the financial impact the stay will have on you. You are likely to spend only a fraction of the amount you would have at a hospital, all while enjoying many of the same perks and resources (Brown, 2022).

In terms of drawbacks, birthing centers only have some general disadvantages. While there is the possibility that your partner will have to be moved to the hospital, the proximity of many centers to medical institutions makes this transfer all the easier. However, this supposes that you find a hospital-adjacent birthing center near you, and these facilities aren't all that common just yet. Apart from this, the financial aspect is the greatest disadvantage to consider, as is your partner's eligibility to deliver in a birthing center.

Given the lack of medical intervention resources present in these centers, only low-risk pregnancies are accepted, as well as those that will have only one birth. While birthing centers do have the resources to keep mothers and babies safe as they are transported to a hospital, the apparatus needed for high-risk pregnancies is only available at hospitals. If you do opt for a birthing center, it's essential that you keep the possibility of moving to a hospital in mind. If any of the complications listed in the section above arise, your partner will have to be moved. Rest assured that the onus won't fall on you to make this call, as the midwife or nurse working with you will let you know if serious medical intervention is needed.

Pain Management

It's possible that you may have heard this before, but labor can be quite a painful experience. Even if things go exactly as planned, bringing another person into this world can provide your partner with a significant amount of pain. When it comes to managing the aches and pains of labor, there are a number of options available to you. It's vital that you explore each of these so you can tailor your birth plan to fit your situation as well as your partner's preferences. Managing the pain of childbirth can be done using both medical and nonmedical means.

Medical Pain Management

Often considered the "mainstream" methods, these pain management techniques are perhaps already known to you. Medication-induced pain relief can range from complete elimination to partial alleviation.

Pethidine

Delivered either intravenously or in the form of an intramuscular injection in the buttock, pethidine provides significant pain relief. The medication's effects typically last between two and four hours. Though not so severe as to warrant concern, pethidine may result in the experience of side effects for both mother and baby.

If treated with pethidine, your partner may experience nausea, disorientation, dizziness, altered sensory perception, and reduced breathing capacity. In some extreme cases, pethidine proves ineffective, and no pain relief is provided. Your newborn may also be somewhat affected by the medication as it passes through the umbilical cord during labor. Potential side effects for babies may also include respiratory problems. This is more likely in cases where the delivery takes place soon after the pethidine has been administered or when several doses have been given (Victoria State Government Department of Health, 2012). Though not ideal, these problems are easily fixed, and doctors will give your baby an injection to reverse the medication's effects. Additionally, there may be some depression in your newborn's reflexes, particularly the sucking reflex used during feeding. The extent of pethidine's side effects on babies is still being researched, and there is as yet no real reason to discount it as a means of pain management.

Nitrous Oxide

You may know this pain management medication by its more fun name: laughing gas. Administered via a mask held up to the face or a tube placed in the mouth, nitrous oxide is perhaps the least invasive means of pain management. Unfortunately, this also means that it falls towards the lower end of the line when it comes to how much pain is relieved. In effect, the gas, which takes seconds to work, can only slightly decrease the pain that comes with each contraction. However, this doesn't make it any less effective, as some mothers will only require this much relief and will not experience pain that needs more intense alleviation.

The use of the gas is preferred by many, particularly as it allows for control of the relief process. The mask or tube is handed to your partner, and she inhales the gas when she feels it is necessary. Side effects of laughing gas include confusion, disorientation, nausea, vomiting, and claustrophobia caused by the closeness of the apparatus to the mouth and face. Notably, this gas may also not succeed in providing any relief at all, a phenomenon that has been observed in one-third of births in which it was the primary means of pain management (Victoria State Government Department of Health, 2012). Though there are some side effects, nitrous oxide remains a popular choice, as it doesn't linger too long within the body, and so its effects are worked out relatively quickly.

Pudendal Block

Moving into the realm of anesthetics now, we find a type of local anesthesia known as a pudendal block. Injected directly into the pudendal nerve, located in the perineum, the block is administered directly before the baby is delivered. Its anesthetic properties allow the pain to recede from the vaginal and rectal regions, which allows the baby to move more easily through the birth canal.

The most common medication used for a pudendal block is lidocaine, as it tends to last longer. However, other anesthetics can also be used and may prove just as effective. When the block is injected, it can take anything from five to 20 minutes before your partner is completely numb in the desired region. As with other local anesthetics, a pudendal block will wear off after a few hours. If more than one dose is required, expect the effects to last a bit longer.

Given that this form of pain management involves a relatively noninvasive injection, the only side effects to take into account are those associated with anesthesia in general. This includes the potential development of a blood clot as well as the possibility that the medication may cross through the umbilical cord and affect the baby. Most commonly, the effect on the newborn is seen in the hours after birth, when they have difficulty breastfeeding. Additionally, as small as the injection site is, the puncturing of the skin does naturally pose the risk of infection. However, these blocks are very common means of pain management and should provide you with no more concern than any of the others outlined in this section.

Epidural Anesthesia

A form of regional anesthesia, an epidural, is perhaps already known to you, given its popularity. Delivered via injection and suitable for use during both vaginal births as well as C-sections, epidurals are the most effective means of pain management for childbirth (Victoria State Government Department of Health, 2012). The epidural block differs from the pudendal block not only because it is injected into the protective, fat-filled area around the spinal cord but also because its numbing effects are much greater. The anesthetic will numb your partner from the waist down, virtually eliminating all contraction-related pain. This relief will usually last for approximately two hours after it has been administered. Take note that if the first dose proves ineffective or if labor is prolonged, additional doses may be required. Naturally, the higher the number of doses your partner receives, the longer it will take for the epidural to work itself out of her system completely.

Epidurals are particularly strong forms of pain relief, and given the relatively large portion of the body they affect, it's natural that a number of side effects may arise. The most common among these is weakness in the muscles of the lower body in the time after childbirth. This weakness may mean that your partner will be confined to the bed or will be immobile for a while. Additionally, your partner may experience feelings of nausea or faintness caused by a drop in blood pressure. This is treated using intravenous fluids, particularly if it starts to affect the baby. If your partner intends to deliver vaginally, consider the possibility that a typical vaginal birth may not be possible. Your partner might find herself unable to push at all because of the extensive numbness the epidural has caused.

Spinal Block

Another form of regional anesthesia administered to the spine, a spinal block, is used most commonly for C-sections, and oftentimes when the cesarean has been scheduled in advance. This form of pain management is delivered via injection, as the anesthesiologist places the block directly into the spinal canal in the lower back. Similar to the epidural, your partner will be numb from the waist down. The spinal block typically lasts for approximately two hours and takes effect almost immediately after it has been administered. Given the similarity between this medication and the epidural, their advantages, disadvantages, and side effects are the same. An important difference to note is that while an epidural may be administered more than once if necessary, a spinal block is only injected once during the labor process.

Combined Spinal-Epidural Anesthesia

A third form of regional anesthesia, combined spinal-epidural (CSE), allows your partner to enjoy immediate pain relief with the possibility of managing her pain as needed. With a CSE, the epidural is administered via a catheter as opposed to an injection. The tube is placed in the lower back, attached to a pump, and remains in place for the duration of labor. Your partner will have control of the pump and will be able to administer a dose of anesthetic when she deems it necessary. As with the spinal block, you can refer back to the benefits, drawbacks, and side effects of the regular epidural to gain some more insight into how this method of pain management works. Epidurals by themselves are popular, but CSE's are becoming more common as they provide both the benefit of immediate ease while still remaining in control throughout the entire process.

General Anesthesia

General anesthesia is rarely used during childbirth, largely due to the fact that the mother will not be actively involved in the labor process. In general, this form of pain management is used only in extreme situations, for instance, when an emergency C-section is required or your partner suffers from excessive bleeding.

Nonmedical Pain Management

Many parents wish to welcome their child into the world without relief from typical Western medications. Though many frown at the idea of making it through childbirth without anesthetics or tranquilizers, there are, in fact, a number of pain management methods that are free of pharmaceuticals and may prove equally effective.

Mindfulness Techniques

Using mindfulness during childbirth involves exercises in breathing and meditation. Your partner can use breath as a means of relaxation and pain management. By taking consistent, deep breaths, your partner will be drawn into the moment and will become more aware of the sensations in her body. This may help her to preempt contractions and to breathe through them when they arrive.

In terms of meditation techniques to use, mantras have proven to be particularly effective during labor. The repetition of simple mantras—"I am strong. I can do this."—can help calm your partner and may make her feel more in control of the process. Some pain relief may come along with this relaxation. Meditation can be used in conjunction with breathing exercises to help center your partner and keep her in control as much as possible.

Distractions

With an extremely straightforward approach, you can populate the delivery room with some sensory stimuli that will help distract your partner from the pain of her contractions. If her attention is diverted away from the pain, she may feel some relief. These distractions can be anything from playing some calming music to perhaps doing some exercises to relieve tension while she can still move around, of course. You can also take your partner's mind off the pain by guiding her through exercises or by helping her divert her focus and fix it on the stimuli you have placed in the room. When the labor process intensifies, you can continue to help by providing constant support and asking her to focus on you, your voice, or your touch as opposed to the pain.

Transcutaneous Electrical Nerve Stimulation

A bit more technical in nature, pain management through transcutaneous electrical nerve stimulation (TENS) involves connecting the nerves in the lower back to a small device that sends electrical impulses into the body. No medication is involved, and your partner remains in control of the device the entire time, making it similar to the use of CSE anesthetic. However, unlike CSE, the TENS pain management method is completely noninvasive and works only on a small group of nerves along the spine. This method poses no risk to either mother or baby and can even be used in conjunction with other techniques in order to provide greater relief.

In addition to the nonmedical pain management options outlined above, you and your partner can look into other, smaller techniques that may also provide some relief. These techniques include the following:

- Aromatherapy.
- Moving around and staying active during labor.
- Hypnosis is more commonly known as hypnobirth.
- Acupuncture and acupressure.
- Submersion in warm water.
- Moving or rocking back and forth on an inflatable exercise ball.

Medical Pain Management: The Pros and Cons

The most prominent benefit of using medication for pain management is that your partner will be all but guaranteed to experience some relief. While some medications may not work as effectively on the first try, many can be readministered as needed, meaning that your partner will feel relief throughout the entire process. Oftentimes, when numbing agents are used during labor, the only sensation left is a dull ache as contractions come and go. Medical options may also mean that the birthing process is less emotionally and physically taxing for your partner. Moreover, with the exception of general anesthesia, medicated births allow your partner to be present and aware the entire time, meaning that you will both be able to experience every moment of your child's arrival.

However, nothing is perfect, and so we must take into account the fact that there are some disadvantages to using medical pain management methods. Chief among them is the experience of side effects and the potential for the medication to affect your baby. Each different medication has its own side effects and will affect each person in a different way. Some women may experience none at all, while others may feel severe nausea, dizziness, or any of the other side effects related to pain medication. Given that these medications are administered so that they may enter the bloodstream, the possibility always exists that they will move through the umbilical cord and be absorbed by your baby while they make their way out of the womb. In instances like these, they may have difficulty breathing after birth and may have issues when attempting to breastfeed. It's important to note that, while not insignificant, these effects shouldn't be permanent, and your healthcare provider will be able to help eradicate them.

Nonmedical Pain Management: The Pros and Cons

If you choose to go the unmedicated route, then the first thing you can look forward to is welcoming your child to the world in as natural a way as possible. Without the presence of pharmaceuticals in your partner's system, the body's natural hormones and endorphins will help her move through the process. The hormones secreted during labor help the process move along as it should, which will allow your partner to deliver in her own time. Endorphins released during childbirth will act as natural painkillers and can help supplement whichever means of pain management you employ. After birth, these same neurochemicals have been known to play a role in fostering parent-infant bonding and helping breastfeeding take place. As with medications, your partner will be alert and present during the birth, and neither of you will miss a second thereof.

On the flip side of the coin, we find a disadvantage to nonmedical pain management. This disadvantage is nothing other than, well, pain. For first-time parents, especially, it can be difficult to gauge just how painful labor will be. If you underestimate the intensity thereof, the experience can be a great deal more traumatizing than expected. Moreover, if labor is particularly painful, the techniques you prepared in advance may prove ineffective, and you will have to find another way of relieving some of your partner's pain.

Remember that there are a great number of variables present during labor, and things may change as the process continues. As such, though you should definitely decide on a method of pain management ahead of time, keep an open mind when it comes to techniques applied when the time comes. Trust your healthcare provider to provide you with honest advice, especially if you have to opt for medicated pain management due to complications. You can stick to your birth plan as far as possible, but there may be extenuating circumstances in which you will have to be flexible.

Choosing a Birth Partner

When it's time to welcome your newborn baby into the world, it's important to know who will be there to share that joyous moment. Naturally, your partner will be there, and hopefully you as well. However, as valuable as your presence is in the delivery room, you may want to consider involving a third party, one to guide your partner through the birth process and to provide support where necessary.

The role of a birth partner is simple enough. A birth partner is someone who steps into a supportive role when labor begins and who remains by the mother's side all the way through to the end of the process. In terms of responsibilities, a birth partner provides support, both practically and emotionally. They provide support and assistance, ensuring that all of your partner's needs are met and that she is as comfortable and safe as possible during labor. The birth partner is well-acquainted with the birth plan and helps your partner adhere to her wishes, as well as deal with any changes or complications that may occur (Nutricia's Medical and Scientific Affairs Team, 2019).

Birth partners are sometimes referred to as "support partners," given that this is the greatest of their responsibilities. Essentially, a support partner is there to hold your partner's hand as she gives birth, to advocate for her choices and well-being, and to ensure that she is being kept safe and taken care of. Oftentimes, a birth partner functions as a spokesperson, communicating your partner's wishes and questions to the birthing professionals overseeing the delivery process. A birth partner will perform different functions as labor progresses. When the process begins, their duties include timing contractions, encouraging your partner to eat and drink as long as is feasible, and naturally, remaining by her side. Later on, the role becomes decidedly more supportive, as the birth partner provides comfort, helps with certain labor and birthing positions, takes the lead in breathing exercises, and does whatever is needed to make your partner feel safe and comfortable. Their presence may extend beyond birth, as they help you and your partner gain your footing as new parents.

It's clear to see that a support partner is an essential addition to your birth plan. Given their importance, it's essential that you carefully consider who you trust with this responsibility. While many people opt to have their partner step into this role, this isn't required. If you will be indisposed at the time of birth, then it's best to have someone else step in. With that being said, it's preferable that you be there to share in that joyous moment with your partner. Aside from this, your presence may very well have implications for the health of both your partner and your baby. Brown (2016) writes that "the children of absent dads are more likely to have a range of health complications and a low birth weight. And moms are more likely to have had complications during pregnancy." These occurrences' origin can be traced throughout the pregnancy, as an absent father will result in more—if not all—the stress of impending parenthood landing squarely on the mother's shoulders. By contrast, if you've been involved the whole time, you will have all the knowledge you need, gained from antenatal classes and doctor's visits. Consequently, you'll know what to expect and can help your partner navigate the stressful experience of labor and delivery.

While you are certainly the ideal candidate for a birth partner, you may not be able to attend due to extenuating circumstances. With that in mind, birth partners other than the father usually fall into one of the following categories:

- Family: Though any family member you trust can fulfill the role of birth partner, it may be advisable to ask someone who has already given birth or who is familiar with the process. You may consider asking your partner's mother, or even your own, to be there to provide support.

- Midwife: You needn't necessarily choose someone to whom either of you holds a close personal connection. You can enlist the services of a midwife, an independent healthcare professional who will be able to provide valuable ante- and postnatal support. If you choose to use a birthing center for delivery, there may already be a midwife present, but you can always have another with you.

- Doula: A similarly independent birthing expert, doulas perform supporting roles in the lead-up to birth, in the moment itself, as well as in the time after. A doula's care often extends quite significantly beyond birth, as they will stay to help you and your partner for a few weeks after your newborn's arrival.

Midwives and Doulas: What You Need to Know

When it comes to birth partners who lie outside the sphere of friends and family, things have a tendency to become muddled. There's a tendency to conflate midwives with doulas, thinking that they provide the same type of support. While there is certainly some overlap between the two, a midwife's functions differ greatly from those of a doula. As such, it's important to know which is which before selecting one as your birth partner, as your needs may be very specific and only manageable by one of the two.

Doula

Doulas fall into one of two categories: birth and postpartum. Depending on which title they hold, a doula will be able to perform certain actions and provide support up until a certain point in the pregnancy and birth journey.

A birth doula, also known as a labor doula, acts as a birth partner during the labor process. They support your partner during labor by applying and helping with various nonmedical techniques, both for pain management as well as for relaxation (Harnish, 2023). Labor doulas perform the tasks assigned to a birth partner, acting as a support system and advocate, communicating the details of the birth plan and the desires of the parents to the healthcare professionals present in the delivery room. The presence of a doula can be invaluable and can make the birthing process easier for both you and your partner. However, it's essential to note that doulas are not trained medical professionals. As such, the doula can only take charge until the time comes for the baby to be delivered. At this point, they will hand it over to a midwife or obstetrician, who will have the medical training required to perform the delivery.

A postpartum doula steps in once your baby is born. Their job is to guide you and your partner through the recovery process after birth. If your newborn has siblings who are older than them, the doula can help your entire family acclimate to the new arrival and learn to cope with the changes that accompany the presence of a new baby in the house. In the recovery period, a doula continues to play a supportive role, taking care of the baby when you need to rest or stepping in to hold it when your attention is drawn away. In addition to this, they can also provide lactation support, helping your partner become accustomed to the practice of breastfeeding. If she is not breastfeeding, a postpartum doula can nevertheless help the both of you get the hang of feeding.

Though you can contract the services of either a birth or postpartum doula, there are many professionals in this field who will be able to work with you before and after delivery. If you are considering making use of a doula, it's extremely important to remember that they are not trained medical practitioners. Though many doulas do undergo formal training, certification isn't required. While uncertified doulas will still be able to play an effective supportive role, they may have little to no knowledge of the birthing process. Regardless of their certification status, you can be assured that a doula will prove to be helpful, as a medical professional will be required to deliver the baby regardless of whether the doula is trained.

Midwife

Covering the entirety of the pregnancy, birth, and postpartum period, midwives are trained medical professionals who work either independently or as members of staff at a hospital. Because they receive medical training as part of the certification process, midwives do not need to work in conjunction with other healthcare professionals. Thus, if you'd like to have your midwife see the birth process from beginning to end, she will be able to do so without the help or intervention of an obstetrician or other medical practitioner.

Midwives Versus Doulas: The Pros and Cons

As with any other component of your birth plan, you have to weigh the advantages of certain choices against the disadvantages these same decisions may present. Choosing a birth partner is no exception, and given their importance during labor, this is one consideration you will have to make carefully. If you are leaning towards contracting the services of a midwife or doula, it's important for you to know what to expect from the experience, both positive and negative.

Should you choose to select a midwife as a birth partner, you can expect the risk of emergency medical interventions, as well as the need for an emergency C-section, to decrease significantly. In addition to this, a midwife's involvement may provide you with less worry, as birth can be a collaborative effort between a midwife and a medical doctor. So, if you'd like the obstetrician in the room along with your midwife, you are more than welcome to do so, and you can be doubly sure that your partner will be kept safe and comfortable. Midwife-assisted births have also been noted for their reduction of several significant risks, including preterm birth, infant death, and the occurrence of third- and fourth-degree tears along the perineum (Hanawalt, 2023).

The greatest disadvantage tied to a midwife-assisted birth is the limited medical intervention they are able to perform. While midwives can perform a number of medical procedures, depending on their training, they may not be equipped to handle greater complications. For instance, should an emergency C-section be required, the midwife will have to hand it over to an OB/GYN, who will be able to perform the procedure safely. There is also the financial aspect to consider. While many insurance companies may cover the costs of childbirth if you work with a CNM in a hospital, an out-of-hospital birth overseen by a midwife may not be covered, and you may not be eligible for reimbursement from your insurance.

Doulas make equally positive contributions to the birthing process. In fact, working with a doula in the lead-up to the birth has been demonstrated to result in better birth outcomes and fewer complications during delivery. Their impact is felt in the immediate postpartum period as well, as many parents find themselves feeling more confident and competent when they begin to parent under the tutelage of a doula (Hanawalt, 2023). The effect of a doula's support mustn't be underestimated, as they will help you through the process of exploring pain management techniques and will assist you with finding the method that will work best for you.

Unfortunately, the greatest disadvantage to making use of a doula is a rather important one. While they are excellent supporters, advocates, and educators, they are not medical professionals. As such, should any serious complications arise during labor, they will not be able to intervene, administer the necessary medications, or perform the necessary procedures. If your partner would like to make use of medical pain management, you will have to supplement your doula's help with that of a medical professional, as the former will not be able to dispense this medication. Finally, finances must be considered here as well. Because doulas are not registered healthcare practitioners, many insurance companies do not cover the cost of their services. However, this has started to change in recent years, so be sure to contact your insurance provider to inquire about coverage and reimbursement.

What to Consider When Choosing a Birth Partner

When brainstorming who you would like to act as support during your partner's labor, the very first thing you have to consider is the person's ability to remain calm in times of distress or when under pressure. They will have to be your partner's rock throughout the entire labor process and must be able to keep a cool head both for support and to explain any changes that may occur.

Being the Best Birth Partner: Tips

As you will most likely be the one to step into the shoes of your birth partner, there are a few things you can do that will make the experience easier for your partner, and ultimately, for yourself as well. Becoming the best birth partner you can be involves the following:

- Maintain a level head at all times. Both you and your partner will experience emotional ups and downs, but you have to stand strong and help her through it.

- Don't wait around to be useful. Be as involved as you can during the pregnancy, and on the day of the birth, help your partner as much as you can. Time her contractions, recording the length and time elapsed between each one.

- Make sure you know what your partner's wishes are. Familiarize yourself with the birth plan thoroughly, and have it at hand during labor. Speak up for your partner and ensure her wishes are being honored.

- Prepare a hospital bag ahead of time. This way, when the time comes to go to the delivery room, you will have everything you need ready to go.

- Keep an open mind, and remember that your partner's well-being is the highest priority. If something isn't going to plan or you are required to divert from your birth plan, ensure that these changes are to your partner's benefit and help her understand why they are occurring.

- Be flexible, and prepare yourself for surprises. No two birthing processes are alike, and you may have to adjust your approach in the moment.

- Check-in with your partner, and make sure you attend to her needs as closely as possible.

- Prepare yourself to put in some effort. You may have to lead your partner through some exercises, help her work through her contractions, or assist in getting her into certain delivery positions. Don't stand back; be assertive and lend a hand as much as you can.

- Remain by her side as much as possible. After the birth, wait until she is settled into recovery before letting friends and family know about the birth. During the process, only leave her side to attend to her needs.

- Know where your limits lie. Though you should certainly be prepared, there will be things that are beyond your expertise. Be aware of the extent of your knowledge, and don't be afraid to speak to a professional to get the help or information you need.

- Look after yourself. Make sure that you stay hydrated, and be sure to eat something when you can. You are your partner's main source of support and won't be of much use if you become exhausted before the baby has even arrived.

Birthing Classes

Though not a compulsory component of your parenthood journey, attending birthing classes is an excellent way of preparing you for the day your child enters the world, as well as for the tasks and responsibilities that await you afterwards. Attendance in these classes can prove to be immensely helpful, especially for first-time parents. Antenatal classes, as they are often called, help you and your partner understand exactly what to expect from the process of childbirth. As you read through this section, keep in mind that the people who will benefit the most from birthing classes are your partner and the person who will be in the delivery room on the day. Although it's recommended that you attend these classes as well, if someone else will act as your birth partner, you may want to consider including them in the educational experience.

Labor and delivery are an important part of any antenatal class curriculum. However, the complete scope of these classes is much wider. A typical birthing class teaches you the following:

- How to recognize the signs of labor.

- How to know when it is time to move to the birthing location.

- How to prepare for labor.

- What are the different stages of labor?

- Ways to calm and support your partner during labor.

- What the different birthing positions are and how to know which one will work best for you.

- How to find your footing as a new parent.

- What to expect from breastfeeding.

- How to decipher the behavior of a newborn and which actions to take.

The social aspect of antenatal classes strengthens their appeal for many parents. You will be attending classes with people who are on the same journey as you. By connecting with them, you can build a support network filled with people who will understand what you are experiencing and who can support you through it all. When attending an antenatal class, you will be able to ask questions regarding specific topics and raise concerns you have regarding labor, delivery, and aspects of pregnancy. However, most birthing classes try to provide you with all the information you need.

Types of Birthing Classes

There are many different types of antenatal classes to choose from. These classes can be divided into two categories. The first set's sessions are known as hospital antenatal classes, while the second set are categorized as independent antenatal classes. Both have specific methods of instruction and depending on the details of their criteria, they yield many of the same benefits. Knowing which options are available to you enables you to choose the type of class that is best suited to your sensibilities, and which fits in best with the other components of your birth plan.

Hospital Antenatal Classes

These classes are tied to a healthcare institution and can be held in either hospitals, clinics, or a doctor's surgery. Taught by doctors, nurses, or other clinical practitioners, hospital antenatal classes are largely formal in nature, giving you a straightforward understanding of what the pregnancy and childbirth processes involve and providing you with guidance regarding the postpartum period as well. More often than not, these classes will take you on a tour of the maternity ward so you can see exactly where your child will be welcomed into the world. Hospital-based classes can consist of a single workshop or a variety of sessions over the course of a few weeks, usually about six.

Independent Antenatal Classes

These classes aren't always tied to a particular institution or to a specific person, such as a midwife or doula. However, independent classes will teach techniques and theories that the person delivering your baby will use. Take note that these classes can take place in a variety of spaces, depending on their curricula. Furthermore, some classes may give you a comprehensive look at pregnancy, childbirth, and parenthood, while others will focus only on teaching you certain strategies to use during pregnancy and labor.

Under the umbrella of independent antenatal classes, we find the following:

- **Lamaze**: Comprising a curriculum that comes out at a total of 12 hours, these classes teach breathing exercises, pain management techniques, and ways of handling labor. Lamaze classes will also provide you with some tips regarding your role as a birth partner.

- **The Alexander Technique**: Originating in the art world, this movement-based technique is designed to make pregnancy more comfortable, to prepare and open up the body for labor, and to practice breathing techniques. While there may be classes tailored to pregnancy and childbirth, you and your partner will still learn a lot by attending a regular class teaching the Alexander Technique.

- **The Bradley Method**: Stretching over 12 weeks, this method provides you with a comprehensive understanding of childbirth while also focusing on maintaining a healthy pregnancy. Classes in the Bradley Method may also focus on your role as a birth partner—especially if something goes wrong—as well as some aspects of infant care.

- **Birthing From Within**: Developed by midwife Pam England, these classes focus on how transformative childbirth can be for the parents, emphasizing the physical and psychological changes that occur (Davies, 2023). Other aspects of the classes include preparing for birth, pain management, and the emotional component. For the latter, the instructor will help you deal with your goals, expectations, and fears tied to parenthood.

- **HypnoBirthing**: Involving very little trance work, these classes teach relaxation techniques that aid in mindfulness during labor and help you unpack your anxieties and worries related to childbirth.

- **Aquanatal classes**: Ordinarily attended during the second or third trimesters, these classes are exercise-based and focus on maintaining your partner's health and fitness without straining her body or potentially injuring ligaments or joints.

- **Antenatal yoga or Pilates**: Similarly to exercise-based sessions, antenatal yoga classes are intended to boost mindfulness while maintaining your partner's health. Additionally, these classes can help your partner prepare for childbirth through bodily relaxation techniques. Antenatal

Pilates similarly prepares your partner's body for the labor process but extends their purview to the maintenance of pelvic floor health and the postpartum recovery period.

It can be difficult to decide which type of class to attend, seeing as each offers its own set of techniques and knowledge. The first thing to consider—after the curriculum itself—is whether the class is worth investing your time (and potentially some money) in. The first box the class ought to tick in this regard is whether it gives you helpful information pertaining to the process of childbirth. Next, consider whether it helps you navigate the medical interventions and procedures that are necessary and which may be avoided. A good antenatal class will also help prepare you mentally, emotionally, and physically for birth. Similarly, a class worth attending will cover a portion of the postpartum period as well, helping you navigate the first days of infant care. Something else to check is whether the class teaches self-care for the both of you once the baby has arrived, as well as whether you learn how to be an effective birth partner. Finally, the very best classes will allow you to connect with other people who have the same experience as you and will give you some tips regarding infant essentials.

Remember to take your own birth plan and birth preferences into account when deciding which class to book. Something that may factor into this is the difference between hospital and independent antenatal classes. With the former, your education will focus mostly on how birth will take place within that specific healthcare institution and which policies the hospital has in place for labor and delivery. Unfortunately, these same classes tend to promote the use of epidurals, sometimes to the point of excluding other pain management techniques. Some hospitals may even describe the delivery process only in the context of epidural use. On a more positive note, hospital antenatal classes tend to cover a wide range of topics and won't necessarily take up a lot of your time. Some institutions offer a single workshop, while others offer a number of sessions over the course of a few months. It's worth noting that these classes are typically large in size and, as such, may provide you with a less intimate, less personal learning experience.

By contrast, independent birthing classes generally aim to empower the expectant parents so they can take control of the birth process and become active participants. These classes tend to explore a wide range of pain relief techniques. Though some may favor natural, unmedicated relief, most of these classes will take you through the options you have for pain management. Similar to hospital classes, independent sessions will cover an extremely wide range of topics. An advantage they have over clinical education is that they don't have fixed curricula. Instead, the instructor usually determines what is taught and to what extent. Independent classes are also smaller, so you may have a more personalized experience. However, on the other side of the coin, we find that these classes won't always explain some of the necessary medical aspects of childbirth. Moreover, independent classes won't always be taught by a certified medical professional, which may result in the aforementioned omission. Finally, if your instructor isn't certified by certain regulatory bodies, your health insurance provider may cover only a portion of the costs or may choose to cover none of the class fees at all.

The Financial Elements of the Birth Plan

As wonderful as becoming a parent is, one of the many worries that accompany this experience relates to your family's finances. Babies are expensive, and planning ahead will save you a lot of stress and scrambling down the line. Below, you will find resources to help you manage your money in preparation for your baby's birth and for the period that follows.

Your Family's Finances: A Nine-Month Plan

Month One

- Start cutting down on any debt either you or your partner have. Even if you can't expunge all of it, reducing the amount owed will go a long way.

- Cut down on your credit card use to avoid racking up more debt.
- Track your spending and build a baby budget (more on that below).

Month Two

- Update your insurance policies so that your beneficiaries are up-to-date. In the process, you can review your coverage and alter it if needed so that you and your family are more comprehensively protected.

Month Three

- Check your credit score and rating, and take steps to improve them if need be.
- If your baby's budget has not yet been completed, the time is now. Lay out all your finances and structure your plan so that you and your partner can save a bit every month. Remember that the goal is to do better than just break even.

Month Four

- Determine how much time off your job will allow you and factor in any changes in income that may accompany extended time away from work.
- Now that you've estimated what your expenses will be once your baby has arrived, set up a savings plan that will allow you to have all the money you need when the time comes.

Month Five

- Explore your childcare options. If neither of you will be staying home with the baby, look into who will take care of them and how much this service will cost you.

- A useful directory can be found on the Child Care Aware website (childcareaware.org).

Month Six

- If you have not already taken out a life insurance policy, the sixth month is the time to do so. According to Batcha & Srinivasan (2023), it's recommended that you "stick to term life, preferably 20 years or less."

- As morbid as it may be, the purchase of a life insurance policy should be accompanied by the drawing up of a will. Ensure that you have an executor, and remember to update the will as your child grows and your family structure changes.

Month Seven

- In the seventh month, you can start to set up a savings fund for your child. If this money is earmarked for higher education, you can use the Upromise savings program to supplement the account's balance.

- When starting up these savings, look into tax-advantaged 529 investment plans. Within the terms of these plans, you can save between $300,000 and $500,000 without paying taxes on this money (Batcha & Srinivasan, 2023).

Month Eight

- Consider that you may be receiving supplies from friends and family, and purchase only the most basic baby care items. Ensure that you are equipped to care for your baby after their arrival, long enough for you to gather any supplies you may still need.

- Births are accompanied by several important documents, including your child's birth certificate and possible savings bonds from people in your life. To keep both of them safe, consider opening a safety deposit box so you know these documents are kept safe and secure.

- By this point in your pregnancy, your eyes are firmly fixed on the future. In keeping with this, consider setting up a retirement fund for yourself and your spouse.

Month Nine

- As the due date approaches, you will want to start taking things slowly in anticipation of your baby's arrival. Stick to your baby's budget and tie up any financial loose ends.

- Within 30 days after your baby's birth, add them to your health and life insurance policies.

How to Build a Baby Budget

The best way to structure your baby budget is by utilizing the 50/30/20 model. In this model, you divide your income proportionally, allocating 50% to needs, including loan payments, bills, and childcare items and services; 30% to wants, which are expenses that allow you a level of comfort and happiness; and earmarking 20% for savings and the repayment of toxic debt, which may include credit cards and payday loans (Renter, 2020). Keep in mind that this framework is an ideal financial structure. Your income and expenses may require you to change the exact percentages. While this is perfectly fine, aim to get the ratio as close as possible.

As you divide your finances according to the 50/30/20 model, it may be useful to take into account what you have now and what you will have once the baby arrives. First and foremost, determine what your priorities are. While saving is an admirable pursuit and having fun is an essential part of life, you have to consider what your family needs to get by. At the same time, you have to consider the future. As such, try to work an amount into the budget that will cover emergency expenses. A good number to aim for is about $500. Once that is secured, you can start to look at your future more earnestly and can begin exploring things such as retirement savings, toxic debt elimination, building your emergency fund beyond that initial amount, and even savings accounts for your child.

Strengthen your baby budget further by practicing how to get by with reduced financial means. Parenthood may cause a shakeup in your household finances beyond the money going towards childcare and supplies. Either you or your partner may be away from work for a while, perhaps with reduced compensation or entirely unpaid. Moreover, one of you may decide to stay at home full-time. To prevent any such changes from becoming overwhelming, practice living this way a few months ahead of the due date. You can set aside the amount you will lose after birth and use it to save while you try to navigate a new lifestyle.

The final two considerations that influence your baby budget similarly relate to the possibility of financial fluctuation. Firstly, take into account that your child-related expenses will change over time. Eventually, diapers and formula will be replaced with tuition fees and money for extracurricular activities. While you can't know exactly what your expenditure will be, getting a rough idea can help you construct a practical, proactive plan.

One-Time Expenses

- Medical bills, specifically those that your health insurance only partially covers or doesn't recognize at all.

- Travel items such as a stroller, baby carrier, diaper bag, and car seat.

- Household items, including bedding and furniture for the nursery, as well as toys and educational materials.

- Items related to nursing and feeding, including a breast pump, milk storage bags, bottles, formula, and cleaning apparatuses.

Ongoing Expenses

- Childcare.

- Food, drink, toiletries, and other necessities.

- Items related to infant care, i.e., diapers, formula, clothing, pacifiers, etc.

- Medical expenses such as inoculations, check-ups, and general healthcare.

Financial Tools to Consider

- Saving for higher education through a Coverdell Education Savings Account, 529 plan, or UGMA/UTMA account.

- Health insurance.

- Life insurance.

- Flexible Spending Accounts (FSAs), which enable you to pay for healthcare and childcare expenses using pretax dollars.

Finally, you have to consider the reality of what your finances may look like at any point in the future. Sometimes, despite our best efforts, we just can't stretch those dollars as far as we want. Though cutting expenses and finding ways to supplement your income are solid solutions, make a note that things such as refinancing loans and mortgages, as well as asking for a raise or searching for a position with higher pay, are also viable options, though the latter may not be the most easily achieved.

Finance Tips for New Dads

- Don't miss out on incredible bargains by dismissing thrift and consignment stores. Their low prices will prove especially helpful when it comes to buying those clothes your baby will grow out of so quickly.

- Lean on your support network whenever you can, and ask for their help to look after the baby during the day. Consider this option when your baby is sick, and you can't afford to take a day off work.

- Turn to your network once more, specifically to other parents, and ask to borrow a couple of items here and there. You can do the same for them down the line, saving both families some money.

- Scale back and start to opt for more affordable options. You may not be able to maintain your pre-baby lifestyle once the little one is here. As such, start looking for deals where you can, and consider downgrading or altering some of the larger expenses in your life to either cost less or benefit the entire family.

Knowing Your Rights

Fathers' rights are expanding in many life sectors, and the workplace is no exception. In the last few years, an increasing number of US states have allowed fathers to take paid family leave. Many of the laws that have been created don't simply make this allowance but guarantee it instead for all those who fall under the legal jurisdiction of that particular state. These states, along with some US cities, now allow workers to take paid sick leave in order to care for their children and family. Crucially, if your workplace allows this, some laws may require your employer to allow the use of this leave for child-related issues (Devi, 2022).

Your fatherly rights in the workplace are protected even on a federal level, as employers are prohibited from discriminating on the basis of sex, which in this case means they cannot default to outdated ideas regarding gender roles and the sex of the family breadwinner. These protections have been extended in certain cities to protect parents of all genders from discrimination and unfair treatment based on their parental commitments.

Though these laws and policies are certainly helpful, you are most likely to find your paternity leave worries calmed by the Family and Medical Leave Act (FMLA). Under this act, you are entitled to a maximum of 12 weeks of unpaid leave that can be used in instances where you must provide care for your family. The FMLA has been expanded to cover the arrival of a child as well and may be used in lieu of paternity leave. Though the leave is unpaid, which is less than ideal, your employer is required to continue providing you with healthcare benefits during those 12 weeks. Apart from this, the FMLA requires your employer to retain you as an employee, meaning that your job must be waiting for you once your leave is up. Should they have filled your post, they are legally required to offer you a position with a salary and benefits of a commensurate value (Devi, 2022). This type of job security can knock at least one worry off your list in the chaotic time that follows a baby's birth.

Take note that there are certain criteria you have to meet in order to be eligible for FMLA leave. This includes the following:

- Working for a covered employer, namely public agencies, public schools, service members, and businesses in the private sector with a minimum of 50 employees.

- Working for an employer whose 50 or more employees all live within 75 miles of the business or institution's location.

- Working for an eligible employer for a minimum of 12 months, either consecutively or in part over the course of several years

- Totaling a number of 1,250 work hours in the 12 months that qualify you for the leave.

If the eligibility criteria are met, FMLA leave should be available to both you and your partner as a form of parental leave. It's worth noting that, as of 2015, FMLA leave was expanded to cover same-sex couples as well. However, it's classified as spousal-care coverage in this instance, so you may want to double-check with your employer as to its use for paternity leave (McDuffey, 2023). Should you wish to make use of your FMLA leave, you must notify your employer as you would with any other type of leave. When you provide this notice, you may also have the option to split the period of leave between paid, and FMLA leave so that you still have some income for the time you are away. Some employers may allow you to use both concurrently, though you will have to clear this with your boss when you request the leave. Though leave may certainly be the most preferable option, if it isn't available to you, inquire about the possibility of adopting a more flexible work schedule or workweek. Several states and cities have signed legislation into law that allows for these types of alterations to workplace models and may just be available where you live.

More on Paternity Leave

By this point, I'd wager that you are strongly considering taking paternity leave if you haven't already decided. If you're still on the fence, take a look at the benefits this time at home with your family will provide:

- Time at home can improve the health of your relationship with your partner, forging a stronger bond and resulting in greater stability within your connection.

- Your presence at home may help to lessen or alleviate the effects of postpartum depression. However, it's important to note that presence alone will not have this effect, and your active involvement in the childcare and child-rearing process is essential to this mitigation.

- Being together as a family in your early days can help shape your family's dynamics, enabling you and your partner to form the foundational approach that will influence your decisions regarding the allocation of domestic work, childcare, and other family matters.

- Your exposure to your child and spending increased amounts of time with them may result in the reordering of your priorities, as your family's importance will become more pronounced.

- Paternity leave and your contribution to child-rearing can help your partner's career progression, as some of the parenting load is lightened. According to (Colantuoni et al., 2021), paternity leave can help to lessen the gender pay gap by increasing your partner's income on a short-term basis while laying the foundation for household financial stability and prosperity in the long term.

- When you return to work, you may even find yourself energized and eager to get back to it. Though paternity leave may present the possibility of a career delay or setback, the familial benefits it yields far diminish the severity of these negatives.

Of all the positive outcomes that result from taking paternity leave, perhaps none match the profundity of its effects on parent-infant bonding. The forging of a connection between the parent and their child is incredibly important, especially in the first months after birth. Naturally, the more time you spend with your child, the better you will get to know them, and the stronger your link will be. Paternity leave facilitates just this. Through your presence and involvement, you are continuously strengthening your infant-parent bond. For instance, holding them against your bare chest has been demonstrated to cause an increase of oxytocin, the bonding hormone, in your bloodstream. Another excellent example of paternity leave's importance can be seen in the fact that children whose fathers are actively involved in their lives from a young age have shown enhanced linguistic, cognitive, and social-emotional abilities (Abdullah, 2022).

Paternity Leave: The Legal Side

Outside of the FMLA, US fathers don't have much in the way of structured, legally protected paternity leave. At least, there is very little being done on a federal level to ensure that you can be with your family in the weeks after you become a father. Wool (2022) reports that only 21% of American workers have employers who provide paid parental leave. There are certain exceptions, such as those workers who are covered by the Federal Employee Paid Leave Act (FEPLA). However, as the name suggests, this act applies only to those employed by the federal government. To qualify for this leave, employees are required to be in federal service for at least 12 months before the commencement of the leave, much like the FMLA. Unfortunately, paternity leave laws don't extend beyond this, at least not in the US. That being said, paternity leave may be protected by your right to leave or, at the very least, by your employer's corporate structure. As such, be sure to check with your boss or HR department to see which options are available to you. Some states and companies have begun to implement paid paternity leave, and you may just qualify.

Birth Plans: A Comprehensive Template

Mother	
Full name	
Due date	
Father	
Full Name	
Relationship to mother	
Healthcare Particulars	
Name of healthcare professional	
Contact details	
Birthing location	
Contact details	

Planned birthing method
- Vaginal.
- C-section.
- Water birth.
- Induction.
- VBAC.

Existing health conditions
- Group B strep.
- Genital herpes.
- Rh incompatibility.
- Gestational diabetes.
- Other:

_____

_____

_____

Preferred means of pain management
- Acupressure.
- Acupuncture.
- CSE.
- Distraction.
- Epidural.
- Massage.
- Mindfulness techniques.
- Nitrous oxide.
- Pethidine.
- Pudendal block.
- Reflexology.
- Spinal block.
- TENS.

Delivery room preferences
- Allowance for video recording and photography.
- Ambient lighting.
- Mood lighting.
- Music.
- White noise.
- Other:

Visitor preferences

- Birth partner present allowed admittance at all times.
- Family allowed after delivery and the first feeding.
- Friends are allowed after delivery and the first feeding.
- None allowed.
- Names of visitors allowed:

Constructing a birth plan is an elaborate endeavor that may take a considerable amount of negotiation, debate, compromise, and practicality. Among the many administrative matters tied to the pregnancy and childbirth processes, a birth plan is by far the most extensive and, simultaneously, one of the most important. As laborious as the task may seem and as overwhelming as all the decisions may be, it's essential that you and your partner construct your plan carefully. A well-thought-out birth plan will provide you with some safety and can help you keep your head on the day of delivery. And considering how chaotic labor can be, you'll be happy to have something coherent close by.

Chapter 4:

Initiating Dad Mode

There's a lot you have to learn when becoming a father. Some of these lessons can be learned on the job, while it's best for others to be committed to memory in advance of your official entry into fatherhood. An excellent example of this is found within the realm of pregnancy nutrition. There's lots of conflicting advice out there, not to mention many, many myths that can get in the way of your parenthood journey.

Let's take a look at some of the misconceptions you can go ahead and ignore:

1. To remain healthy, more calories are required throughout pregnancy: Though there is nothing wrong with eating some more food, increasing caloric intake during pregnancy isn't essential to your baby's development. In the first trimester, your partner can stick to her pre-pregnancy dietary habits. In the second trimester, the number of calories required per day increases by approximately 340, with this number growing to 500 in the third trimester (Pike, 2022). It's important to consider that these numbers are averages and that your partner's needs may differ depending on unique factors present in her pregnancy.

2. Caffeine should be avoided at all costs: As with most other foodstuffs, caffeine can prove to be harmful when consumed in excess. The concerns surrounding caffeine intake are largely centered around the possibility of it moving through the placenta and into the baby's bloodstream. This may happen as pregnancy results in the slower metabolization of caffeine. However, drinking caffeinated beverages is safe in moderation.

Your partner can drink one or two cups of coffee or tea per day.

3. Seafood may prove harmful to your partner and baby: Seafood poses some risks given the mercury naturally found in fish. However, this risk is present for everyone, pregnant or not. While your partner should avoid undercooked dishes such as sushi, eating seafood in moderation poses no risk, as the mercury levels will be negligible. Many healthcare professionals actually recommend adding seafood to the diet during pregnancy, as it is nutritionally rich and contains healthy proteins and omega-3 fatty acids.

4. A nine-month-long embargo should be placed on cheese: This rule really only applies to certain types of cheeses, and dairy products, in general, are safe nutritional territory during pregnancy. To ensure the safety of your partner and baby, stick to hard, pasteurized cheeses. Steer clear of softer cheeses and those that are not pasteurized—the latter counts for dairy as a whole. Softer cheeses are more likely to contain harmful bacteria, which may result in illness, so it's best to stick to the hard stuff (Pike, 2022).

5. Meat is the cornerstone of a healthy pregnancy: If your partner is tempted to enjoy a variety of meats during her pregnancy, that's her prerogative. However, if she would prefer to steer clear of this food group, both she and the baby will be just fine. Following a plant-based diet will provide your partner with the same nutrients they would get from steak, chicken, and all the rest. Eggs, yogurt, and meat substitutes made from soy are chock full of the same proteins and nutrients.

Car Seat Installation

Among the many places you will have to adapt to ensure your baby's safety, your car ranks among the most important. Keeping your infant secure during car journeys is essential for you, for them, and for other travelers on the road. There are two main types of car seats: forward-facing and rear-facing. However, you may find seats that are convertible, meaning they can shift from one direction to another. Whichever one you choose, always read the user manual before installation, and follow all safety tips and instructions provided therein.

Installing a Car Seat

1. Place the seat in the middle section of the backseat. If it will not fit there, place it behind either the driver's or passenger's seats.

2. Install the base using either the LATCH or seatbelt method. Take note that you should use one or the other and should not anchor the seat's base with both. If you are using the LATCH method, look for the anchors near the bottom of the backseat. Attach the forward-facing base to these anchors, referring back to the manual to ensure its proper connection. If you are using the seatbelt method, place the base in the same way, then thread the seatbelt through the belt path. You can lock the belt by pulling it out completely before threading it back in. Refer to both the seat and the car manual to ensure this is done correctly, especially if the belt will not lock this way.

3. Press down on the base to tighten its connection to either the anchors or the belt. Should the manual recommend additional attachments, you can connect them now.

4. Ensure the stability of the base by grasping it at the belt path and shaking it slightly. The force used should be equivalent to

that of a handshake. It's important to note that the seat is allowed to move if you test it, but you shouldn't do so for more than one inch. If it does, recheck the attachments and refasten the base.

5. You can now simply click the seat or carrier into the top of the base and finish the installation by adjusting the handle by lowering it from its raised carrying position.

Ensuring Proper Installation

Throughout the installation process, you can refer back to the car seat's manual to ensure that you are implementing the necessary safety precautions. In addition to these measures, you can also call in some external help to ensure proper installation. You can contact your local firehouse and have them inspect your seat's base as well as the security with which the carrier is attached. Alternatively, you can peruse the National Highway Traffic Safety Administration (NHTSA) directory to find a car seat inspection station. If you'd like to consult a certified professional, you can locate a technician near you using the National Child Passenger Safety Certification Program.

Car Seats: Dos and Don'ts

- Don't buy or use car seats that appear old or have sustained visible damage.

- Don't look for the perfect car seat, as it doesn't exist. Instead, look for the seat that will suit your child. Criteria to consider include whether your child can fit inside comfortably, whether it will be able to be properly installed in your car, and whether it will maintain its stability when the car is moving.

- Ensure that the car seat is anchored as much as possible. In addition to using the attachments of the LATCH or seatbelt method, you can also use a tether. The tether will tie the seat to an anchor point in the vehicle, providing an added measure of stability.

- Ensure that the seat is installed at the correct angle so that your child's head and body will not move excessively during journeys.

Keeping Mom Safe and Healthy

When your brain shifts into dad mode, most of those paternal faculties will be focused on preparing for your baby's arrival as well as for your introduction to fatherhood shortly afterwards. While this is commendable, there is a part of this cognitive shift that should account for the well-being of the person who will be bringing your baby into the world. Take note that most pregnant women will be able to fend for themselves and will take the necessary safety precautions. Any and all help you provide is intended to supplement what your partner already does and to help cover areas she may have overlooked.

Nutrition

During the antenatal months, there are certain foods your partner should steer away from, as well as some that can prove beneficial if incorporated into her diet. Note that your partner shouldn't restrict her food intake to the latter group but rather use these items to supplement her existing diet.

What to Eat

During pregnancy, it is essential that your partner consumes enough vitamins along with adequate amounts of iron, calcium, and protein (Bjarnadottir, 2018a). The foods that will provide these nutrients include the following:

- Avocados.

- Berries, especially strawberries, raspberries, blueberries, acai berries, and goji berries.

- Dried fruits, for instance, prunes and dates.

- Eggs.

- Fiber-packed whole grains such as oats, barley, wheat berries, brown rice, and quinoa.

- Fish liver oil.

- Green vegetables, broccoli, spinach, kale, and lettuce in particular.

- Lean cuts of beef, pork, and chicken.

- Legumes and pulses, including lentils, soybeans, beans, peas, chickpeas, and peanuts.

- Pasteurized dairy products, especially gut-healthy yogurts.

- Vitamin-rich starches such as sweet potatoes.

- Salmon.

What to Avoid

Certain foodstuffs can prove harmful to both your partner and your baby. As such, the items listed below should be avoided at all costs during pregnancy:

- Alcohol.

- Beef, chicken, pork, and fish that are raw or undercooked.

- Fruits and vegetables that haven't been washed or prepared properly.

- Fruit juice has a high sugar content.

- Leftovers that have been stored for more than one day.

- Meat is cut from an animal's organ, such as the kidney or liver.

- Processed meats such as sausages, salami, pepperoni, hot dogs, lunch meat, and any other deli meats.

- Raw eggs and the foods that contain them, namely cookie dough, uncooked batter, runny scrambled eggs, tiramisu, eggs Benedict, hollandaise sauces, as well as many homemade sauces and dressings.

- Raw or undercooked sprouts, including clover, radish, alfalfa, and mung bean sprouts.

- Seafood that contains high levels of mercury, including tuna, orange roughy, tilefish, swordfish, and mackerel.

- Smoothies or juices made from raw products.

- Soft cheeses.

- Unpasteurized dairy products.

What to Limit

Between the extremes of good and bad, we find a group of foods and drinks that fall somewhere in the middle in terms of their level of benefit or disadvantage. Though not entirely healthy nor helpful, your partner can still consume the following, albeit in moderation:

- Fish should be eaten in moderation, as larger portions thereof may lead to the ingestion of mercury.

- Food and drink containing retinol (vitamin A).

- Healthy fats and oils should not amount to more than six tablespoons per day. Even then, only plant oils such as sunflower, canola, olive, and safflower are recommended.

- Only 200 mg of caffeine a day is permissible. This amounts to one 12-ounce cup of coffee or tea.

- Though beneficial in many ways, dried fruits should not be eaten in excess due to their high sugar content.

Food Safety During Pregnancy

According to Dean & Kendall (2012), "[p]regnant women are at increased risk for getting some foodborne infections because of the hormonal changes that occur during pregnancy." They elaborate further by explaining that these hormonal shifts, while essential to the baby's development, may make your partner vulnerable to illnesses carried by foodborne pathogens. These pathogens can very easily permeate the placenta and infect the developing fetus. This can cause complications that may result in developmental issues, premature labor, miscarriage, or stillbirth.

The best way to avoid these dangers is by practicing safe food practices. These actions involve the following:

- Washing hands before and after handling food.

- Washing hands after working outdoors or handling animals.

- Thoroughly cleaning all utensils, cutlery, cutting boards, and kitchen surfaces before and after cooking.

- Storing perishable foodstuffs at a temperature between 35- and 40-degrees Fahrenheit.

- Thoroughly cooking raw items such as meat.

- Rinsing fruits and vegetables before consumption.

Medication

Navigating the use of medication during pregnancy can be just as challenging as that of food and drink. Right off the bat, it's worth noting that, due to the side effects they all carry, no medicine can be classified as entirely safe for use during pregnancy. This counts for prescription as well as over-the-counter medications. Crucially, the use of medicine cannot be discontinued during pregnancy, as many chronic conditions require treatment even during the antenatal months. As such, there is no overwhelming cause for concern regarding the regulated use of medication during pregnancy. While certain medicines do pose a risk in terms of complications or defects, this is not a given.

Unfortunately, given the number of variables present, we cannot conclusively state whether medication has an adverse effect on pregnancy. Moreover, we cannot conclude that the opposite is true either. What we do know is that the use of medication should always be preceded by a visit to a healthcare practitioner. If your partner was on prescription medication before her pregnancy, she would have to consult a doctor to find out how this influences her medicinal regimen. It is possible for your partner to continue using medication while pregnant and for it to have no adverse effect at all. It all comes down to which medicines are taken and in what dose. Naturally, taking too many pills will prove harmful, but some pharmaceuticals can be dangerous even in moderation.

Speaking of moderation, it is perfectly alright for your partner to take prenatal vitamins, such as vitamin B6. However, she needn't consume the entire supplement aisle, as this can be just as detrimental. It's recommended that your partner also takes folic acid, as much as 400 mcg per day, until week 12 of pregnancy (Newman, 2023). Folate, from which folic acid comes, helps to stimulate red blood cell production, which may help avoid anemia. Additionally, during the prenatal period, folate can help the progress of fetal development and forms an essential component of the process of cell division. Should your partner wish to use natural, holistic medications, note that they should also be prescribed by a professional, just as conventional medication would be.

General Safety

- Substances such as nail polish remover and paint thinner should be avoided. The chemicals present in these, and other solvents can adversely affect the fetal developmental process.

- Climbing on ladders or on top of surfaces should be avoided at all costs.

- When traveling, ensure that your partner is able to stand up and stretch her legs every now and then. Furthermore, all travel should be discontinued after the 28th week of pregnancy.

- If cats count among your household pets, take the task of changing kitty litter off your partner's hands. Handling animal excrement, especially that of felines, exposes your partner to a dangerous parasitic infection known as toxoplasmosis (Wahlberg, 2021).

- Spa treatments should be undertaken with great consideration, as some may have severe adverse effects. Your partner should avoid saunas during pregnancy and ought to steer clear of any bodily treatments involving harsh chemicals, such as peels and microdermabrasion.

- Certain spa treatments can be enjoyed, albeit with some precautionary measures in place. These treatments include manicures, pedicures, hair removal, massages, and body scrubs.

Babyproofing Your Home

Ensuring that your home is safe for your baby to inhabit is essential, and given how much work babyproofing entails, it's recommended that you start the process well before your infant arrives. You can begin making the first adjustments about three months before your partner's due date. This way, most of the work will be out of the way by the time of the birth. If there are still some things left to do, it's recommended that you have it all done by the time your baby starts to crawl, which will be around six to 10 months after birth (The Bump Editors, 2014).

Babyproofing: A Comprehensive Checklist

Making your living environment safe for your child is an extensive undertaking, and there are many things that will require your attention, many of which you may not have thought of initially. To that end, use the checklist provided below to ensure that each area of your home and its surroundings have been outfitted to keep your infant safe and secure.

Living Areas

- Cover cables or tuck them behind furniture.
- Anchor large pieces of furniture to the walls.
- Place guards around heaters and fireplaces.
- Secure the contents of china and ornamental cabinets by fitting their doors with childproof locks.
- Hide remote controls and other smaller items that babies may place in their mouths or wave around. Alternatively, place them on higher surfaces out of your infant's reach.
- When using tablecloths, be sure to tuck their edges away so that the baby cannot reach them. Alternatively, use shorter clothes or forgo them entirely.

- If curtains or blinds have hanging cords, tuck them away or install safety tassels and cord stops.

Kitchen

- Tuck away cords and cables, and ensure that no part of an appliance extends beyond the edge of the counter.
- Place guards around the edges of the stovetop, and fit the oven door with a guard or childproof lock.
- Set up a gate or other barrier at the kitchen entrance to prevent your baby from wandering in while food is being cooked.
- Store all cleaning products and loose kitchen implements in cupboards or drawers fitted with childproof locks.
- If you keep poisons, pesticides, or other chemical agents in your kitchen, similarly lock them away, but also be sure to avoid storing them in food containers.

Laundry

- Ensure that all buckets and other open-top containers are empty or put away.
- Store all detergents and softeners in a cupboard fitted with a childproof lock.
- If using cloth diapers and a diaper pail, ensure that the pail's lid is able to shut firmly. Store the pail on an elevated surface where your baby cannot reach it.
- After use, firmly shut the washer and dryer doors.

Bathroom

- Fit the toilet lid with a childproof lock or clasp.
- Any cleaning products, medications, and grooming products should be stowed away in a cabinet, which should be secured with a childproof lock.

- Set a cap on the temperature to which your water heater can rise, and go no higher than 120 degrees Fahrenheit.
- Place a non-slip mat or non-slip stickers at the bottom of a bathtub.
- Fit childproof covers over faucets.

Nursery

- Keep all non-sleeping paraphernalia out of the cot. Store these items in drawers or on shelves away from your baby.
- When assembling the crib, measure the space between the slats to ensure that they are no more than 2 3/8" apart. When placing the mattress in the finished crib, check that there are no gaps between the bedding and the framework.
- When your baby starts standing on their own, remove mobiles and other hanging items. You can either place them higher up or get rid of them entirely.
- Fit a childproof lock on the side of the cot that can be dropped.
- Do not hang items on the cot.
- If you have cats, consider placing a cat net over the top of the cot.
- If the nursery is air-conditioned, avoid extreme temperatures, both hot and cold.
- Place a thick rug underneath the changing table.

Hallways, Landings, and Stairs

- Install stair gates at the top and bottom of staircases. You can also fit these gates at either end of a hallway if you like.
- If banisters or railings have spaces bigger than 2 3/8" gaps between the slats, fence them off.
- Ensure that all carpets are firmly fixed to the floor and that no part of them juts out.

Doors

- Place doorstops underneath or behind each door to prevent your child from opening or closing them.
- Fit childproof locks on doorknobs and handles.

Backyards

- Determine if any plants in the garden are poisonous or harmful. Remove these plants entirely or place them out of your baby's reach.
- Ensure that all barbecue supplies are out of your baby's reach, and consider moving a portable barbecue to a fenced-off area.
- Secure shed and garage doors with childproof locks.

Outdoor Areas

- Fence all pools, balconies, decks, and patios. Install childproof gates into these fences so that access to the area isn't lost entirely.

Becoming a father is a big event in anyone's life, and there are many stops to be made along the road to becoming a good dad. However, it's worth keeping in mind that your efforts will be supplemented by good old-fashioned paternal instinct. And the things that instinct doesn't account for, you will pick up with practice. It may not be entirely easy to switch into dad mode, but once you're there, you'll never look back.

Chapter 5:

The Lowdown on Prenatal Check-Ups

If there is one thing we've established by now, it's that education is paramount to the process of preparing for and entering fatherhood. This learning takes place in many settings and on many occasions, and there's an excellent chance that you will never feel more informed than after attending a prenatal check-up with your partner. And while the focus will most certainly be on your partner and baby, there are some elements of the check-ups that concern you more heavily. For example, through a simple blood test, there is a wealth of information to be discovered about your unborn baby's health. Additionally, many dads-to-be are now required to undergo a health screening during one of the prenatal check-ups. The importance of these visits extends far beyond what we might assume.

Why You Should Be Present During Prenatal Visits

Naturally, it's essential that you are as involved as possible throughout the pregnancy, but prenatal visits are especially important. A lot of information is shared during these visits—information that applies to both your partner and baby and will inform how you approach the way forward. And while these appointments are learning opportunities for you, your presence there is largely in the capacity of a support person. Accompanying your partner to a prenatal visit enables you to help your partner remember all the tips, tricks, and facts that your healthcare provider will be supplying. Additionally, should there be some difficult news to receive, you can be there to comfort your partner. In those moments when she feels overwhelmed or distressed, your presence means you can reassure and encourage her, letting her know you'll be there all the way. More than anything else, attending these visits is an opportunity for you to take an active role in your partner's pregnancy and to share in this experience, which culminates with both of you becoming parents to a brand-new baby.

Your attendance at these visits can help in ways you may not even be aware of. For instance, the support you provide during an antenatal check-up can help make your partner feel relaxed and secure. Subsequently, this may decrease the levels of stress hormones to which your baby is exposed in utero. Additionally, taking on an active role means that your partner will value your opinion on pregnancy-related matters more. So, if there is something you're concerned about, your expression of this worry will go over better, as she knows you understand the ins and outs of the pregnancy and speak from a place of concern, love, and knowledge. Finally, paternal attendance at antenatal visits has been known to increase feelings of preparedness, as dads feel more knowledgeable about current and future pregnancy developments (Redshaw & Henderson, 2013).

How Often Should They Be?

With most pregnancies, prenatal visits will follow the same schedule. Healthy, uncomplicated pregnancies require attention from healthcare professionals, but neither your partner nor baby will need overly close supervision or additional help. However, for pregnancies that have complications or in which other health problems are present, the regularity of these visits will vary. That being said, if your partner progresses through pregnancy as is considered typical and there are causes for concern, you can expect to attend approximately 10–12 prenatal visits over the course of 40 weeks (Raising Children Network (Australia), 2023a). From weeks four through 28, you will accompany your partner to a prenatal check-up once every four weeks. From weeks 28 to 36, you will meet your healthcare provider once every fortnight. Finally, from weeks 36 to 40, prenatal check-ups take place weekly.

We know that no two pregnancies are exactly alike and that there are a number of personal variables that may influence the lead-up to the birth as well as the event itself. In terms of prenatal check-ups, we've already established that high-risk pregnancies or pregnancies influenced by chronic illness may influence the regularity of visits to the doctor. Alongside these, there are a number of other risk factors that may result in an increase in the frequency of your visits to your healthcare provider, including:

- Pre-existing, long-term health issues, such as elevated blood pressure, diabetes, anemia, and lupus.

- Being age 35 or older, pregnancies beyond the mid-thirties have an elevated risk of producing birth defects (Kam, 2012).

- Complications arise during pregnancy, such as preeclampsia, gestational diabetes, and pregnancy-related high blood pressure.

- The danger of preterm labor will be indicated either by its occurrence during previous pregnancies or by a number of signs present during the gestational period.

- Multiple births, such as twins or triplets, require additional guidance and help from healthcare providers.

What Happens During a Prenatal Visit?

During prenatal visits, the primary goal is to ascertain how your baby is doing and how your partner's body is coping with the pregnancy. In both instances, your healthcare provider will determine whether everything is progressing as it should and whether there is anything that warrants concern or intervention. The latter happens only when necessary, and most prenatal visits follow a regular process from the first through third trimesters.

Typically, you can expect blood pressure measurements and urine tests to be conducted during each check-up. Though not a component of every visit, your partner may be asked to undergo some blood tests, something you yourself may also be asked to do. A record will be kept of your partner's weight and its change throughout the pregnancy, a recording that goes hand-in-hand with the measurement of her abdomen, where the baby is developing in the womb. At some point during the second trimester, a glucose tolerance test will be conducted to determine whether your partner has, or is at risk for, gestational diabetes.

Prenatal check-ups will check in on your baby's well-being as well. In addition to tracking their development and growth, healthcare providers will check the fetal heartbeat during each visit and determine via ultrasound if there are any problems to take note of. An ultrasound will also give you an indication of your baby's position in the womb and will provide you with a picture of your soon-to-be newborn. In the interest of monitoring and protecting your baby's health, your partner will undergo several different rounds of testing. Each of these diagnostic measures is intended to detect the presence of potentially harmful infections, including hepatitis B and the group B streptococcus bacterium.

The Ideal Prenatal Visit Schedule

The First Trimester (Week One to 12)

The First Visit

Your first antenatal appointment will take place at roughly four weeks if your partner suspects or knows she is pregnant. If you only discover the pregnancy after the fourth week, don't worry; simply schedule a check-up for the earliest possible date. Of all the prenatal visits you will have, the first will potentially be the longest. This is because your healthcare provider will need to gain an accurate, comprehensive picture of your partner's physical and mental condition, as well as determine whether any lifestyle choices may play a role in the pregnancy. Your partner will also be asked to supply the names of any medications she is taking, as well as disclose the use of substances such as nicotine, alcohol, and other drugs. Ordinarily, the progress of the pregnancy will be ascertained through the use of an ultrasound.

At the first prenatal check-up, confirmation of the pregnancy will be obtained, as well as how far along it has progressed. Additionally, your partner will undergo a physical examination that measures her weight, height, and blood pressure. This may also include a pelvic exam. Both you and your partner will be asked to provide your medical history, as well as that of your family, and to do so with as much detail as possible. If your partner is experiencing any discomfort or issues, such as excessive breast tenderness or morning sickness, this will be addressed if mentioned to your healthcare provider.

Other tests administered during the first visit include a urine test to check for urinary tract infections, a blood test to determine blood type and Rh status, as well as the presence of anemia, hepatitis B, hepatitis C, chlamydia, syphilis, and HIV. Though not compulsory, your partner may be offered a cervical screening to check for HPV and cervical cancer. Your partner will also be tested for immunity against diseases such as chickenpox and rubella if this has not been noted in her medical history.

On the lighter side of things, you will also be furnished with a due date at this first appointment. All future check-ups will be scheduled according to this date to ensure that tests, scans, and examinations are performed at the correct stage of the pregnancy. Finally, that first appointment will include discussions regarding lifestyle changes and options during pregnancy. If your healthcare provider does not volunteer this information, ask about nutrition, prenatal vitamins, dentist appointments, sex, exercise, travel, and vaccinations. Any other factors related to you and your partner's lives that may have an impact on the pregnancy must be shared so that your healthcare provider can help you find solutions or make changes if need be.

Other Check-Ups During the First Trimester

At each of the other appointments during the first trimester, you can expect your partner to undergo blood and urine tests, as well as a measurement of her blood pressure. If the due date was not determined at the initial visit, the check-up between the 11th and 14th weeks will allow for its calculation. During this ultrasound, your healthcare provider will also be able to let you know if you will be having multiple births. Additionally, your partner will be weighed at each check-up, your baby's cardiac activity will be monitored, and any swelling of your partner's hands or feet will be addressed and treated if necessary. At approximately week 12, your doctor will use a Doppler machine (an ultrasound) to help you hear the fetal heartbeat for the first time.

Your healthcare provider may offer or recommend a number of different tests during the first trimester. They may include the following:

- Chorionic villus sampling (CVS) between weeks 11 and 13, which tests for chromosomal abnormalities.

- A nuchal translucency scan between weeks 11 and 14 tests the risk for the development of Down syndrome.

- Noninvasive prenatal testing (NIPT) at week 10 tests for Down syndrome and other developmental abnormalities.

The Second Trimester (Week 13–26)

During the second trimester, you can expect the length of the check-ups to become shorter, though they will still contain many of the same components. At each visit, your partner's weight and blood pressure will be taken, and urine as well as blood tests may also be conducted—although only if necessary. Additionally, each check-up during this trimester is marked by an abdominal palpation, in which your partner's abdomen is measured as a means of tracking the baby's growth. Your baby's fetal cardiac activity will also be monitored from this point onward.

Your healthcare provider will also check in with your partner to ensure that her overall health is still satisfactory and to address any problems that may have arisen. If any tests were conducted during the first trimester and their results have not yet been shared, you will likely receive them during your first check-up in the second trimester. Should your partner have tested negative for her Rh status, a blood test may be done to determine the fetal blood type. Knowing your partner's Rh status is incredibly important, as she will need to receive treatment if her blood type is incompatible with the baby's. This is necessary in case some of the fetal blood crosses over into your partner's bloodstream. If this happens, your partner's body will create antibodies to fight off the blood that isn't hers. Should these antibodies then cross through the placenta, it may lead to serious health complications or even death.

As development is well underway by this point in the pregnancy, your partner may also be asked about fetal activity, such as kicks or fluttering in the region of the womb. At approximately week 19 or 20, your healthcare provider will perform an ultrasound to check the progress of development. At this point, if you so wish, they may also be able to reveal the baby's sex. Around week 25, if this is your partner's first child, the fetal movements will start to be tracked, something that will continue for the rest of the gestational period.

Some tests, including the CVS and nuchal translucency scan, may be recommended during the second trimester. In addition to these, your partner may also be subjected to the following screenings:

- A blood glucose tolerance test was performed between weeks 24 and 28 to determine whether elevated hormone levels make gestational diabetes a concern.

- An amniocentesis, in which amniotic fluid is extracted to test for chromosomal abnormalities, may be conducted between weeks 15 and 20. If your healthcare provider suspects an issue earlier, this test may be performed earlier (Healthdirect Australia, 2023a).

- A quad test around weeks 15–20, which focuses on your baby's brain, neural tissues, and spinal cords to suss out any potential risks as well as any developmental delays or complications. Note that this test cannot diagnose a condition but will indicate whether more tests are required.

The Third Trimester (Week 27 to Birth)

In the final trimester, you will be seeing your healthcare provider more often. First fortnightly, then weekly in the final month of pregnancy. As is standard practice, your partner's blood pressure will be annotated, as will her weight and the baby's development (abdominal palpation). She may also be asked to submit a urine sample during each check-up. Urine is tested during the third trimester to detect urinary tract infections as well as symptoms of high blood pressure. The baby's heart rate will be measured and recorded during each appointment, as will their movement in the womb.

Your partner may also be asked about any contractions she has had or is having, as well as any fluids excreting from the vaginal area. When it comes to contractions in the third trimester, your partner is likely to experience Braxton Hicks contractions, which, though painful, aren't a sign that labor has begun. These contractions are uterine tightenings and help prepare your partner's body for labor (Cleveland Clinic, 2022a). They may cause you some worry, particularly if they occur close to the due date. However, you can monitor the contractions, and if they are irregular in their pattern and go away once your partner shifts her position, it's merely a case of Braxton Hicks.

From the 34th week onward, the baby's presentation (their physical orientation in utero) and station (the distance their head has moved into the pelvis) will also be recorded. The extent of your partner's cervical dilation will also be noted and tracked as the pregnancy approaches its end. As the birth nears, you will be discussing its logistics more frequently with your healthcare provider. You will discuss your birth plan as well as how you are equipped for parenthood after the birth. In anticipation of the big day, your healthcare provider may also provide you with some antenatal counseling to help prepare you for all the changes and responsibilities you are about to face.

In the third trimester, your healthcare provider may advise or carry out the following tests and medical procedures:

- An anti-D immunoglobulin injection if your partner's blood type is Rh-negative. More than one injection may be administered, depending on necessity.

- A Tdap vaccination against whooping cough (pertussis), diphtheria, and tetanus.

- A vaginal swab for group B streptococcus (GBS).

A typical human pregnancy lasts 40 weeks, or 41 at most. Should your partner not yet have given birth past the 41-week mark, your weekly visits to your healthcare provider will shift in focus to cover possible methods of inducement. If this deviates from your birth plan, it's worth remembering that the longer your baby remains in utero past the normal end of the gestational period, the greater the risk of complications for them and your partner becomes.

Questions to Ask During Prenatal Appointments

It's natural to be curious about pregnancy, birth, and all related experiences, especially if this is your first time becoming a father. As such, it's perfectly alright for you to ask questions during prenatal check-ups. In fact, it's encouraged, as you may cover something your partner missed or may have different concerns given the perspective from which you are experiencing the pregnancy. With that in mind, here are some questions you can ask the next time you visit your healthcare provider:

- What are the best resources for me to learn from during this time?

- Which tasks and duties can I take over during the pregnancy?

- Is sex advisable and safe during pregnancy?

- Are there specific exercises or techniques I can participate in, either as health measures or methods of inducement?

- Will you be delivering the baby? If not, who will be there in your stead?

- How is the hospital, birthing center, or clinic equipped to deal with emergent medical situations and interventions?

- When would it be advisable to ask for intervention during labor?

- Is there a birthing method you can recommend?

- How will the delivery procedure work in terms of logistics, and who will be present in the room?

- Are there extra steps we can take in order to avoid complications?

- If our child has genetic, developmental, or other health issues, how can we proceed after the birth?

These are just examples of the types of questions you can ask. Remember that these check-ups are not only an opportunity for learning but also for getting some help. Share any concerns you have regarding the pregnancy, as well as any suggestions you may have (within reason). If there is a specific aspect of the pregnancy or birthing process you are curious about, don't hesitate to ask. The more you participate, the better prepared you will be for the day.

Family History and Genetic Testing

Prenatal genetic testing is an increasingly common practice and involves both you and your partner being tested for genetic abnormalities or disorders. This is used to determine the risk of either or both of you transmitting a hereditary disorder to your unborn child (Dungan, 2022). Genetic testing involves an examination of both of your families' medical histories, though it may include the taking of blood or tissue samples for analysis. This type of testing is entirely voluntary, and while healthcare providers will recommend it for some pregnancies, anyone can request a prenatal genetic test.

There are two types of prenatal genetic testing: screening and diagnostic. The former is entirely noninvasive and provides results that indicate whether a potential risk for genetic disorders exists. These tests do not provide a conclusive diagnosis. By contrast, diagnostic tests are more invasive and yield conclusive results regarding the presence of birth defects or hereditary conditions. These tests are usually recommended for women aged 35 and over, those who have chronic or autoimmune disorders, or who have delivered children with birth defects in previous instances.

If you are considering having such a test performed, it's important that you weigh the advantages against the disadvantages. Fortunately, there isn't very much to consider. Genetic testing is in no way bad for you, your partner, or your baby. Most tests are mildly invasive, involving only a blood sample or some tissue taken from the inside of a cheek. Some tests may be more invasive, particularly those aimed at making a formal diagnosis. However, these are only performed in instances where the healthcare professional has deemed it necessary, and every precaution is taken during the procedure.

On the whole, genetic testing can have a number of advantageous outcomes. In addition to the easy method of testing, obtaining these results can help you discover more about your familial medical history. If there is some confusion regarding this part of your life, the answers provided by this test should clear things up and can even give you some indication of what you can expect moving forward, health-wise.

Moreover, there are many risk factors that aren't linked to hereditary patterns, race, or ethnicity (DerSarkissian & WebMD Editorial Contributors, 2022). You may be carrying a genetic mutation that no one else in your family does. By getting these tests done, you can become privy to this information and make informed, careful decisions regarding yourself and your family.

On the flip side, you have to consider the fact that no test, diagnostic, or screening, will ever be 100% accurate. Sometimes mistakes are made, and you or your partner may erroneously be identified as carriers. Conversely, you may be mistakenly told that there is no risk of your baby developing congenital disorders when you are, in fact, a carrier. Becoming a parent is already stressful enough, and either experience will only serve to compound your worry. On that same note, there is no way of knowing how severely any genetic abnormalities will affect your child. The impact could be extensive or possibly negligible. You will only be able to determine the extent of its effects after the birth, which will also increase the tumult of your emotional state in the lead-up to your baby's arrival.

Though it's always a good idea to weigh the pros and cons, when it comes to prenatal genetic testing, there are some questions you and your partner can mull over independently of the factors outlined above. These include:

- How will the results influence our family? Some relatives may react contentiously to learning you (and possibly they) are carriers of genetic disorders.

- How will the results influence us as individuals? Gaining this knowledge can influence your perspective on your impending parenthood, for better or worse.

- How will we proceed from here? If there is a chance you have passed down a disorder to your child, you will need to consider how you will deal with it if such a condition develops. The information may also be overwhelming, and it may be a good idea to ask your doctor to refer you to a genetics counselor.

You will recall that all prenatal genetic tests are done on an entirely voluntary basis. However, while some people may choose to take these tests based on their own research or desire, there's a chance that your doctor may recommend you undertake screening or diagnostic tests. There are a number of factors that can influence the necessity of this test. You may be advised to have these tests done if either you or your partner are of French-Canadian, Cajun, Eastern, or Central European Jewish descent, specifically Ashkenazi. Other ethnic groups who are often referred for testing include people of African-American, Southeast Asian, and Mediterranean descent (Masters, 2022). Testing will also be recommended if either one of you has a family history of genetic disorders.

Types of Prenatal Screening Tests

Carrier Screening

Masters (2022) defines a genetic carrier screening as "a medical test that determines whether you or your partner is a "carrier" for certain genetic diseases and the odds that your child will inherit them." If you are identified as a carrier, it means that your DNA carries a mutation that presents the possibility of carrying a disorder down to your child. Crucially, you don't need to have the disorder yourself to be a carrier, as the mutation may be inert in your system. This type of prenatal genetic test involves the testing of both you and your partner, as the potential genetic condition may come from the chromosomes your child inherits from either one of you.

Carrier screenings test for a variety of genetic aberrations and disorders. Some of the most common genetic disorders your DNA will be tested for are:

- Alpha-thalassemia is a blood disorder resulting in decreased levels of oxygenated blood cells in the body.

- Beta thalassemia, a blood disorder, similarly resulting in lower levels of hemoglobin in the body.

- Cystic fibrosis is a respiratory disorder in which the airways are clogged by mucus, thereby trapping bacteria within the respiratory system.

- Familial hyperinsulinism, resulting in elevated levels of insulin.

- Fanconi anemia group C, a disorder originating in the bone marrow, decreases the total number of blood cells in the body.

- Fragile X syndrome is a developmental disorder characterized by the lack of a protein essential to the process of neural development.

- Gaucher disease, which prevents the proper processing of lipids, results in elevated levels of harmful fats in the body.

- Glycogen storage disease type 1A, wherein glycogen, a sugary substance, isn't properly processed and builds up in the body.

- Maple syrup urine disease is the inability to process a number of amino acids.

- Niemann-Pick disease type A or B. The former enlarges the liver and spleen, leading to issues with the respiratory system as well as growth. The latter, while less severe, similarly results in the enlargement of the spleen and liver.

- Sickle cell disease is an umbrella term for several blood disorders that affect the shape of red blood cells.

- Spinal muscular atrophy impacts neurological and motoric function due to damage inflicted upon the neurons in the spinal cord.

- Tay-Sachs disease, in which lipids cannot be fully processed, results in a buildup of fatty materials in the brain cavity.

Screening for Abnormal Chromosomal Numbers

This test detects aberrations in the number of chromosomes inherited from the parents, either extra or missing chromosome sections. Abnormal chromosomal numbers can lead to disorders such as Turner's or Down syndrome. There are two types of screening tests performed for this purpose. They are:

- Cell-free fetal DNA screening, also known as NIPT, is a method in which chromosomal abnormalities are sought out in small quantities of fetal DNA found in your partner's blood. This test can only be performed from week 10 onwards.

- Serum screening is an analysis of protein levels in your partner's blood to determine the risk for chromosomal abnormalities. There are a number of subtypes of this test, all of which are only performed during or after the 11th week of pregnancy.

Screening for Physical Abnormalities

Performed via ultrasound or the examination of blood samples, this test analyzes your baby's phenotype, which constitutes their physical characteristics as determined by their genetics. If physical abnormalities are present, they are analyzed to determine whether they are genetic in origin. There are four types of screening tests done for this purpose, namely:

- Nuchal translucency measures the thickness of the back of the baby's neck via ultrasound. This screening is performed between the 11th and 14th weeks of pregnancy.

- Maternal serum screening, also known as AFP screening, measures the level of alpha-fetoprotein in your partner's blood. The sample was analyzed between weeks 15 and 22.

- A quadruple or multiple marker screening, where a blood sample is tested for four different substances. This is also done between weeks 15 and 22.

- A fetal anatomy scan, which is an ultrasound done between the 18th and 20th weeks, analyzes the development of the baby's physical structures.

Prenatal diagnostic tests may be more invasive and involve the analysis of cells obtained from the chorionic villi or the placenta.

How to Be the Best Support Person for Your Partner

Though a prenatal check-up is a chance for you to learn about pregnancy and birth, remember that the majority of the focus is on your partner and baby. As such, there are a number of dos and don'ts to keep in mind when you visit the OB/GYN.

- Don't try to lighten the mood with jokes, especially about the setup or equipment in the room. If you're nervous, your partner most likely is as well. Comfort her instead of making "witty" remarks regarding the implements that will be used on her in a moment.

- Come prepared with a list of questions. Write down everything you want to know, no matter how odd or random it may seem.

- Don't pull focus. Unless you're lying on an inspection table with a paper gown on, this isn't your moment. Speak when appropriate, but remember your supportive role.

- Pay as close attention as possible. Both of you are learning, and your healthcare provider will be sharing essential information during check-ups.

- Unless you have an excellent reason, don't miss, or skip a check-up; your partner needs you there.

- Express your excitement when appropriate and become involved in the discussion.

- Don't attempt to make light of the process or downplay the importance of your parenting journey. The both of you are going through a big change, and acknowledging it better equips you to deal with it.

- Despite phenomena like dad brain and sympathetic pregnancy symptoms, remember that your partner's body is changing much more than yours. Be respectful of this, don't dismiss any issues she brings up, and ask how you can help ease her physical experience.

- Double-check what your insurance covers. While they should cover the majority, if not all, of prenatal check-ups, take a look at what your policy says so that you know you will be able to attend the number of check-ups and get the help you need.

If it seems like the list of things you have to consider before becoming a dad is growing longer, you wouldn't be incorrect. However, remember that things like these check-ups are essential and will be your greatest source of reliable information throughout the pregnancy. Though it may seem overwhelming to navigate all the medical jargon and advice your healthcare provider gives you, lean into all these visits have to offer and make the most of the resources they provide you. More than anything else, remember that you are there as the pillar of the person carrying your baby. However scary it is for you, it's probably much worse for her, so be present during visits, hold her hand, and let her know that you're invested and that the two of you will tackle this together.

Chapter 6:

A Peek Into the Womb

As you will learn not too long after your child's birth, newborns are fascinating beings. For instance, did you know that newborns already possess the ability to swim? Not only do they know how to hold their breath underwater, but they can even make rudimentary swimming motions with their arms and legs. Staying in the realm of physical abilities, newborns are born shortsighted, having clear vision that extends only between eight and 12 inches in front of their face. Another one to note is that a newborn's stomach is only about as big as a hazelnut. Also, they have more bones than adults. You've probably heard this one before, but it remains fascinating that a baby enters the world with 300 bones in their body, a number that will be brought down to 206 as they mature (Logan-Banks, 2016).

And, perhaps most interesting of all, babies actually have the ability to "cry" in utero. A study performed by Gingras et al. (2005) in New Zealand determined that by the 20th week of pregnancy, a baby can perform all the physical movements involved in crying. This includes opening their jaws, extending their tongues, moving their mouths, making their chins quiver, swallowing, and altering their breath patterns to become more complex. Clearly, a number of fascinating things take place while your baby is developing in the womb. With that in mind, let's take a look at what actually happens in utero over the course of nine months.

A Weekly Breakdown of What's up With Baby and Mommy… and What You Can Do to Help

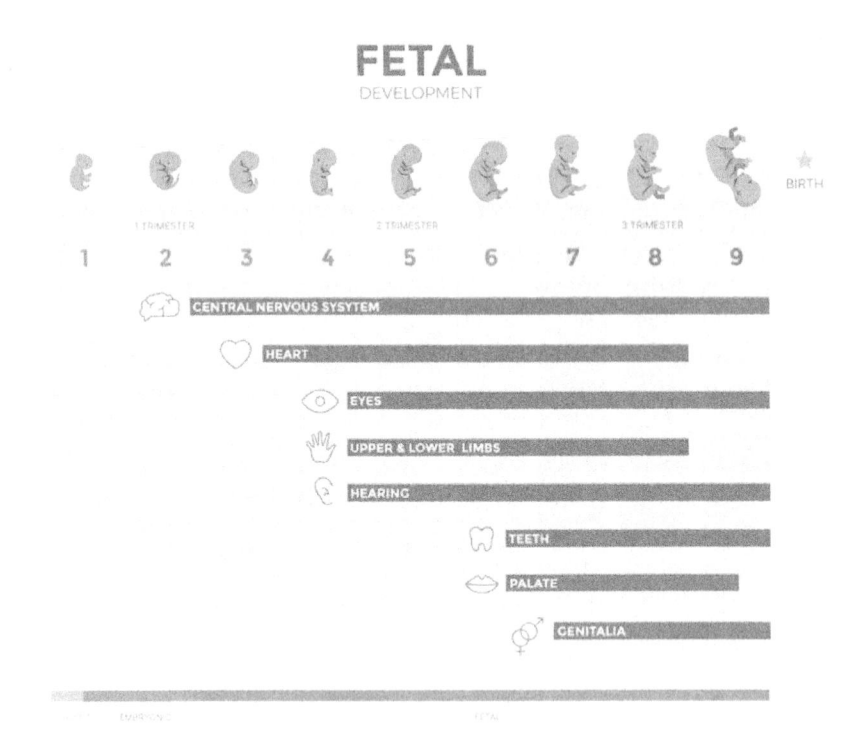

FETAL DEVELOPMENT

1 2 3 4 5 6 7 8 9
1 TRIMESTER — 2 TRIMESTER — 3 TRIMESTER — BIRTH

- CENTRAL NERVOUS SYSYTEM
- HEART
- EYES
- UPPER & LOWER LIMBS
- HEARING
- TEETH
- PALATE
- GENITALIA

EMBRYONIC — FETAL

In the nine months that make up the gestational period, there's an awful lot going on. So far, our focus has been on how impending parenthood manifests in your life and world. Now it's time for us to take a closer look at what actually happens that leads up to becoming a father. As each week passes in your partner's pregnancy, something new is happening that furthers the process of fetal development. Moreover, each week brings with it new symptoms and changes in your partner's body. These are both things you will have to consider and navigate as you prepare to become a dad. Something that's also worth noting is that different stages of development are denoted with different labels for what will eventually be your baby. From conception through to the fourth week, the technical terms used are "zygote" and "blastocyst." After that, in weeks five to seven, they become an embryo. From then onwards, you, your partner, and your healthcare provider can use the terms "fetus" and "baby" interchangeably, depending on your personal preference (Marple, 2019).

Week One

Technically, the first week of pregnancy takes place before conception has even occurred. This is a time of internal preparation within your partner's reproductive system. Her body will start to secrete additional hormones to foster ovulation, which will facilitate the release of an ovum for fertilization. In this first week, your partner isn't regarded as being *technically* pregnant just yet. As such, she will only experience typical menstrual symptoms. Naturally, that doesn't stop you from providing her with hot water bottles, some calming beverages, and plenty of TLC.

Week Two

In the second week, ovulation occurs, and the fallopian tubes release an ovum. If a sperm cell does come into contact with an ovum, fertilization takes place between 12 and 24 hours after the initial penetration. It's worth noting that certain sources may report ovulation as the only occurrence during week two, with conception taking place in week three. Others maintain that both occur in the second week, with implantation taking place in week three. For our purposes here, we will be using the latter timeline. However, in these first few weeks, you may not even be aware of the pregnancy, so you shouldn't bother yourself with the nitty-gritty concerning the exact timeframe for fertilization and implantation.

Because week two contains the moment of conception and the pregnancy officially starts, there are some signs you can be on the lookout for. However, take note that they may be hard to spot, as the signs are tied to the typical menstrual cycle. As the body secretes preparatory hormones, your partner's breasts may grow. While this can be a sign of pregnancy, given how early it is, you will likely not notice it.

Week Three

This part of the pregnancy is commonly known as the germinal stage and is the shortest of all the different gestational periods. The zygote travels downwards and implants itself into the lining of the uterine wall. All the while, its cells multiply. By the end of the third week, the zygote is firmly attached to the uterine lining and has become a blastocyst. Additionally, it starts secreting hormones that will alert the body to pregnancy and catalyze the range of internal processes that will occur over the following nine months. At this stage, the blastocyst is a microscopically small clump of cells.

With the pregnancy now underway, your partner will start to experience some changes. The first will be undetectable to either of you, as it constitutes those cellular multiplications mentioned above. The second, however, can be monitored. As the zygote implants itself in the uterine wall, some blood may be excreted in a process known as "implantation bleeding," which may be accompanied by some abdominal cramps (Harris, 2022). A little blood and pain are normal; however, should it increase in intensity or duration, take your partner to a healthcare provider immediately. If the symptoms remain within typical parameters, provide your partner with ginger ale and any other pain relief she needs.

Week Four

In the fourth week, the placenta and amniotic sac begin to take shape. For your own reference, the size of the blastocyst is about as big as a speck of glitter. If crafting is outside your wheelhouse, it may help to picture it being roughly the size of a poppy seed. If you are more mathematically minded, that means its length is between 0.014" and 0.04", with its weight coming in at about 0.04 ounces. At the end of this week, it graduates from being a blastocyst to a fully-fledged embryo.

Near the end of the first month of pregnancy, symptoms and signs begin to manifest. In week four, you and your partner may begin to suspect pregnancy, as she will experience nausea, fatigue, and frequent urination, and her breasts may become sensitive and enlarged. Your suspicions may be confirmed by an at-home pregnancy test, though a false negative can also be reported given how recently conception will have taken place.

Week Five

Five weeks in, and your partner may still be unaware of the pregnancy (chances are you will be, too). Coming in at an astounding 0.04 ounces and 0.05", the embryo is now closer to a sesame seed in size. Despite its small measurements, changes are happening rapidly as the cells that will eventually become a heart emit pulses, and the circulatory system starts to take shape. Those heart cells will flicker approximately 110 times per minute. Additionally, the neural tube—which comprises the spinal cord, brain, and other central nervous system tissues—begins to develop. Though resembling a tadpole more than a baby, the embryo is now fully on track to grow into a tiny person.

Week Six

In the week that ear canals begin to form, and the heart starts to pump blood, beating 80 times per minute, the embryo grows to be 0.125", with the weight remaining largely the same at around 0.04 ounces. Other developments include the emergence of rudimentary eyes, arms, and legs, as well as the nose, mouth, brain, and intestinal system. Embryos at this stage will be equal in size to a lentil. Though still so small, the embryo's effect on the body will now become more apparent. Nausea and fatigue will continue, and your partner's hormonal changes may lead to sudden drops in blood pressure. It's at this point that folic acid should be introduced as a prenatal vitamin. Harris (2022) writes that the recommended daily dosage of folate is 600 micrograms.

Week Seven

When week seven rolls around, there are still some tadpole-esque qualities present. However, these will soon fade away as the soft embryonic cartilage is replaced with the first semblances of bones. The embryo will also have doubled its six-week size, still weighing in at 0.04 ounces but measuring a whopping 0.5". Other advancements made during this week include the development of the kidneys and tongue and the embryo's growth spurt, resulting in a size close to that of a blueberry.

In the seventh week, both you and your partner may have a rough time. She may experience crankiness, mood swings, malaise, and morning sickness.

Week Eight

Though it isn't yet palpable, this is when the fetus starts to move around in utero. This movement can be chalked up to the emergence of neural pathways that will carry impulses throughout the body. The eighth week also sees a giant leap forward in terms of respiration, with breathing tubes now connecting the throat to the (still-developing) lungs. Speaking of respiration, the umbilical cord is also fully formed and carries oxygenated blood to the circulatory system.

Week eight is especially impressive, as the foundation for each and every one of the body's organs and internal systems has been formed, meaning they're all on their way to becoming functional physiological components. Additionally, the eyes can now be clearly discerned, as can one of the last tadpole-like embryonic qualities: webbed hands and feet. The mover and shaker that are the fetus now measure a full 0.63", still weighing 0.04 ounces. If you'd like to put that into visual terms, it's about the size of an app icon on your phone.

Your partner may experience some pelvic pain this week, especially if she stands up. Additionally, you may notice some light bleeding. This is typical for the first trimester, but only within reason. Should it become excessive, seek medical help.

Week Nine

As your partner nears the end of the first trimester, the fetus clocks in at 0.90", just smaller than a wireless earphone. In addition to this jump in length, the ninth week sees the weight increase to about 0.07 ounces. There's also some good news in terms of physical developments, as the embryonic tail is a thing of the past by week nine. In contrast to this disappearance, we see an increasingly apparent manifestation of anatomy. Things are moving along, and the fetus will have earlobes by this point. The body is also starting to take on a more human-like shape, and the very early forms of muscles, taste buds, and teeth begin to arrive.

Your duty during week nine is to ensure that your partner remains hydrated. Pressure in the region of the bladder will lead to an increase in bathroom breaks, so be sure to supply her with plenty of fluids. Note that this week forms part of what many consider to be the most difficult period of pregnancy. As such, take care of your partner in any way she needs, ensuring she takes her prenatal vitamins, drinks plenty of fluids, and doesn't overdo it.

Week 10

During the 10th week, we see some wonderful progress, almost as wonderful as the cocktail sausage the fetus now matches in size. In the same week that the head rounds, the neck develops, and the eyelids close over the eyeball, the fetus' growth continues, this time lengthening to 1.22" with a weight of 0.14 ounces. Bones and cartilage both enjoy significant developmental progress this week, as do the teeth. It's during this week that smaller details also begin to arise. Fingernails appear at the ends of fingers, as do their counterparts on the toes; the skin is no longer translucent, and the limbs are even able to make bending movements. The amphibian phase is now fully over, with webbed hands and feet a thing of the past. Other external changes include the initial development of genitalia as well as the pinnae of the ears.

Week 11

Motility only increases in the 11th week, with the fetus, as the joints begin to work, and the fists are made and loosened. The mouth also starts to begin making opening and closing motions. The bones continue to harden, and the fetus' face becomes more clearly visible. Almost all the biological building blocks are now in place, with the diaphragm also stepping into action with hiccups. This week, when the fetus starts to make facial expressions, there is still impressive growth. You can picture the fetus about the size of a golf ball, weighing 0.25 ounces and measuring a full 1.61".

In all likelihood, week 11 will mean some trips to the store for you. Food cravings, which may already be present, will become more intense this week. While you can most certainly help your partner get what she needs, be sure to monitor what she craves. If this shifts from craving food to something like pica (meaning she wants to eat inedible items such as dirt, ash, or clay), some dietary changes are in order. Both of you can incorporate more iron, fiber, and folate into your diets. Chives are a quick fix, so toss them into a dish should you notice this shift.

Week 12

The final week of the first trimester is marked most significantly by impressive developments in the digestive system. At the same time, reflexes start to activate, and fingers as well as toes can now be curled, while the mouth can now be used to make suckling motions. Impressively, the first trimester is closed out with all organs, bones, muscles, limbs, and internal systems present in one form or another. Internal progress is especially apparent, with the liver's first secretions of bile as well as the functioning of the urinary and circulatory systems becoming more prominent. A lot is happening in terms of digestive and excretory structures. As such, it's only appropriate that we compare the fetus' size to that of a donut hole: 0.49 ounces and 2.13 inches. Though still small, your partner's body will be noticeably changed by the fetus during this week. In addition to symptoms such as gas, constipation, and an elevated heart rate, her hips will begin to widen in order to accommodate the growth taking place.

Week 13

In the first week of the second trimester, the fetus' vocal cords experience significant development, as do their veins and organs, which can now be seen through the skin. Moreover, the fingers are now not only equipped with nails but with prints as well. This week's reference size is for all the soon-to-be dads with green thumbs. Approximately 2.91" long and 0.81 ounces heavy, the fetus' closest size equivalent is a mini cactus. The second trimester brings with it a host of changes to your partner's body. Though many of the first trimester symptoms, such as morning sickness, will abate, physical changes are still continuing.

Week 14

The second-trimester growth spurt continues as the fetus lengthens to 3.42" in week 14, accompanied by a heavier weight of over an ounce, more specifically, 1.52 ounces. That's about as big as your average lemon. This uptick in growth comes along with the firing of some of the first brain impulses, meaning that facial expressions and motility become more pronounced. The now-opaque skin starts to thicken, and hair grows from the scalp. By the end of the 14th week, the external genitalia will have completed their development.

Week 15

Permanent shifts are made this week as organs like the intestines and ears move to the positions they will permanently inhabit after birth. Though respiration still occurs through the use of amniotic fluid, the lungs are well on their way to becoming fully-formed. Movements are also more pronounced, and the fetus may even begin sucking one or both of the thumbs. Another neural development occurs in that the fetus can now sense light even behind still-shut eyelids. In terms of size, growth continues as the fetus reaches 3.98" and 2.47 ounces by the end of the week. On average, that's equivalent to a standard apple.

From week 15 onwards, you can be on the lookout for Braxton Hicks contractions. These will be painful for your partner, so provide whichever methods of relief she needs. However, you will also have to monitor the nature of the contractions. Should the hourly number exceed four or a mucosal discharge be excreted, visit your healthcare provider immediately.

Week 16

The fourth month of the pregnancy comes to an end, and the ears have become functional enough to start picking up sounds. The lips also fully form during this week as the head moves to become more upright, the ears near the end of their positional migration, and both legs enjoy significant developmental progress. The hair on the scalp continues to grow, and the pattern of the hairline can become visible in week 16. Pivoting from the health-forward size comparison of week 16, this week's visual aid—weighing 3.53 ounces and measuring 4.57" in length—is the French delicacy that is an éclair. Physical changes continue, and the fetus' increased growth may lead to your partner gaining approximately one pound in every remaining week of the pregnancy.

Week 17

Moving right into the size developments, we see the fetus end the first week of the fifth month at 5.12" and 4.94 ounces, more-or-less the same as a turnip. The root-vegetable-sized fetus' former cartilage skeleton is now hardening into bone, and a significant quantity of fat has been gained this week, with vernix settling on the skin. Your partner will also experience some changes in her appearance as week 17 brings that famous pregnancy glow. However, on a less bright note, she may also experience disorienting lucid dreams, which may be linked to stress or anxiety regarding impending parenthood.

Week 18

In the 18th week, the fetus' skin becomes covered with a protective layer of peach fuzz called "lanugo" (Cleveland Clinic, 2020). Neural activity experiences an uptick as a sleep-wake cycle may be established for the first time, and protection is provided to the nervous system in the form of myelin around the nerves. Movement also increases, this time to the extent that it may be felt. Your partner may experience bodily pain as a result, feeling pangs in her legs and tailbone as well as in muscles throughout the body. In keeping with referring to foodstuffs as a metric for size, the bell pepper-sized fetus ends this week at 5.59" and 6.70 ounces.

Week 19

Sensory development is the headline of week 19, with all five primary senses experiencing significant improvement in their evolution. Along with this comes the appearance of hiccups, demonstrating the further strengthening of the diaphragm. Size-wise, you're looking at a pint of ice cream (or frozen yogurt, if that's more your speed), which translates to 8.47 ounces and 6.02".

Week 20

The fifth month comes to an end with some work happening in the digestive system. The swallowing reflex has developed by this point, and meconium is being produced. This is the substance that will constitute the baby's first postpartum bowel movement. Roughly the size of your average banana, you can measure the fetus at 6.46" and 10.58 ounces. The brain region responsible for the management of the senses continues to see significant expansion and strengthening. From this week onwards, you and your partner can begin to track the uterus' movement towards the ribcage, which will happen at a pace of roughly one centimeter per week. Additionally, you may find that your partner's mood lightens, partially due to reaching the halfway mark and partially due to the lessening of some symptoms.

Week 21

As your partner moves past the halfway point for a typical pregnancy, the fetus' limb movements become increasingly frequent, and you'll enjoy a boost in strength and coordination as well. Sensory centers in the brain, as well as receptors throughout the body, continue to develop and refine. Speaking of senses, you can get out the hot sauce bottle for this week's measurement, with the fetus now coming in at 10.51" and 12.70 ounces.

Week 22

In the 22nd week, the fetus' face is adorned with eyelashes and eyebrows. However, while these features have appeared around the eyes, the pigment of the fetus' iris has yet to appear. Motoric development also takes place this week, with grasping becoming an increasingly easier task. The fetus may be able to reach up and touch their ears, as well as reach out to touch the umbilical cord. At 15.17 ounces and 10.94", the fetus is comparable in size to a regular smoothie. During week 22, a number of health issues may arise, specifically in the vaginal region. Yeast infections may present at this point, though they may also show up in the weeks immediately preceding or following this one.

Week 23

The senses continue to develop in week 23, and hearing, in particular, sees an increase in strength. As the pregnancy progresses, the fetus gets ready for birth and for life after. In the 23rd week, fat is packed into the body in anticipation of entering the world. Appropriately, this week's measurement visual aid is a burrito, coming in at 1.10 lbs and 11.38".

Week 24

For the second week in a row, a milestone is reached. About seven days after the fetus moves over the one-pound mark, their lungs become fully developed, though they are still only suited for in-utero respiration. Externally, the skin is becoming more opaque by the day, though it may still be thin and see-through in some places. At the end of the sixth month, the fetus' measurements can be estimated at approximately 11.81" and 1.32 pounds. They are now just about as big as an ear of corn. Physical symptoms may be especially pronounced in week 24 and may include muscle aches, heartburn, fatigue, and dizziness.

Week 25

Fat continues to pad the body, smoothing out the previously creased skin. The follicular pattern that was presented earlier is now filled in as textured, pigmented hair begins to grow from the scalp. Just below the hair, the brain and its attached nervous system are quickly becoming more sophisticated and active. In week 25, when the nostrils open for the first time, the fetus weighs 1.46 lbs and is 12.50" long. For reference, this brings us back to the root-vegetable family, as the fetus is similar in size to a rutabaga. Many of the symptoms your partner will experience are carried over from the previous week, and she may still experience dizziness and fatigue. Bodily pain also remains an issue, with the aches moving into the legs, hips, and back.

Week 26

The pigmentation process, which started with the hair, continues in week 26 as melanin is produced to color the eyes and skin. The lungs also see some progress in the production of surfactant, a substance intended for postpartum respiratory aid. Respiration through the amniotic fluid continues. Other systems are also beginning to increase their action as the eyes open, and neural waves can be detected in the brain. In terms of size, you can use a bottle of soda (the fancy kind) for comparison, as the measurements stand at 14.02" and 1.68 lbs.

The 26th week will not be kind to your partner's sleep cycle. She may experience discomfort when trying to settle in for the night. You can help ease this by propping pillows up against her back and ensuring that she sleeps on her side. More than just being uncomfortable, sleeping on her back may prove dangerous to the fetus, as the uterus' positioning can clamp down on and block the blood flow in a major artery.

Week 27

Soon after the fetus' eyes open, the reflex of blinking will become operational. Other significant changes are observed, firstly in the strength of the lungs, which are now able to function outside the womb, albeit not without assistance. Secondly, the brain is making great strides. Not only is there an uptick in activity, but a regular sleep-wake pattern is established in the 27th week. As long as we're using vegetables to envision the size, take a look at a head of cauliflower; specifically, one measuring 14.41" and 1.93 lbs.

We opt for the large cauliflower because the pregnancy may be causing some significant discomfort at this point, first in the form of an elevated heart rate and feelings of being flushed. Worse than this is the pain that presents at week 27, specifically shooting back pain known as sciatica. You will have to keep your partner as still as possible, as the worsening of this pain may cause the levels of amniotic fluid to decrease. Walking, bending over, and lifting objects are some of the movements that cause this. It's essential to keep an eye out for this pain, as 50–80% of women report this experience during pregnancy (Freutel, 2016).

Week 28

When the seventh month of pregnancy draws to a close, your partner may feel increased movement as the fetus begins to shift in position, turning its head downwards in anticipation of the ever-nearing birth. Additionally, eyesight improves at 28 weeks. This week, the size statistics will change to 14.80" and 2.22 lbs. We'll close out the second trimester with one final vegetable equivalent, this time an eggplant, but a large one.

Pain is ever-present, this time in the form of leg cramps and body aches. Braxton Hicks contractions may also return around this time and will likely be greater in intensity than before. Keeping your partner calm and relatively still continues to be important, though ensure that she doesn't remain in the sun too long. In week 28, watch out for low blood pressure and dizziness. The sun may exacerbate these symptoms, so make sure she relaxes somewhere out of its reach, preferably with lots of liquids nearby.

Week 29

In the final trimester, developments are finishing up with the aim of preparing the body for life outside the womb. At the 29-week mark, the developmental focus is on the lungs and muscles. The head also continues to expand as the brain grows, though the skull won't fuse until well after birth. In honor of the approaching joy that nears with this trimester, we compare the measurements of 15.2" and 2.54 lbs with a delicious—large—sundae. If you're having trouble choosing a specific type, go for a banana split.

Despite the relief and happiness that may come with the arrival of the last trimester, be prepared for some significant symptoms to present and persist. Following the previous weeks' battle with pain and dizziness, your partner's body may start to self-regulate, leading her to become more tired, which hopefully leads to better sleep and longer naps during the day. While this does present a chance for some much-needed recharging, be aware that frequent urination will persist, if not increase, during week 29.

Week 30

By the middle of month eight, the fetus' internal temperature regulation will kick into action. As the overall growth continues, special attention is given to the brain, which rapidly increases in size and ability during this week. To retain a sense of whimsy for this final stage of the pregnancy, we'll use a garden gnome as a visual aid this time. In week 30, the fetus resembles an outdoor decoration, measuring 15.71" and 2.91 lbs. This week, you may take your partner indoors more regularly, as frequent trips to the bathroom continue to form part of the pregnancy symptoms present at this point. As the uterus expands, she may also feel some pressure on her diaphragm, leading to difficulty breathing.

Week 31

Brain development remains a key occurrence, as the fetus is now able to process stimuli and information more efficiently and expansively than before. Fat continues to pad the body, and the head can now be turned from right to left. Thumb-sucking may become more common, and overall growth continues. This latter event means that the week 31 size statistics are recorded as approximately 16.18" and 3.31 lbs. If you go to the movies during this week and buy a large popcorn, you can use it to imagine the size of the fetus.

Week 32

The end is near, and so the growth continues. According to Marple (2019), the fetus will "gain one-third to half their birth weight in the next seven weeks." The skin is now entirely opaque, and nearly all the internal organs have all but completed their development. Notably, the brain and lungs still have some way to go before birth. In week 32, the fetus weighs 3.75 lbs and is 16.69" in length, making it about as big as a large lunch box, potentially the one you take to work every day.

Week 33

In the first week of the ninth month, the bones are becoming more dense, and the immune system starts to take shape. Also, the fetus measures 17.20" and 4.23 lbs, approximately the size of your smaller-than-average chihuahua. Rounding out the relatively uneventful week

33 is the occurrence of abdominal contractions, though these shouldn't be too severe.

Week 34

This week, both the lungs and CNS experienced significant development, with both maturing and increasing in strength. Externally, the vernix coating the body thickens, and overall growth continues. By the end of this week, at 17.72" and 4.73 lbs, the fetus will be about as big as a cantaloupe.

Week 35

The impressive progress seen in the previous week continues as the liver is now able to perform some of its processing functions, and the kidneys have become fully functional. With just over a month left of the pregnancy, the fetus' weight continues to increase in preparation for birth. By the end of week 35, they weigh 5.25 pounds and have a length of 18.19", roughly the same size as a honeydew melon. It's worth noting that the brain's growth also continues, though it is still significantly smaller than it ought to be at the time of birth.

This close to the due date, your partner will definitely be feeling the weight of another living organism in her body. Take as much work and effort off her hands as you can, as even small tasks may result in shortness of breath and tiredness. If she insists on doing something or you cannot take over, ensure that she takes breaks whenever she feels the need, even if this extends the duration of the task.

Week 36

As month number nine comes to a close, the fetus loses their lanugo, though the head on their hair continues to come in. During this week, some of the vernix will also thin out as the amniotic fluid no longer poses such a great risk to the fetal skin. With so little time left in the pregnancy, preparations are being made for their arrival. The bones continue to become stronger, and their position may change in anticipation of moving through the birth canal. Moving away from foodstuffs for a moment, this week, we can take the numbers 18.66" and 5.78lbs and use a throw pillow from the living room as a close equivalent.

Week 37

Movement increases in the final month of pregnancy. Internally, both the brain and lungs continue their development. If any toe- or fingernails have yet to reach the end of their appendages, they will do so during this week. Given how close the due date is, the fetus will also move lower into the pelvis. By week 37, the fetus' figures come in at 19.13" and 6.30 lbs. In keeping with our desire to move away from edible comparisons, you can think of them as being about the same size as the light kettlebells you find in the gym.

Week 38

In order to reach a healthy birth weight, fat continues to be added to the body. This is close to the due date, and most development is coming to an end. However, one thing that won't be finalized is the pigmentation of the irises. Though they will have color by week 38, the specific hue may change until the end of the first year of life. This week, the fetus will be about the same size as a toolbox, measuring 19.61" and 6.80 lbs. Given the significant size of the fetus, your partner may suffer from quite extensive fatigue as well as a decrease in her overall mobility. Some experiences of bodily pain may still persist, specifically in the regions of the neck and back. Eating small, nutrient-rich snacks or meals can help with some quick-acting pain relief, though it is by no means a cure.

Week 39

At week 39, the fetus is considered to be fully developed. The term commonly used is "full-term," denoting the readiness for birth to occur as the gestational period comes to an end (Cleveland Clinic, 2020). Crucially, though development is finished, the fetus will continue to gain weight as long as it remains in utero. As the term comes to an end, the fetus is closest in size to a beach ball, with a length of 19.96" and a weight of 7.25 lbs. Discomfort may persist and intensify this close to the due date, particularly in the pelvic region. You can help your partner relieve some of this through the use of exercises you learned in antenatal classes. More importantly, she should be as relaxed as possible, so take as much from her hands as possible so that she can retain her strength for the delivery date.

Week 40

In the week that the delivery ought to take place, a gallon of milk is the closest equivalent to the fetus' size, being a size of 20.16–21" and 7.63–9lbs. Development has been completed at this point, though growth continues.

Week 41

Fetal growth will continue through the 41st week. While pregnancies beyond the 40-week mark aren't uncommon, you and your partner will most likely be paying a visit to your healthcare provider to discuss delivery options should labor not begin by the end of this week.

Week 42

In week 42, your partner is well past the average due date, and fetal growth will still continue. At this point, discomfort may be very intense, and your healthcare provider will discuss options pertaining to inducement, as pregnancies lasting 42 weeks become increasingly risky for both mother and baby.

The Three Trimesters: Advice for Dads

Trimester One

- Your partner's sense of smell may become stronger during pregnancy, and strong odors may contribute to morning sickness. As such, cut down on perfumed products such as soaps and detergents until this has passed in the second trimester.

- You know how important nutrition is throughout pregnancy. Help your partner recover lost nutrients, vitamins, minerals, and electrolytes by preparing some healthy meals for both of you. If you'd like, you can do this in advance so that this food is readily available when needed.

- Liquids containing ginger can help with nausea and vomiting, and heartburn can be avoided through the elimination of fried and spicy foods, as well as chocolate.

- Help your partner combat fatigue by constructing an easy exercise routine. This needn't be more than a walk around the block, as long as it's sustainable. You can continue this routine for as long as is appropriate.

- Do whatever you can to lighten her load. Everything from chores to errands can fall under your purview for these nine months since she needs her strength to grow an entire person.

- Be patient when hormonal mood swings happen. Hear her out and support her as much as you can. If needed, give her some space to work through her emotions and step in with support when she is ready.

Trimester Two

- Physical changes become more pronounced during this trimester, something about which your partner may feel self-conscious. Help her work through these feelings. Keep a supportive, reassuring attitude to remind her she is doing just fine.

- To reduce the risk of illness and infection, especially UTIs, practice thorough hygiene in all shared spaces. The bathroom, in particular, should be subject to good, regular cleaning.

- You can provide some pain relief through the use of hot compresses and massages.

- If your partner is experiencing nasal congestion, you can give her fluids. If this doesn't work, set up a humidifier to help lessen these blockages.

- Remain involved, especially when it comes to tracking the progress of the pregnancy. For instance, Zalewski (2021) writes that "weight gain and swelling are normal; sudden weight gain could indicate preeclampsia." If changes are manifesting too quickly or intensely, consult your healthcare provider. It may be helpful to keep a chart or journal to keep track of changes pertaining to growth and other important things such as blood pressure, bleeding, and pain.

Trimester Three

- In the final trimester, comfort is the name of the game. Supply as many pillows, blankets, backrests, snacks, and fluids as you can. An excellent way of getting your partner to relax while relieving some pain at the same time is by drawing a warm bath and encouraging her to soak as long as she likes.

- Follow your healthcare provider's advice to a T when it comes to food and drink, as some foods may cause heartburn while others may lead to discomfort. You can continue to prepare and consume the same types of healthy meals and snacks you prepared during the first trimester.

- Massage can still be used as a measure of pain relief. Additionally, doing some light exercise can help to reduce bodily swelling, and keeping the legs elevated can reduce swelling in either limb as well as the ankles.

When Your Baby's Due Date Has Passed

While no due date can be set in stone entirely, it is generally a reliable metric for determining when your baby will arrive. Also known as an "estimated date of delivery" (EDD), a due date is usually calculated using either the timeframe of the last menstrual cycle or by determining the baby's maturation via ultrasound imaging. However, despite the use of relatively reliable, sound mathematics, no EDD is fully guaranteed, as any number of factors may delay or expedite the baby's arrival. In the case of the former, the conversation surrounding the pregnancy shifts. Once your partner passes her due date, her pregnancy transitions from one considered full-term to one termed either "post-term," "prolonged," or "overdue." Note that this term is generally used in cases where the gestational period has extended beyond 42 weeks, though the exact timeframe can differ between countries and healthcare professionals, with some considering a pregnancy post-term from the onset of the 41st week (Institute for Quality and Efficiency in Health Care, 2008).

Frustrating as it may be the cause of an overdue pregnancy is rarely known. In some instances, there are genetic factors that may be at play. In others, moving into the post-term can be tied to a similar delay in a previous pregnancy. However, given how divergent the specifics of each individual pregnancy are, there is no singular, conclusive cause we can point to. It's also worth noting that while moving past the due date will be frustrating for all involved, you don't need to worry about it in advance. The Institute for Quality and Efficiency in Health Care (2008) reports that around 35 in 100 women will go into labor naturally within the first two weeks after the EDD. For only 5 in 100 women, the delay is extended, and should intervention be considered?

This rarity extends to the delay in birth, which proves to be harmful. The 41st week is especially innocuous, though things do change after that. In that first week, however, both mother and baby should be doing just fine, though your partner may experience some discomfort and fatigue. If the EDD has passed, tests will be done to determine whether intervention is necessary. Should these reflect that there is no cause for concern, you may be advised to wait out this week.

Once the 42nd week arrives, the main concerns are the increased risk of infection within the womb and the increased likelihood of complications arising during delivery. Additionally, from this week onwards, there is some concern that the placenta may begin to lose some of its functionality. In the very rare instances where pregnancy is extended beyond week 42, the risk of stillbirth also sees a not-insignificant increase.

From week 42 on, your healthcare provider may start recommending inducement. Factors that may influence this recommendation include:

- Whether complications have arisen that are concerning, but not so much so that a C-section is warranted.

- The emergence of high blood pressure, or preeclampsia.

- There are notable changes in the baby's vital functions or growth.

- Labor has started, but no contractions are felt, and the process is progressing too slowly.

Unless medically necessary, you can still choose not to have labor induced. However, it's worth noting that after the 41st week, being induced can significantly lower the risk of stillbirth or infant death.

Should you choose to have the process started, you can either do so with medical help or by using some traditional, at-home methods. In the latter category, we find strategies such as going for long walks, having sex, acupuncture, hypnosis, drinking tea made from raspberry leaf, and making use of homeopathy. By contrast, medical inducement typically takes the form of any of the following:

- The application to the cervix of hormones known as prostaglandins is typically in the form of a gel.

- Prostaglandins and oxytocin can also be taken orally, intravenously, or via vaginal suppositories, should the gel prove ineffective.

- The insertion of a balloon catheter to open the cervix.

- An amniotomy in which the amniotic sac is opened with a small incision.

- A membrane sweep, in which a finger is used to separate the amniotic sac from the uterine wall.

Inducing labor at this stage has negligible disadvantages. Once your partner has passed her due date this far, she is likely to want to give birth as soon as possible. While it may not be the exact plan you had in place, it's crucial that you rely on the advice of your healthcare provider when amending your birthing plan in this way.

Your Sex Life During and After Pregnancy

Given how much we've discovered will change during pregnancy, it should come as no surprise that your sex life will also be affected by the prospect of impending parenthood. That being said, note that there may be no change at all, neither for yourself nor your partner. This is also perfectly normal, and your sex life continuing as usual is no cause for concern. However, some changes may happen, many of them related to desire and libido. As much as 60% of women have reported a lower sex drive during pregnancy due either to feelings of physical discomfort, severe pregnancy symptoms, or simply an overall lack of desire to engage therein (Levine, 2022).

Hormonal changes may also have an effect, especially in the first trimester. Should this happen, you can expect your partner to potentially become more interested in sex during the second trimester, when the hormone levels are somewhat lower. However, as the third trimester brings pain, discomfort, fatigue, and malaise, you may find your amorous activity dipping low again. Crucially, you may also be the reason your sex life may become more dormant. Many men worry that sex will hurt the baby (it won't) or feel that sexual activity may interfere with aspects of fetal development. Others still simply find themselves less in the mood, potentially due to their partner's difficult experience with pregnancy symptoms.

Though infrequency is what many of our minds may jump to when placing sex in the context of pregnancy, the opposite is also possible. Many people find their libidos elevated during this time. You may find your partner's fertility and femininity very alluring during this, and she may feel the same sense of sensuality about her pregnant body. Increased blood flow to areas such as the vulva, genitals, and breasts. Additionally, both of you may feel a sense of liberation that comes with the ability to discard birth control for a while. For many couples, this means greater room for exploration and an elevated level of physical intimacy.

Whichever way it goes for you and your partner, note that there is no right or wrong experience with sex during pregnancy. If you find that your activity lessens, that's fine. Conversely, if your sex life is more engaged than ever, then by all means, make the most of this time. As long as your communication remains open and honest and no one feels compelled to do something with which they feel uncomfortable, there is no reason your sex life should become an issue at all.

Sex During Pregnancy

Should you and your partner engage in sex regularly during the gestational period, there are some things you will have to take into consideration. This includes the following:

- Libidinous fluctuations are unpredictable, and the nature and frequency of your sex life may change quickly and drastically.

- As the pregnancy progresses and the shape of your partner's body changes, you may have to try some new positions. See this as an opportunity to mix things up and explore things that may potentially be pleasurable for both of you.

- Keep in mind that the release of oxytocin and endorphins during an orgasm may help to calm your partner. As such, work to make the experience as pleasurable as possible for everyone.

- Though this is true of all relationships, regardless of pregnancy, remember that sex isn't guaranteed. There are a lot of changes happening in your partner's body, so respect her decision to cancel your night's sexy plans or retract her consent after sex has started.

- Your partner's genitals and breasts may be especially sensitive or tender during pregnancy, so while you can use this to her advantage, be careful not to overstimulate any part.

- You needn't worry about sex causing a miscarriage, no matter how vigorous. Miscarriages result from a host of other causes, among which sex does not rank.

- Condoms and femidoms may still be necessary if either one of you has a sexually transmitted infection (STI).

- Sex is largely harmless during pregnancy, but you may be dissuaded from partaking in it by your healthcare provider. Instances in which this may happen include when your partner has unexplained vaginal bleeding, is leaking amniotic fluid, the placenta moves to cover the cervix to some degree, or the cervix opens prematurely.

- You should also note that sex will not bring on labor. Though it may result in the experience of Braxton Hicks contractions, especially near the EDD. Furthermore, while popularly believed to be effective, there is no real proof to support the notion that sex will act as a means of natural inducement for an overdue pregnancy.

- Finally, on a lighter subject, you don't have to worry about your child remembering when you and your partner had sex while they were in utero. They will have no recollection and may not even be aware that anything is happening. Should your partner orgasm, there may be a spike in fetal movement, but that is due only to the elevation in heart rate that comes with the moment of climax.

Sex After Pregnancy

Once the little one has arrived in the world, you can expect to wait at least six weeks before sex becomes a viable option again. This is the typical period that elapses after birth, though it's advised that you and your partner move at your own pace. She may feel up for or want to engage in sexual activity as soon as possible, or she may perhaps want to wait longer. A desire to delay a return to sex can be due to a number of reasons, ranging from sensitivity in the vaginal region to insecurities regarding her postpartum body. Whatever the reason, be supportive and respect her decision.

The important thing to remember as you try to get your sex life going after birth is that your partner has experienced what is essentially a bodily trauma. Recovering from childbirth can take some time and may result in difficulties regarding sex. In addition to feeling tired from caring for a newborn and having to endure physical recovery, your partner's hormone levels take a dip, which may lessen the amount of vaginal lubricant produced. This may make sex uncomfortable or downright painful (Raising Children Network (Australia), 2022). Again, support your partner as she makes her recovery, and don't try to expedite the process, especially if she has expressed hesitance or fear.

It's possible that your view on pregnancy may be forever changed after reading this chapter, which isn't necessarily a bad thing. If anything, you should now understand exactly what your partner will experience over the course of nine months, if not longer. As unsettling or worrying as some of this information may be, remember that it empowers you to be her strongest pillar of support and to help her through what can be an extremely tough time, both physically and emotionally. Pregnancy won't always be the glorious origin of life experience many make it out to be. There may be instances where it becomes an onerous load to bear, and things may become heavy for both of you. Remember that the more you know, the more you can do, and the lighter both your loads will be.

Chapter 7:

Overcoming the Challenges of Pregnancy

When considered as a whole, we see that pregnancy contains many facets that are pure joy. However, as with most things in life, this experience has its darker aspects too, and though we'd like to believe that our partners' pregnancies will go off without a hitch, it's all too possible that things may go wrong. As morbid as it may seem, it's worth knowing what the worst-case scenarios may be and preparing how to deal with them. One of the most common challenges your partner may face is that of postpartum depression (PPD), though there are a host of other difficulties that may cross your path during or after the gestational period.

According to Carberg & Langdon (2019), approximately one in every 10 women will experience PPD, with this number rising to one in seven in some studies. Furthermore, despite its prevalence, their article reports that nearly half of all PPD cases aren't formally diagnosed or treated. This disorder is a strange thing to navigate, as it typically lasts no longer than six months, though a number of different factors may lengthen its duration. It's important for you to know these things, as depressing as they may be so that you can provide support for your partner and call in for help when you are out of your depth. This importance becomes much clearer if we consider that 80% of PPD patients make a full recovery, something you can help make happen if you know what's going on.

Pregnancy Complications

Within the context of pregnancy, complications refer to any mental or physical conditions that may affect your partner and baby either during the gestational or postpartum period. Complications often arise during pregnancy, though they can manifest before or after as well (Centers for Disease Control and Prevention, 2022). Pregnancy complications can be caused by any number of things, including changes that happen as the fetus develops, as well as preexisting health conditions. Some of the more common complications you can keep an eye out for include:

- Anemia, a condition characterized by decreased red blood cell levels.

- Anxiety disorders, in which your partner struggles with feelings of worry, fear, and panic. Treatment for this and any other mental health issues that arise during pregnancy is essential, as your partner's overall health has a direct impact on that of your baby. Note that anxiety disorders often present comorbidly with depressive disorders.

- Congenital disorders, such as those covered in Chapter 5.

- Depression, specifically episodes that last for more than two weeks. This complication poses a significant threat, as depressed people often neglect their own well-being. In this case, this can have an impact on the fetus' health and development, especially if your partner's depression causes her to skip meals or the taking of prenatal supplements.

- Diabetes, which may be type 1, type 2, or gestational diabetes.

- Ectopic pregnancy, in which the zygote implants in the lining of the fallopian tube as opposed to that of the uterus. These pregnancies will need to be medically terminated, as the fetus cannot develop outside the uterus.

- High blood pressure, which may be either chronic or gestational hypertension.

- Hyperemesis gravidarum, characterized by intense vomiting and nausea, is more common than is typical, even in cases of severe morning sickness.

- Infections can be anything from a yeast infection to an STI or HIV.

- Placental placement issues, either placenta previa (where the cervix is covered by the placenta, either partially or fully) or placenta accreta, where the placental attachment goes awry, with the placenta growing too deeply into the lining.

- Preeclampsia, which can manifest by the halfway point, can also appear within the first six weeks of the postpartum period.

- Preterm labor describes deliveries taking place before the 37th week of pregnancy.

- Stillbirth, which differs from a miscarriage in that it takes place after the 20th week of pregnancy. In most cases, the cause of this complication cannot be determined.

- Vaginal bleeding. Though this may be common at some points during pregnancy (see Chapter 6), excessive or sustained bleeding should be addressed with a visit to a healthcare provider.

Should your partner be diagnosed with any of these complications, it's entirely normal for her to become worried or fearful. Though most conditions are treatable, pregnancy complications can be overwhelming. Once this news has been delivered, it's time for you to step into your role as a supporter once more. Here are some dos and don'ts when providing support:

- Don't make your support inconsistent or conditional. Be there for your partner as much as you can, being a non-judgmental pillar on which she can lean.

- Don't make assumptions or offer explanations as to the cause of the complications.

- Don't wait for your partner to ask for help. You know her well and know what will upset her. Be proactive and step in before things get too bad, letting her know you'll be there all the way.

- Foster healthy communication by asking open-ended questions and giving her the time and space to express her feelings.

- Acknowledge the truth of the situation, and don't tiptoe around the issue or its effects.

- Though you can certainly offer words of encouragement and comfort, make sure you listen more than you speak.

- Provide her with a safe space in your company, and keep it that way even when neither of you knows how the path ahead will look.

- When appropriate, share your own feelings so that she knows she isn't suffering alone. It's more than okay for the two of you to lean on each other.

Postpartum Depression

We've already encountered PPD in some measure, but the truth of the disorder is much more than a handful of statistics. The very first thing to note is that there is a difference between baby blues and PPD. Postpartum hormonal changes are a major contributor to the extremely common condition known as baby blues. Baby blues, a mild form of depression, leads to feelings of restlessness and anxiety and may result in a lot of crying. By contrast, PPD is a longer-lasting, more severe mental condition (Johns Hopkins Medicine, 2019).

PPD lasts much longer than a week or two, which is the typical duration of baby blues. Moreover, PPD is debilitating. The trauma of childbirth may naturally lead to an emotional rollercoaster. However, if your partner's feelings of sadness, anxiety, restlessness, etc. impede her ability to continue her day-to-day functioning, it's likely she has developed PPD. While depression is largely an internal event, there are some signs you can keep an eye out for. Should any of the following present themselves in your partner, consider consulting a mental health care professional:

- She no longer enjoys the things before the baby's birth, nor does she take particular joy in interacting with the newborn.

- She regularly expresses doubt in her ability to be a good parent.

- She has trouble making decisions.

- Her sleeping patterns have changed independently of childcare, meaning that she has trouble staying awake even when rested or cannot bring herself to sleep even when the baby is in bed.

- She shuts down and isolates herself, refusing interpersonal interaction in favor of a solitary activity or simply doing nothing.

- She presents a significant reluctance to leave the house.

- She experiences drastic weight loss or demonstrates other signs of neglecting her well-being.

The manifestation of PPD requires you to support your partner to a greater extent than before. The first way of doing so is by helping her realize she has a problem. You have to get her to recognize that her behaviors and thoughts are maladaptive and that she needs help. Once she has realized this, you can encourage her to seek professional help. Consequently, you can help by supporting her through whatever course of treatment is recommended. Help facilitate her recovery by doing what you can to help her follow the doctor's advice. You can also show your support and understanding by tackling specific things you know she is struggling with. In doing so, you not only help her out but also let her know that you see what she is going through and that her experience matters to you.

Some general tips for handling postpartum depression include the following:

- Don't shy away from addressing her depression, and don't gloss over her expressions of self-doubt or negative self-talk.

- Lower the expectations you have of your partner right now, and remember that she is navigating both mental health issues and the task of being a new parent.

- Regularly remind her that she is loved and that you are there for her. It may not appear to have any immediate effect, but it will make a difference in the long run.

- Take care of yourself so that you don't burn out while trying to care for her.

- Understand where your limits lie. You cannot fix her or provide everything she needs.

Miscarriage

Having a miscarriage is a concern for every expectant mother, and the actual experience of losing a pregnancy is devastating. Though each situation will be different, you will find some general tips below describing what you can do to help your partner navigate this intensely difficult and painful experience:

- Provide your partner with some extra TLC, and be mindful not to become withdrawn.

- Share your own thoughts and feelings so that she understands she isn't alone in this.

- Take into consideration that your partner may not only be grieving the lost child but also the life she had imagined for them.

- Do research into the signs and symptoms of depression, and keep an eye out for when grief may potentially transition into something more.

- While you shouldn't just ignore the issue, excessive discussions also aren't necessary. Talk about it when your partner wants to and when both of you feel comfortable enough to discuss the loss.

- When some time has passed, help your partner find some healthy coping mechanisms. There are no requirements other than the fact that it should take her out of her own head for a while.

- Don't try to provide comfort by looking to the future or mentioning a possible next pregnancy.

- Ensure your partner knows that she can express her feelings when around you, and hold space for her to work through what she is thinking and experiencing.

- As with grieving any other loss, give her time.

It's important to note that while the information above outlines how you can support your partner, you should allow yourself space to deal with the loss as well. Don't shove your feelings aside in favor of attending to your partner's. Acknowledge what has happened, and support your own journey of grief as much as hers.

Problems and Stress Related to Relationships

For all its wonder, pregnancy can elicit significant feelings of stress in both you and your partner. At one point or another, the two of you may find yourselves chafing against one another, something caused largely by the changes your lives are undergoing and the stress that comes along with attempting to navigate them.

In the antenatal months, you may find contention bubbling up time and time again. The first source of this may stem from feelings that emotions regarding pregnancy aren't shared in equal measure. Your partner may feel that she is more excited about the prospect of parenthood than you, and vice versa. Alongside this, you may also find that your partner feels you are unable to truly comprehend her experience, as she is undergoing those physical and emotional changes alone.

Additionally, many couples find the matter of sex to become an issue during pregnancy. We've already addressed this to an extent, but it's worth mentioning again, as a decrease in sexual intimacy can take its toll on a relationship, with many people feeling as though intimacy between them and their partner has vanished entirely. Other issues you may encounter during pregnancy include conflict regarding the baby's name, feelings of disbelief regarding the prospect of becoming a parent, your partner finding you to be too clingy or overprotective, and an array of anxieties. For the latter, it can be anything from your partner worrying you no longer find her attractive to anxiety relating to assuming the responsibility of parenthood and worrying that pregnancy symptoms are proving detrimental to your connection.

The postpartum period may bring with it several difficulties of its own. Most commonly, parents experience friction stemming from irritability caused by exhaustion and the overwhelming task of caring for a newborn. Because your attention will be focused on the baby, your relationship may take a hit in terms of the quality time you spend with your partner. A great source of conflict in the time after birth is the division of labor. In many relationships, women are still tasked with performing the majority of the household duties, all while recovering from childbirth. For many couples, the financial strain that comes with parenthood can drastically affect the quality of their relationship. Finally, you may find that your tiredness and constant occupation leads to a breakdown in communication, which will lead to a host of problems down the road.

Understanding which issues may arise during pregnancy is the first step, with the second being taking the time and effort to work out these kinks in your relationship. To that end, you may want to consider the following:

- Ensure that your communication in the pre- and postpartum periods remains open and honest. Create a safe space for one another to express your thoughts, feelings, and concerns. Subsequently, listen without judgment.

- With difficulties regarding names, step away from the conversation if it gets heated or repetitive. Return when both of you are calm and ready. Then, talk through your reasons for wanting a certain name and allow your partner to do the same. Be willing to compromise.

- Try to remain calm as much as you can, as getting agitated may only serve to worsen things.

- If sex becomes an issue, talk through what the exact problem is. Should the issue be tied to pleasure or a desire for physical intimacy, find other ways for the both of you to get what you need. If it is simply about closeness and intimacy in general, brainstorm alternatives to sex that will still bring you close to one another.

- Finances are a big issue, but they should already be part of your prenatal preparation. Refer to the section in Chapter 3 discussing finances to see how you can structure your expenditures as a new parent.

It's worth noting that relationship problems arising during pregnancy don't cancel out existing issues between you and your partner. If anything, the added stress may exacerbate these problems. It's essential that you address each of the negative aspects of your relationship, regardless of when they originated.

As this chapter draws to a close, you may be beginning to realize just how much of a team effort pregnancy is. Though your partner is the one experiencing physical changes, you may find that both of you experience emotional or mental challenges in equal measure. As such, remember to keep an open mind and to speak up when necessary. Though you can't be everything for your partner, being there as much as you can will help. If the prospect seems overwhelming, keep in mind that relationships are a two-way street and that your partner will be there to hold your hand, too. Neither of you will go through this alone, and realizing that can make all the difference in the world.

Chapter 8:

Remembering the Other Person in Your Pregnancy Journey

Thus far, our focus has largely been on your partner, the changes she will experience, and how you can be a pillar of support during good times and bad. While this isn't necessarily a bad thing—pregnancy will take its toll on her—it's important that the care you provide for your partner doesn't come at the expense of the care you ought to provide for yourself. It can be tempting to try and do it all as a father, but no one can be everything to everyone, not healthily. As we move into this chapter, you would do well to keep the words of Lamott (2015) near the back of your brain: "Almost everything will work again if you unplug it for a few minutes, including you."

Postpartum Depression in Men

Surprising though it may sound, the experience of postpartum depression isn't limited to women, with as many as one in every 10 new fathers experiencing this form of depression. Referred to as paternal postnatal depression (PPND), this condition describes a debilitating change in a father's emotional state and functionality within the first year of parenthood (Berendzen, 2023). PPND largely looks the same in men as it does in women, though there are some differences.

This form of depression can develop during pregnancy, as with women, though men have been shown to be most vulnerable to its manifestation in the first trimester. Should PPND only occur after birth, it's likely to do so three to six months after the fact.

Additionally, some basic facts to know about PPND include the following:

- PPND can manifest as either mild symptoms or a condition severe enough to warrant diagnosis. The National Childbirth Trust (2022c) reports that between 10% and 12% of new fathers' depression will receive a formal diagnosis, while as much as 25% will experience mild, temporary symptoms.

- Due to a variety of societal and cultural factors, PPND mostly goes undiagnosed. Crucially, a similar lack of clinical attention is present with PPD as well.

- Between 25% and 50% of dads whose partner struggles with depression experience similar psychological troubles.

- There are many risk factors present with PPND, with age being a significant one among them. Fathers aged 25 and under are at greater risk for the development of depression.

- PPND may have an impact on your child's development. Depression in fathers has been linked to issues regarding social, behavioral, and emotional maturation.

- Though they differ greatly in some aspects, therapeutic treatments for PPND are largely the same as for PPD.

One of the most prominent differences between PPD and PPND lies in their origin. The continuation of hormonal fluctuations after delivery is thought to contribute to PPD in women. However, while hormones may also contribute to the experience of PPND, it's a drop in testosterone levels that occurs soon after the baby's birth that's most notable. Fluctuations in estrogen and cortisol also occur during the postpartum period. Along with this particular change, we see that the timeline of each disorder differs. Women often reach the severest extent of their symptoms within the first few months of the postpartum period. By contrast, this same peak may only occur for men closer to the end of the first year.

Interestingly, the presentation of the two different depressions is also different. Men tend to externalize the disorder, engaging in anger and risk-taking behaviors. Women experience PPD more internally, retreating into themselves. Understanding the difference between these types of depression is important, as is knowing which aspects of your life and personhood make you more vulnerable to its occurrence. Risk factors for PPND include:

- Preexisting mental health issues.
- Severe complications or trauma during the birth of your child.
- Financial stress.
- Problems with alcohol and substance use.
- Provider pressure.
- Cultural expectations regarding your role in your child's life, especially if you deviate from these norms.
- Lack of sleep.
- Strain or stress in your relationship.
- Fears about parenthood and the changes it brings.
- Your baby is experiencing health issues.
- A less-than-dependable support network.

Risk factors alone aren't enough to tell you whether there is cause for concern. As such, keep an eye out for the following signs and symptoms:

- Throwing yourself into work or, conversely, withdrawing from it.
- Impulsivity is coupled with risk-taking behaviors.
- Suicidal ideation.

- Irritability.

- A lack of motivation.

- Sudden outbursts of rage or violence.

- Difficulty concentrating.

- Physical issues such as indigestion and pain in your stomach, head, or muscles.

- Exhaustion.

- Lack of appetite.

- Insomnia.

- Noticeable, sudden weight loss or gain.

Should you suspect that you may have PPND, rest assured that the condition needn't be permanent, as there are a number of different interventions available to you. The first thing to do is to speak with your partner and the people who make up your support system. Expressing your feelings and having a safe space to work through them can work wonders. Beyond that, you can also engage in some self-help techniques, including mindful practices such as yoga and meditation. Keep in mind that you can always seek professional help. If you do, note that treatment will likely consist of therapy sessions with a mental health care professional and that you may be prescribed medications should the need arise.

Coping With Miscarriages and Loss

Losing a pregnancy is always devastating, both for your partner and for you. For many men, the impulse is to ignore their own pain and grief in favor of tending to their partner's. While there is certainly nothing wrong with helping your partner through this difficult experience, glossing over what you are going through isn't exactly a healthy means of coping. Though it may be difficult to do so, you have to acknowledge how the miscarriage is affecting you, too. You are allowed to grieve the loss you have suffered and to experience all the thoughts and feelings that come along with it.

After a miscarriage, it's important that you continue to care for yourself. Make sure you get plenty of sleep and that you continue to exercise regularly while maintaining a balanced, healthy diet. While this may prove helpful to an extent, it amounts to a cotton ball over a large wound in the long run. The only way to truly feel better is to work through your grief. You can do this by opening up to the people in your life, whether friends, family, or even your partner. If this makes you uncomfortable or you feel they won't understand, don't be scared to consult a professional.

The truth is that there is no right or easy way to work through this kind of loss. As such, do whatever feels right in order to process your grief. If that involves shouting at the universe or crying for hours on end, then that's just what you need to do. Crucially, don't withdraw from or hide your pain. You aren't alone in this, and reaching out to those who will love and support you may prove to be the greatest source of comfort and the most potent contributor to your recovery.

Support Groups for Fathers

Father support groups are pretty much what the name suggests. They are spaces, either physical or virtual, in which dads are able to communicate with one another about, well, being dads. Experience or the number of children isn't important in support groups, as their purpose is to help men learn the ins and outs of fatherhood from one another, particularly through learning about parenting from different perspectives (Galla, 2020). In addition to having the goal of education, support groups aim to provide dads with a safe space in which they can share their parenting triumphs and defeats, as well as in which they can connect with other dads whose experiences resemble their own.

The need for a support group may not be apparent from the get-go, but it is advisable that you seek one out even if you feel prepared for parenthood. Keep in mind that parenting is something you learn by doing, and the dads in a support group will potentially have done quite a bit, thus making them a treasure trove of information. Fathers nowadays want to be more involved in their children's lives, but they may not have people in their lives they can look to as models for positive parenting behaviors. By joining a father support group, you will find the role models you are looking for and may even build a support network that can help you become the dad you've always wanted to be. In addition to these positive aspects, there are a number of other benefits presented by father support groups, including:

- They offer the opportunity for connection and present you with many potential new friendships, particularly with people whose life trajectory resembles yours.

- Because not everyone in the group will have the same experience or perspective as you, you stand to gain guidance from a variety of different avenues. You may not know how to solve a problem with your approach, but a support group dad who sees it another way may just have the answer.

- Father support groups can provide you with valuable resources, both in terms of guidance and literature. As your child grows, the knowledge you need to have will change. In these groups, you can find recommendations for learning resources.

You can find father support groups in a number of different ways. In-person groups meet at the same location and with the same frequency, usually once or twice per week or per month. A quick online search will let you know which of these groups can be found in your area. However, if you are unable to attend in-person meetings or simply prefer virtual spaces, you can join an online support group. These groups may also have regularly scheduled meetings or have chat spaces open 24/7. There are a large number of online father support groups out there, though some are better known than others. The most popular online father support groups include forums such as the National Fatherhood Initiative, MensGroup, Fathers4Kids, and Dads

Group. Note that if you can't find a group that appeals to you, there's nothing stopping you from reaching out to friends, family, and community members to start your own!

Self-Care Tips

By now, it should be apparent that taking care of yourself is an important part of being an effective, involved father. Though you may sometimes feel guilty for doing something just for you, remember that the stronger your physical and emotional state, the better your parenting abilities will be, as will your presence in your relationship. It's also worth noting that some self-care activities can make you more involved in the parenting process, which in turn can make you feel like a better, more hands-on dad.

Some easy-to-implement self-care strategies include the following:

- Taking responsibility for parenting tasks without needing to be prompted by your partner.

- Spend quality time with your child by playing, singing, reading, or just enjoying one another's company.

- Don't allow sexist, uncomfortable gender roles to limit you. When it comes to parenting and your presence in the home, do what feels right to you, and don't let antiquated ideas limit your involvement.

- Take advantage of any opportunities your work provides for paternity leave, as it will allow you to be there after birth and gain your footing as a father.

- Stay healthy by eating a balanced diet and exercising regularly. The latter can also be used as opportunities for infant-father bonding, as you can take your baby along on a walk or a jog through the park.

- Actively make time for you and your partner so that you can reinforce your connection.

- Take care of your physical appearance by keeping yourself tidily groomed.

- Try to find some inner peace and stabilization through mindful practices like yoga and meditation.

- Keep your brain active and strong by doing some puzzles or other cognitively stimulating activities.

- Engage in your hobbies whenever you can. If you don't have any, find some passions that will provide you with some me-time.

- Take naps when you can.

- Don't feel afraid or ashamed to accept help from your support network when it is offered.

Your preparational journey towards fatherhood is nearly complete, and given everything you've learned thus far, you may feel awkward or guilty about paying attention to your own needs. This counts for both the antenatal and postnatal periods. However, in those moments, it's worth remembering that your efforts as a dad will mean so much more if you are fully there, emotionally as well as physically. It's natural to want all the attention to be focused on your partner, as this is a monumental time for her. Keep in mind that it's just as big for you. More importantly, keep in mind that your desire to be a good father is the driving force behind your presence here. Once you consider that, it should be all the easier to realize that a healthy, balanced, and stable father is the best kind of father to be.

Chapter 9:

Preparing for Your First Day as a Dad... and Beyond

Nine long months have passed, and finally, the day is here! After today, your partner's due date, you will forevermore be a father. However, before you go trying to use every tip you've learned at once, take a moment to familiarize yourself with what will happen on the day. First and foremost, note that only 5% of babies are born on their actual EDD (*Interesting childbirth and delivery facts*, 2006). So, even if today's marked on the calendar, don't count on popping the confetti just yet. Some other facts you can fill your head with to distract from your excitement include the fact that your child will be born without kneecaps and that they will be able to recognize your partner's voice and scent from the moment of their arrival. Also, your infant is a pretty tough cookie, possessing a wealth of strength comparable to oxen, particularly in their legs.

Why You Should Attend the Birth

Chances are, if you've made it this far, your intention to be there for the moment of your child's arrival is fairly strong. However, regardless of how determined you may be to attend the birth, it's always a good idea to know *exactly* why your presence is such an important part of the birthing process. The first component of this importance can be found in the fact that just being there means something to your partner. You have been a part of this journey from the very beginning, and seeing it through all the way to the end means you are the final piece of the puzzle. Even though you may not be able to do something specific, by giving your partner the ability to see and touch, you will provide comfort and support.

Furthermore, Dlugosz (2013) reports that a father's presence during their child's birth signals their commitment to the parenting process. The same study found that your presence makes the birthing space feel safer, as your partner has someone there who will support her without judgment and for whom she won't need to justify her feelings or experiences. Finally, all things considered, being in the room and holding your partner's hand when she delivers your child is the very least you can do. Regardless of your level of involvement throughout the pregnancy, know that your partner has been tasked with so much more.

D-Day Hospital Bag Packing Checklist

Once D-Day (with the "D" meaning delivery) rolls around, there are a number of supplies you will need to get you through the birth process as well as the recovery time afterward. All of these items can be packed in a designated hospital bag a few weeks before the EDD. No item is compulsory, and you are more than free to pack the bag according to your specific needs and circumstances. Additionally, if your partner will not be spending the night in recovery at the birthing location, you will only need packing supplies for the duration of labor and the few hours before you return home. Your partner will most likely take care of her bag's items as well as the baby's. As such, you can focus on your own supplies and those of another support person, should there be one.

Supplies for Birthing Coaches and Partners

- Identification and any documents you may need to present when checking your partner in.
- A phone charger.
- Cash.
- A pillow.

- Toiletries.
- A change of clothes, preferably something lightweight and comfortable.
- Snacks and beverages.
- A recording device, should you wish to capture the birth on video.
- Something to keep you occupied during the wait. You can pack the same type of entertainment as your partner, bringing things you can do together as well as some diversions just for you.

While you should certainly stock up on necessities for your trip to the birthing location, be careful not to overdo it. One change of clothes will be more than enough. Moreover, you don't have to haul your entire nursery to the delivery room. While you can certainly bring a few diapers and other items you deem essential, rest assured that your healthcare provider will furnish you with some supplies as well. Finally, should you wish to bring valuables with you (cash, jewelry, electronics, etc.), be mindful of the fact that the delivery room will be a flurry of activity, especially in the final stages of labor. As such, try to avoid packing things you definitely don't want to lose but cannot keep track of the entire time.

You can start to gather your hospital bag supplies as early as you'd like. However, it's recommended that you pack no later than the end of week 38. In high-risk pregnancies, this is pushed up to the end of week 35 (Kashtan, 2023). That being said, don't bring too much. You can check ahead of time what size bag (and how many) you will be allowed to bring to the birthing location. Many institutions have guidelines and may even be able to give you some tips if you ask. One such tip you can get now is that your hospital bag can be anything from a backpack to a duffel bag, as long as its contents make you prepared for the day. And for an extra touch of preparedness, pop the bag in your car's trunk or backseat once it has been packed. That way, it'll be ready to go when you are. If you aren't driving to the birthing location, place the bag by the door or in a place where you can't miss it.

How to Help During Labor and Delivery

While your presence on the day of birth is important in and of itself, the value you bring to the delivery room will increase exponentially if you understand how the process will proceed and how you can lend a hand. This starts with recognizing the signs of labor. The childbirth process will most likely start with physical symptoms such as persistent pain, specifically in the region of the lower back. Contractions will come along with this, increasing in frequency and intensity as labor progresses. In addition to these symptoms, your partner may find that some discharge is excreted from the vaginal area. This will be both the mucus plug and the amniotic fluid. Take note that in the case of the former, labor may still be some ways away, though it is an indicator that the process has begun. You may know the latter better as your partner's "water breaking." Once the amniotic fluid has been released in this way, you can count on labor not being too far behind. It's worth noting that your partner's water may only break quite some time after contractions have started, though this isn't always the case (Cassell, 2021).

When the day comes, contractions will be the best way for you to keep track of how labor is progressing and to know when it's time to move to your birthing location. You will be timing the contractions, starting at the onset of one and counting in seconds until the beginning of the next. Keeping track of the contractions' duration and interval will help you determine when it's time to grab the hospital bag and go. The further apart your partner's contractions are, the longer the labor process still has to go. When they become closer and more intense, you need to start considering heading for the door. For a more precise estimate, use the 4-1-1 rule, meaning there is a contraction at least every four minutes, and the pain lasts for at least one minute, establishing a regular pattern over a period of one hour. If your partner's pregnancy is more high-risk or there are other health issues, you may wish to use the 5-1-1 variation of the rule, changing the interval from four to five minutes.

More often than not, you can use contractions and the water breaking alone to determine when it's time to go. However, there are certain instances in which you can forego the typical process and head directly to your chosen birthing location. These instances may indicate that complications have arisen or that your partner or baby may potentially be in distress. Go to the hospital immediately if your partner experiences vaginal bleeding to a greater extent than constitutes spotting. You can also keep an eye on the amniotic fluid. If it is colored or has a strong, unpleasant odor, it may indicate a cord prolapse or the contamination of the amniotic fluid. Finally, you should travel to a healthcare practitioner immediately if your partner reports significant decreases in fetal movement.

Barring any complications, the idea is that you go to your birthing location when your partner moves into active labor. This is the second of three distinct stages in which labor takes place. The first stage comprises three distinct phases: early, active, and transition. The early phase typically lasts approximately 12 hours and largely involves your partner's contractions steadily growing in intensity and frequency. By the time this phase concludes, your partner's cervix will be dilated by about three centimeters. Following this is the six-hour active phase, during which contractions last between 40 and 60 seconds. Along with an increased frequency, your partner's contractions will be much more intense, and dilation will increase to between four and seven centimeters. The first stage of labor concludes with the transition phase, lasting anything from minutes to hours. Contractions are now 60 to 90 seconds long, much closer together, and extremely intense. As the first stage draws to a close, your partner's cervix will dilate to the full 10 centimeters (Winder, 2015).

The second stage of labor can similarly last only a few minutes, though it may also be stretched out over the course of several hours. The typical duration of this stage is a minimum of 15 minutes, though it should come as no surprise if it lasts up to three hours. Contractions in this stage are the same length as those in the transition phase, and your partner will start to push once her cervical dilation reaches 10 centimeters. Subsequently, labor concludes with the third stage, which begins once your baby has been welcomed into the world. This stage is characterized by the delivery of the placenta and lasts approximately five to 20 minutes.

Labor and Delivery: Some Handy Tips for Dads

- Ensure that your partner doesn't expend essential energy during early labor. Encourage her to rest and relax in order to conserve her strength for the later stages and phases.

- If you plan on recording the birth, clear the angle of the shot with your partner ahead of time and remain out of the healthcare practitioners' way while you capture the special moment.

- Understand that childbirth is a messy, primal process, and make peace with the fact that your partner may not be at her best during this time.

- Don't take what is said during the labor process too personally. Your partner may lash out due to pain or stress, but that doesn't truly mean anything bad. Take these remarks with a heavy pinch of salt.

- Support in whichever way you can, whether you feed your partner ice chips, describe the contraction monitor's activity or help her change positions during the first stage of labor.

- Don't be afraid to ask questions. You can do this if you are unsure of something, but you should definitely speak up if your partner is confused or curious.

What Happens if You Don't Make It Out of the House

Over the course of the preceding nine chapters, we've explored just how important planning is as you make your way towards fatherhood. However, we all know what they say about the best-laid plans. Because we have to take into account that the universe may throw you a curveball on the day of your baby's birth, it's worth knowing what to do should you and your partner be unable to move to your chosen birthing location. This information only applies if you don't have a home birth or if you cannot reach the intended location of the birth and is by no means a guide to delivering a baby. Should you be required to deliver your child, these steps can help. Even so, you should seek medical attention as soon as possible after the baby has arrived. You can prepare for this occurrence by gathering the necessary materials ahead of time and storing them somewhere accessible.

If you cannot make it out of the house for the delivery, take the following steps:

- First and foremost, call emergency services for help. Stay on the line with them as long as possible so they can provide you with guidance.

- If your partner's labor is progressing quickly and she has entered the second stage, it's advisable that you prepare for the possibility of a home delivery.

- Gather the supplies needed, including surgical gloves, clean plastic sheeting, clean shoe laces, cotton balls, scissors, cold packs, a hot water bottle, a baby-sized bulb syringe, sterilizing alcohol, and hand sanitizer.

- Keep your partner calm and comfortable as much as you can. Remember to wear gloves when handling bodily fluids, and keep any animals and kids out of the makeshift delivery room.

- You can prepare the bed for delivery by placing a shower curtain or other length of plastic (such as a clean tarpaulin) over the sheets. Place another sheet on top of the plastic, and pad the bed with pillows and other soft items for comfort.

- If your partner expresses that she has an insuppressible urge to push, position yourself where you can see the baby exit the birth canal.

- Guide her through the process by helping her regulate her breathing as she pushes. Remind her to push gently, even when compelled to use more force.

- The head will come out first, followed by the shoulders and the rest of the body.

- Next, you will need to clip the umbilical cord. Should it be wrapped around the infant's neck, simply loosen it so that the head can slip through or so that you can pull it over the head.

- Making a double knot, tie a shoelace tightly around the cord, approximately three inches from the infant's abdomen. Place a second knot about two inches above the first. Snip the cord between the two knots.

- When the placenta is pushed through the vaginal canal, there will be some blood and other fluids, which you can staunch by firmly pressing on your partner's abdomen below the navel.

- Once the process has been completed, give your partner some fluids and something light to eat. Seek medical attention for her and the newborn as soon as you can.

The Apgar Score

Named after its creator, Dr Virginia Apgar, this test is an assessment of your newborn's medical need for medical attention immediately after birth. The results are used to determine their overall health and whether any medical intervention is necessary (Healthline Australia, 2019). The Apgar test is performed at both one and five minutes after birth, with each individual score quantifying different successes. The first score measures how the infant has tolerated the birthing process. The five-minute score measures how well the baby is acclimating to life outside the womb. It's worth noting that the results aren't in any way indicative of your child's health prognosis for life. Instead, it is meant as an immediate assessment tool to determine what your baby needs in the time following their birth.

The Apgar test is comprised of five different criteria, namely:

- Appearance refers to your newborn's skin tone. Typically, the skin tone will shift from blue to pink once oxygenated blood circulates through the body.

- Pulse, which measures the heart rate as well as the organ's ability to pump blood.

- Grimace refers to your infant's reaction to stimuli. This criterion is also known as reflex irritability.

- Activity: measuring the newborn's movement and muscle tone.

- Respiration is determined by the volume and length of your baby's cries. This criterion checks to see how strong their breathing effort is.

Apgar scores are relatively easy to interpret. Each criterion is given a score out of two, with zero being the worst and two being the best result. These scores are tallied to provide you with an overall score out of 10. Typically, a score of seven or higher is considered indicative of good postpartum adaptation. Lower than this, and your healthcare provider may wish to monitor your baby further or administer some form of treatment. There's no need to worry if your newborn doesn't score a perfect 10, as this rarely happens. In fact, the Cleveland Clinic (2022a) reports that most infants score between seven and nine, with 90% achieving a score between seven and 10.

The Newborn Screening Test

Newborn screening (NBS) involves a panel of tests performed between 24 and 48 hours after birth. NBS tests to determine whether your baby has serious conditions or disorders that may be rare but are treatable for the most part (*Newborn screening tests for your baby*, 2015). The tests can be conducted using either a one-screen or two-screen model. The former involves once-off testing a day or two after birth, while the latter performs a first screening in those first days with a second set of tests conducted one to two weeks postpartum.

Typically, NBS is comprised of three components, namely:

- Blood spot screening, in which some blood is taken from the baby's heel.

- Hearing screening, in which earbuds or earphones are used to determine the strength of the baby's aural sense.

- Heart screening, also known as pulse oximetry screening, is a process in which a sensor is used to test for critical congenital heart disease.

A newborn screening is a fairly comprehensive set of tests, and the NBS ordinarily tests for specific conditions. Note that while it may vary depending on where you live, your baby's NBS will screen for:

- Biotinidase deficiency
- Congenital adrenal hyperplasia
- Congenital hypothyroidism
- Galactosemia
- Hearing loss
- Homocystinuria
- Maple syrup urine disease
- Medium-chain acyl-CoA dehydrogenase deficiency
- Phenylketonuria

- Sickle cell disease

Variations in NBS are extended to your options as parents with regards to the logistics of the screening as well. While most states in the US have instated NBS as a mandatory postpartum health screening, there are some states in which you may be able to refuse to have the panel performed. Note that this is very much dependent on your state's laws. In some cases, you will only be able to refuse the NBS for reasons related to religion, while others may allow you to refuse the screening for any reason provided. Another option you may find presented to you pertains to the storage of your infant's blood sample. While not common practice in all states, you may be given the option to have the sample destroyed, stored, or preserved and used for research purposes. You can find out more about which options are available to you regarding the NBS by contacting the newborn screening program that has been set up in your area or state.

Along with knowing what your options are, there are some other questions you ask either in anticipation of the screening or once it has been conducted. Note that some of the questions can be posed before your baby's birth so that the NBS may be incorporated into your birth plan. These questions include the following:

- Will we have to request the NBS, or will it be conducted automatically?

- Can either I or my partner accompany the baby during the screening?

- How long after the screening will the results be available?

- How will we receive the results?

- What course of action will be taken should the results be abnormal or out-of-range?

- Can we consult with a healthcare provider regarding the way forward?

- Are the costs tied to the NBS covered by insurance?

While there is little you can do in preparation for the NBS, there are some steps that can be taken should the results prove to be less than desirable. The first thing to note is that abnormal results don't necessarily equate to a diagnosis, and it may merely be indicative of a need for further testing. Most likely, if the results indicate that something is amiss, your healthcare provider will perform a second diagnostic test. With this second test, normal results will indicate no need for further action or screening. Should the results be unusual or indicative of an underlying condition, you will be given more specific guidance and assistance by your healthcare provider.

Taking Your Baby Home

Bringing your baby home from the birthing location can be an auspicious moment in your journey as a family and will certainly be a sentimental one. Because this is the first step you will be taking together as a family, don't feel as though you have to rush home, especially from the hospital. Ensure that your partner and baby are both doing fine and that all of your questions have been answered before you go. If there is something about which you feel unsure or that you think warrants attention, ask one of the medical professionals who will be all around you.

When it comes to actually taking your little one home with you, two things are paramount to making a successful journey home: clothing and car safety. In the first category, it's important to remember that a newborn doesn't have the same abilities for temperature regulation as you. As such, they require an extra layer of clothing in order to be comfortable (Milbrand, 2023). Outside of this, you should dress your newborn as you would yourself, keeping them in comfortable, weather-appropriate clothing. If you will be carrying them in a blanket, regardless of the season, remember to keep it from covering their face, as this may lead to accidental suffocation. In terms of car safety, you are required by law to take your newborn home for the first time in a car seat, whether in your own vehicle or that of another person. See the "Car Seat Installation" section of Chapter 4 for a refresher regarding the installation and use of a car seat.

A bit of planning you may have to do ahead of time concerns the introduction of your baby to your home environment, specifically to any other living beings inhabiting the space. As this book is intended to help first-time dads, we won't concern ourselves with introducing the newborn to older siblings. We will, however, look at what you can do if you have a household pet. To ensure that your pet isn't overwhelmed by the new arrival, bring a piece of clothing or a blanket home from the hospital before you bring the baby back. Ensure that the thing you select is used for your baby so that it carries its scent. Place it near your pet so that they may become accustomed to the smell of the newcomer. However, remember that it is best not to leave a newborn alone with a pet, no matter how well the two get along.

The Newborn Body

We've learned enough about the fetal developmental process to know that the body of a newborn differs significantly from that of a human at any other age. As such, there are some things you will have to approach in a specific way to keep your baby clean, comfortable, and healthy, including:

- Washing their neck and face daily, using lukewarm water, a mild baby soap, and a washcloth. Should redness or blotches arise on their face, rest assured that baby acne is a very common occurrence.

- Wiping their eyes with warm water in which you have wetted a cotton ball. Use separate balls for each eye, wiping from the inside to the outside of the eye.

- Washing their hair, no more than three times per week. Use a baby shampoo, brushing the hair daily using either a soft toothbrush or a hairbrush for infants.

- Unclogging the nostrils using an infant-sized nasal bulb syringe. Babies will usually blow their own noses, but the nasal passages may become blocked. Should this happen, you can fill the syringe with nasal spray or saline solution before irrigating through each nostril.

- Clipping their nails after a bath, using either baby nail clippers or a pair of blunt-edged scissors designed for the same task.

- Bathing them a maximum of three times per week in the first year of life. Remember to wait at least a day after birth before bathing your baby. Once this time has passed, use lukewarm water and unscented soap for a bath lasting no more than 10 minutes. If you'd like to apply lotion to their body afterwards, ensure it is hypoallergenic.

- Changing their diapers as necessary and ensuring that the region is properly cleaned and dried.

- Performing daily cleanings of the genitalia with warm water. Take note that both testicles and vulvas will be swollen for a while after birth due to the presence of maternal hormones. In the case of the latter, there may also be some bloody discharge, though this should last no more than a few days.

- Waiting for your baby's legs to straighten out, which they will do in the period between six and 18 months of age.

Postpartum Visiting: The Early Days

In the days and weeks following the birth, you will essentially be your house's bouncer and your partner's security guard. It's perfectly reasonable to want some time alone as a family so that you can get to know one another within this context before allowing outsiders to join the party. You can include this in your birth plan or construct your approach after the birth. Don't be afraid to stagger the introduction of visitors or limit the number of people you allow to see the baby at once. A good method would be to start with your immediate family, followed by the baby's godparents. After that, you can allow visits from friends and extended family members. Keep in mind that accepting visitors isn't compulsory, and you can absolutely stop the stream any time you'd like. If you have a few people over and discover you would like some more time as a family, you are at liberty to let people know that visits won't continue just yet. Should some of the people in your life be foaming at the mouth for news and statistics concerning the baby, consider sending out a mass email or text letting people know the baby's birthday, size, sex, and name. How you introduce your child to others is entirely up to you, so feel free to do as much or as little as you feel comfortable with.

Bonding With Your Baby

Once your baby is safely home, one of the best ways for you to bond with your newborn is at feeding time, when it's just the two of you and your focus is entirely on that moment. However, your parent-child bond can be forged and strengthened outside of this one activity. While the methods outlined below are aimed at postpartum bonding, know that you can start forging a connection with your baby during pregnancy by talking or singing to them. After they have entered the world, the two of you can connect by means of the following:

- Bathing with your baby in body-temperature water. Lay your baby on your chest so that both of you can enjoy a moment of soothing relaxation.

- Skin-to-skin contact, in which you can place the baby on your bare chest as you recline in a comfortable chair.

- Comfort your baby with the dulcet tones of your voice by reading to them whenever possible. For newborns, the reading material can be anything you have at hand, and you can move to age-appropriate books as they mature.

- Taking your baby along when you go for a walk or jog. When they are older, you can place them in a jogging stroller, child's bike seat, or bike trailer.

- Wearing your baby in a carrier as you move around the house or when out and about.

- Establishing a specific ritual at the end of the day that allows you to transition from work to family mode. This can be as simple as taking a deep, cleansing breath before picking your baby up and spending a few minutes in each other's company.

- Carrying on traditions from your own childhood or creating new ones alongside your child.

Newborn Sleep

As we know, while sleeping patterns may emerge in utero, your newborn is unlikely to have a structured sleep schedule immediately after birth. Though they do require a significant amount of sleep, they won't fill their quota for overly long stretches of time. However, you can establish certain habits and routines that may help them fall into some sort of pattern, especially at night. These bedtime rituals will help calm them down and may even help them achieve sleep quicker and more easily.

These rituals include establishing a clear difference between the level of activity during the day and when it's time to go to bed at night. While you can keep your baby occupied and stimulated during the day, you can intentionally calm them down at night. This includes lowering the lights, moving more slowly, and speaking in softer tones. Furthermore, try to establish a firm routine, meaning that you prepare them for bed and put them down at the same time each night. You can add to their schedule by allowing them to take naps during the day, allowing them to get adequate rest. However, make sure to pay attention to your child's sleep needs. You will see them do this naturally, with most babies assuming a napping schedule on their own, having a rest at nine in the morning and two in the afternoon by the age of nine months (Milbrand, 2023).

Newborn Poop

For many people, poop duty is one of the first things that comes to mind when they think of parenthood in its early days. While it certainly won't be pleasant to take care of your newborn's excrement, there is some knowledge to be gleaned from its frequency, color, and consistency, all of which are linked to your baby's well-being.

First and foremost, it's important to know that the frequency of your newborn's pooping may vary, and that this variation shouldn't worry you. Some infants will excrete feces after each feeding, while others may only do so every few days. However, should your baby go four days or more without pooping, it may be indicative of an underlying health issue. If this is the case, contact a healthcare professional as soon as possible.

Next up is the importance of color. We've already encountered the term "meconium," which is used to describe your baby's first poop after feeding. This is the only instance in which black feces are acceptable. Meconium will also be thicker than typical baby poop and may have a tarry texture. After this first time, if your baby's fecal matter is black again, it is a cause for concern, as their stomach may be bleeding. Ensure that the poop isn't dark green, as this isn't necessarily something bad. Green feces, both light and dark, may only contain the bile produced in the liver. You can use a light to inspect whether the poop is green or black and take action accordingly.

On the topic of concerning colors, should your baby's excretions be white or gray, medical attention is required as soon as possible. If the color is this light, your baby may have issues with digestion and their liver. By contrast, unless it's bloody, red stool doesn't always indicate something bad. This discoloration is most often caused by medications or red-tinged foods. However, if the stool contains blood, it may be a sign of bleeding in the intestines or an allergy. Shades of green, brown, and yellow are also perfectly acceptable and are the typical hues you'll find in baby stools.

Finally, you have to take note of the consistency of your newborn's poop. Once your child starts to feed, their poop will take on a less viscous consistency. Over time, as your baby starts to consume solid foods, their feces will become more solid, and the color will also change. While they are still consuming breast milk or formula, the consistency will be seedier, softer, and more pasty. It will also be close to liquid and will remain runny until they start consuming solid foods. Any of these textures is perfectly normal, and though there may be some variations, if the feces consistently have these characteristics, nothing's gone awry. If that changes, consult a healthcare professional.

Newborn Illness

In babies, one of the symptoms you should be most concerned about is fever, as it may be tied to a large number of illnesses. Milbrand (2023) reports that any fever is reason enough to call your pediatrician. Furthermore, you should call the doctor if your baby is three months of age or younger and their fever reaches 100.4 degrees Fahrenheit. For babies older than this, this maximum is lowered to 102 degrees Fahrenheit. In addition to a fever, you should call the doctor if you notice any of the following:

- Bloody stool or vomit.
- Difficulty breathing.
- Seizures.
- Diarrhea.
- Vomiting (more than is typical of spitting up).
- Your baby becomes limp or unresponsive.
- An inability to stop crying.
- Presents signs of dehydration.
- Discharge from the ears.
- A rash.

- A cold that persists or worsens.

- Refuses milk or formula for several consecutive feedings.

Should you notice any of the signs or symptoms mentioned above, there are a few things you should have on hand when calling the doctor. This includes the names and dosages of any medications they are taking and their immunization records. You should also make mention of any preexisting medical conditions your baby has, as well as the temperature you recorded before calling.

Deciphering Your Newborn's Cries

This may come as a surprise, but babies tend not to have a way with words for the first time. As an alternative, they cry a lot. You may become concerned by the frequency and intensity of their cries. Though the cries may sound the same, there are other clues you can look for. A hungry cry will be accompanied by physical movements such as wriggles or stretches, and they may suck their fingers as a means of signaling hunger. Cries tied to sleepiness will be accompanied by yawns and eye-rubbing. If something really is wrong, you will hear the difference in tone and intensity immediately.

Growth Progress

Because the literature concerning early childhood describes so many different milestones your baby is meant to achieve, you may become concerned if they don't adhere to the timeline set out by these books. Remember that the ages aren't set in stone and that they usually cover a range of months or years. Moreover, each child is unique. While some milestones will be hit early and easily, others may take some more time. Both occurrences are fine as long as you see them making progress.

Take Turns

Remember that the baby will be just as much yours as your partner's. As such, you can mitigate your fears regarding fatherhood by playing an active role and working through your worries. Divide each of the responsibilities down the middle to ensure that both of you get enough time with your child. Additionally, taking the reins soon after childbirth can help your partner recover and deal with the stress she has undergone.

Don't Forget About Your Partner

Remember to check in with your partner to see how she is doing after the birth. Don't let romance or intimacy fade. While you may not have the opportunity or time to do things exactly as you did before, simply being there for one another will help maintain your connection. Remember that intimacy exists in many forms. Talk to your partner, sharing your emotional experiences and encouraging them to do the same.

Postpartum Preeclampsia

It's a commonly held belief that the risk of developing preeclampsia disappears once the baby arrives. Regrettably, this isn't the case. The risk of blood pressure issues arising remains a possibility in the first six weeks after birth, regardless of whether elevated blood pressure was an issue during pregnancy. By keeping an eye out for the warning signs, you can help your partner avoid a potentially fatal occurrence. Seek medical intervention if your partner reports changes in vision, such as seeing spots, nausea or vomiting, abdominal pain, shortness of breath, headaches, or swelling in her hands and face. If you measure her blood pressure at home, seek help if the reading reaches or exceeds 140/90 (*Postpartum preeclampsia*, 2023).

Baby Blues

Many first-time mothers experience baby blues if not full-blown postpartum depression. According to Auteri (2015), "9% to 16% of postpartum women experience postpartum depression. And a much larger number of postpartum women (60% to 80%) experience the plain old baby blues." Provide your partner with as much support and love as you can. Don't try to label or manage her feelings but allow her the space to work through her emotions.

Postpartum Perception

Because parenting is a learning process, many first-time moms worry that if they make mistakes, other people will think of them as terrible mothers. If your partner expresses this type of concern, the first thing you can do is hear her out. Allow her to vent her frustrations, then gently remind her that no one expects her to have everything down pat within two days of the baby's arrival. Eventually, both of you will learn how to be parents, but it won't happen overnight. If you feel that others are judging you as well, let her know. More importantly, let her know that she isn't alone in this and that the two of you are learning the ins and outs of parenthood together.

Emotional Changes

For many moms, their sudden, intense focus on their baby may mean that they worry about losing their sense of self. This is why it is essential that you are involved from the start. By fulfilling your role as a father, your partner will have the mental and emotional capacity to retain her sense of self. If you see that your partner is having a hard time, take on some of her chores so she can step back and be more present.

Breastfeeding Concerns

For many first-time moms, breastfeeding is a sort of rite of passage. However, if your partner has difficulty breastfeeding or if the experience is unpleasant, she may become dismayed. In advance of your baby's arrival, discuss alternatives to breastfeeding, such as the use of baby formula. Should breastfeeding prove difficult or impossible, you will know which course of action to take. Note that your partner should not breastfeed if she doesn't want to, as negative experiences with this form of feeding may affect the baby. If there are genuine health concerns, consult a lactation specialist, who will be able to provide you with a plan for the way forward.

New Dad Parenting Hacks

We close out the final chapter of this book with things that every new parent wishes they had: Some helpful parenting hacks. Ideally, you will be able to take the information below and apply it to your own life to make the parenting process easier—if only slightly. As with so many other techniques in this book, feel free to use these hacks as a framework through which you can construct your own fatherhood fixes.

Helpful new dad parenting hacks include:

- If your baby is seemingly crying without stopping and without reason, consider checking their socks. Oftentimes, the threads of the socks may wind themselves around your baby's toes. Apart from relieving some discomfort, by checking their socks (or putting them on inside out from the start), you can prevent the threads from cutting off the circulation to one of their toes.

- Save some money on expensive changing pads by buying a cheap yoga mat and cutting it into rectangles, providing you with changing pads that are spongy, reusable, and easy-to-clean.

- If you become frustrated with the snaps on your baby's clothes, consider swapping them out for zippered garments.

- Deal with the cradle cap by rubbing some coconut oil into your baby's scalp before gently brushing their hair. The oil moisturizes the scalp and provides it with a pleasant scent.

- If you are having difficulty with burping techniques, place your baby on their back, take their feet, and move their legs as though they were pedaling a bicycle. This antagonistic movement will stimulate the intestine to release any trapped gas.

- Save money on umbilical cord diapers by simply taking a regular diaper and folding it down the waist so that it lies below the umbilical stump.

- To avoid accidents (and unnecessary stress), trim their fingernails with a nail file.

- Lessen the mess at changing times by unclasping the onesie before pulling it up to the shoulders and taking it off.

- You can also cut down on mess during diaper changes by opening a new diaper first and placing it under your child's bottom before sliding off the old diaper.

- Meconium may be difficult to clean, but you can make the process easier by applying some lotion—or coconut oil—to your baby's bottom.

- Teach your child to sleep under noisy circumstances by switching on a fan or playing some music from your phone while they nap.

- Add an extra level of efficacy to the bedtime process by hanging darkening or blackout curtains in the nursery.

- When you're out and about with the baby, free up a hand or two by clipping the things you need to your baby carrier.

The process of labor and delivery can be equal parts terrifying and thrilling, and the hope is that your preparation will make the latter feeling stand out more. In addition to this, bringing your baby home for the first time is exciting, and you may look back on the days that follow as some of the most blissful in your time together as a family. That bliss will be greatly heightened if you know what to expect and how to take your first steps as a dad. Despite your research and preparation, you may not feel entirely prepared. However, rest assured that this chapter contains all you need to conquer any difficulties those first days may present, and you can refer back to it anytime you need a refresher.

Conclusion

Nine chapters and dozens of parenting tips, tricks, techniques, and facts later, our time together comes to an end. Over the course of this book, your pantheon of fatherly knowledge has been greatly expanded, if not constructed for the very first time. We've covered everything from determining what type of father you'd like to be to how you can tackle all of the paperwork that comes with preparing to be a father, as well as on the day of your baby's arrival. With any luck, you will have supplemented the theory presented here with things you have picked up through your own lived experience and the words of wisdom you've received from other dads in your life. Even if you haven't, I'll bet you're more prepared for fatherhood than you think.

As you move forward and step into the role of dad for the first time, remember that parenting is an ever-changing experience. Much like a job, you'll never really stop learning, regardless of your child's age. However, while most of your education will happen through practical experience and that specific type of trial-and-error that comes with the parental territory, preparing for fatherhood will give you a baseline of knowledge to fall back on. With that being said, keep in mind that every parenting experience is different, as is the domestic circumstance in which you will be applying the knowledge you've gained. As such, remember to cut yourself some slack. You won't be the perfect dad from day one, but you're bound to become better as time goes on.

Another thing to keep in mind is that this isn't a one-man operation. Whether you will be raising the baby with your partner, with the help of your chosen family, or with the help of your support network, there will be someone there to lend a hand and provide a word of support. And should there ever be an instance in which you can't find what you need from the people in your life, rest assured that there is a wealth of information at your fingertips, particularly within the pages of this book. Return to these chapters whenever you feel the need, and know that you can do so for issues both big and small.

A final word of parenting wisdom before we part ways: Nothing will help you become the father you want to be more than confidence. In the world of parenting, confidence can only be won if you feel like you know what you are doing. With that goal in mind, take what you have learned here and equip yourself with the skills and tools you need to step into this parental role with ease, expertise, and confidence. If you believe you can be a good father, there's no reason why that thought can't be translated into reality. You have what it takes; all you need to do is take the first step.

It takes a village to raise a child, and sometimes that village may look a bit different from what we imagine it to be. As such, if you feel that this book has been of use to you on your path to fatherhood, you can help empower another first-time dad by leaving a review and letting other fathers-to-be know of the skills, knowledge, and confidence they stand to gain. Who knows? You may just start a chain reaction that creates the most well-equipped generation of fathers the world has ever seen.

References

A guide to being the best birth partner you can. (2018, June 6). Bounty. https://www.bounty.com/family/family-dynamics/guide-to-being-the-best-birth-partner-you-can

Abdullah, M. (2022, June 15). *How paternity leave helps dads and babies bond.* Greater Good. https://greatergood.berkeley.edu/article/item/how_paternity_leave_helps_dads_and_babies_bond

Achwal, A. (2019, November 6). *7 things new moms worry about most and how to handle them.* Firstcry Parenting. https://parenting.firstcry.com/articles/brand-7-things-new-moms-worry-about-most-and-how-to-handle-them/

Adams, K. (2019). *Budgeting for a new baby.* Investopedia. https://www.investopedia.com/articles/pf/08/budgeting-for-baby.asp

Allen, N. (2022, May 27). *21 ways to prepare for fatherhood, from the practical to the emotional.* Mindbodygreen. https://www.mindbodygreen.com/articles/preparing-for-fatherhood

Aman, L. (2020, October 31). *21 things dads should do during labor.* These Hungry Kids. https://thesehungrykids.com/things-dads-should-do-during-labor/

American Academy of Pediatrics. (2019). *Car seats: Information for families.* HealthyChildren.org. https://www.healthychildren.org/English/safety-prevention/on-the-go/Pages/Car-Safety-Seats-Information-for-Families.aspx

An essential guide on what to eat during pregnancy. (2020, December 15). Family Health Centers of San Diego. https://www.fhcsd.org/prenatal-care/what-to-eat-during-pregnancy/

Auteri, S. (2015, January 22). *10 common fears all first-time moms have.* Mom.com. https://mom.com/baby/17197-10-common-fears-all-first-time-moms-have

Baby blues and postpartum depression: Mood disorders and pregnancy. (2019). John Hopkins Medicine. https://www.hopkinsmedicine.org/health/wellness-and-prevention/postpartum-mood-disorders-what-new-moms-need-to-know

Baby poop guide. (2018). Children's Hospital Colorado. https://www.childrenscolorado.org/conditions-and-advice/parenting/parenting-articles/baby-poop-guide/

BabyCentre UK Editorial Team. (2022, October). *Childproofing checklist: Before your baby crawls.* BabyCentre UK. https://www.babycentre.co.uk/a536364/childproofing-checklist-before-your-baby-crawls

Barnett, C. (2019, October 15). *Healthy father, healthy family: Six self-care tips for new dads.* The Fashionisto. https://www.thefashionisto.com/healthy-father-healthy-family-six-self-care-tips-for-new-dads/

Barth, L. (2020, June 11). *Is pregnancy brain real?* Healthline. https://www.healthline.com/health/pregnancy/is-pregnancy-brain-real

Batcha, B., & Srinivasan, H. (2023, January 25). *Here's a nine-month plan to get your finances in check before baby arrives.* Parents. https://www.parents.com/pregnancy/considering-baby/financing-family/a-nine-month-plan-for-getting-your-familys-finances-in-order-pre-baby/

Bell, J. (2020, February 11). *Dad bod & dad brain: How a man's brain changes when he becomes a father.* Big Think. https://bigthink.com/neuropsych/neuroscience-of-fatherhood/

Bell, S. (2021, December). *How your sex life will change as a dad-to-be.* BabyCentre UK. https://www.babycentre.co.uk/a1005112/how-your-sex-life-will-change-as-a-dad-to-be

Ben-Joseph, E. P. (2018, June). *Bringing your baby home.* Nemours KidsHealth. https://kidshealth.org/en/parents/bringing-baby-home.html

Bendapudi, N. (2020, March 16). *Hospital antenatal classes vs lamaze childbirth classes.* IBU Family. https://www.ibufamily.org/post/hospital-antenatal-classes-vs-lamaze-childbirth-classes

Benefits of having a private midwife. (2019, June 18). MyBump2Baby. https://www.mybump2baby.com/benefits-of-a-private-midwife/

Berendzen, J. (2023). *Male postpartum depression.* UnityPoint Health. https://www.unitypoint.org/news-and-articles/male-postpartum-depression--unitypoint-health

Birth methods: Which one is right for you? (2020, May 20). Mustela USA. https://www.mustelausa.com/blogs/mustela-mag/birth-methods-which-one-is-right-for-you

Bjarnadottir, A. (2018a). *A guide on what to eat during pregnancy.* Healthline. https://www.healthline.com/nutrition/13-foods-to-eat-when-pregnant

Bjarnadottir, A. (2018b, July 18). *15 foods and drinks to avoid during pregnancy — what not to eat.* Healthline. https://www.healthline.com/nutrition/11-foods-to-avoid-during-pregnancy

Bogle, J. (2021, August 10). *11 ways dads can practice self care and why they should (yes, even you!).* The Dad. https://www.thedad.com/dads-self-care/

Bose, J. (2021, November 13). *Coping with stress as a new dad.* DadPad. https://thedadpad.co.uk/ask-dadpad/new-dad-coping-with-stress/

Brennan, D. (2021, September 1). *What are the advantages and disadvantages of a hospital birth?* MedicineNet. https://www.medicinenet.com/advantages_and_disadvantages_of_a_hospital_birth/article.htm

Brown, C. A. (2016, July 7). *Dad's presence at birth leads to a healthier baby and mom.* National Fatherhood Initiative. https://www.fatherhood.org/championing-fatherhood/dads-presence-healthier-baby-mom

Brown, M. (2022, December 15). *Delivering at a birth center.* What to Expect. https://www.whattoexpect.com/pregnancy/birth-center/

Brown, S. (2003, November 11). *How to change a baby's diaper.* Verywell Family. https://www.verywellfamily.com/how-to-change-a-diaper-289239

Buckner, S. (2023, July 18). *Paternity leave, FMLA, and state leave laws.* Findlaw. https://www.findlaw.com/family/paternity/paternity-leave.html

Burgess, C. (2021, May 25). *10 things dads-to-be need to know about pregnancy sex.* Emma's Diary. https://www.emmasdiary.co.uk/blog/things-dads-to-be-need-to-know-about-pregnancy-sex

Calming your new-mom fears. (2020, October 2). The Lactation Network. https://lactationnetwork.com/blog/how-to-deal-with-new-mom-fears/

Carberg, J., & Langdon, K. (2019). Statistics on postpartum depression. PostpartumDepression.org. https://www.postpartumdepression.org/resources/statistics/

Cassell, A. (2021). *How to support a woman in labor: A childbirth cheat sheet for partners.* BabyCenter. https://www.babycenter.com/pregnancy/relationships/a-childbirth-cheat-sheet-for-dads-to-be_8244

Centers for Disease Control and Prevention. (2018, July 19). Centers for Disease Control and Prevention. https://www.cdc.gov/pregnancy/meds/treatingfortwo/facts.html

Centers for Disease Control and Prevention. (2019a). *Toxoplasmosis: Pregnancy FAQs.* Centers for Disease Control and Prevention. https://www.cdc.gov/parasites/toxoplasmosis/gen_info/pregnant.html

Centers for Disease Control and Prevention. (2019b, October 1). *Signs your child is hungry or full.* Centers for Disease Control and Prevention. https://www.cdc.gov/nutrition/infantandtoddlernutrition/mealtime/signs-your-child-is-hungry-or-full.html

Centers for Disease Control and Prevention. (2022, April 4). *Pregnancy complications.* Centers for Disease Control and Prevention. https://www.cdc.gov/reproductivehealth/maternalinfanthealth/pregnancy-complications.html

Changing face of fatherhood - more family time. (2021, June 7). MensLine Australia. https://mensline.org.au/being-a-dad/changing-face-of-fatherhood-more-family-time/

Cherney, K. (2020, April 16). *Pain relief in labor: Natural vs. medicated birth.* Healthline. https://www.healthline.com/health/pregnancy/pain-relief-in-labor

Chertoff, J. (2018). *30 pregnancy facts that may surprise you, plus 5 myths.* Healthline. https://www.healthline.com/health/pregnancy/pregnancy-facts

Children's Bureau. (2018, June 7). *A father's impact on child development.* All4Kids. https://www.all4kids.org/news/blog/a-fathers-impact-on-child-development/

Chubb, C. (2022, January 2). *The ultimate first year baby budget.* WealthKeel Advisors LLC. https://wealthkeel.com/blog/first-year-baby-budget/

Cleveland Clinic. (2018a). *Medicine guidelines for pregnancy.* Cleveland Clinic. https://my.clevelandclinic.org/health/drugs/4396-medicine-guidelines-during-pregnancy

Cleveland Clinic. (2018b). *Types of delivery for pregnancy.* Cleveland Clinic. https://my.clevelandclinic.org/health/articles/9675-pregnancy-types-of-delivery

Cleveland Clinic. (2019a, July 22). *Miscarriage: Risks, symptoms, causes and treatments.* Cleveland Clinic. https://my.clevelandclinic.org/health/diseases/9688-miscarriage

Cleveland Clinic. (2019b, September 16). *Yes, postpartum depression in men is very real.* Health Essentials from Cleveland Clinic. https://health.clevelandclinic.org/yes-postpartum-depression-in-men-is-very-real/

Cleveland Clinic. (2020a, April 16). *Fetal development.* Cleveland Clinic. https://my.clevelandclinic.org/health/articles/7247-fetal-development-stages-of-growth

Cleveland Clinic. (2020b, November 25). *When to call the doctor for your newborn baby.* Health Essentials from Cleveland Clinic. https://health.clevelandclinic.org/when-to-call-the-doctor-for-your-newborn-baby/

Cleveland Clinic. (2022a, May 10). *Braxton Hicks contractions: Overview & what they feel like*. Cleveland Clinic. https://my.clevelandclinic.org/health/symptoms/22965-braxton-hicks

Cleveland Clinic. (2022b, May 24). *Apgar score*. Cleveland Clinic. https://my.clevelandclinic.org/health/diagnostics/23094-apgar-score

Cleveland Clinic. (2022c, June 27). *Baby blues vs. postpartum depression*. Cleveland Clinic. https://health.clevelandclinic.org/baby-blues/

Cleveland Clinic. (2022d, September 9). *Pregnancy genetic testing: What it is, options, benefits & risks*. Cleveland Clinic. https://my.clevelandclinic.org/health/diagnostics/24136-pregnancy-genetic-testing

Cleveland Clinic. (2022e, November 14). *Pregnancy complications*. Cleveland Clinic. https://my.clevelandclinic.org/health/articles/24442-pregnancy-complications

Cleveland Clinic. (2023, March 10). *Labor pain relief: Options & side effects*. Cleveland Clinic. https://my.clevelandclinic.org/health/articles/4450-labor-pain-relief

Colantuoni, F., Diome-Deer, W., Moore, K., Rajbhandari, S., & Tolub, G. (2021, March 5). *Paternity leave benefits extend beyond personal*. McKinsey & Company. https://www.mckinsey.com/capabilities/people-and-organizational-performance/our-insights/a-fresh-look-at-paternity-leave-why-the-benefits-extend-beyond-the-personal

CoParents Team. (2016, December 13). *Is there such a thing as paternal instinct?* CoParents.com. https://www.coparents.com/blog/baby/is-there-such-a-thing-as-paternal-instinct/

Couple relationship during pregnancy: Changes & challenges. (2018, August 27). International Forum for Wellbeing in Pregnancy. https://www.ifwip.org/couple-relationship-during-pregnancy/?cn-reloaded=1

Dale, C. (2023, May 19). *Pregnancy symptoms in men are real—and they have a name.* Parents. https://www.parents.com/pregnancy/signs/symptoms/pregnancy-symptoms-in-men-couvade-syndrome/

Davies, A. (2023, June 22). *Your comprehensive guide to childbirth classes.* The Bump. https://www.thebump.com/a/childbirth-classes

Davies, J., Green, A., Madden, D., Burns, J., Burchett, N., & Clark Elford, R. (2021). *Becoming dad: A guide for new fathers.* https://www.mentalhealth.org.uk/sites/default/files/2022-06/MHF-Becoming-Dad-A-guide-for-new-fathers.pdf

de Bellefonds, C. (2014, September 16). *How to burp your baby: Basics, tips and positions.* What to Expect. https://www.whattoexpect.com/first-year/baby-care/how-to-burp-your-baby/

de Bellefonds, C. (2022). *What is pregnancy brain?* BabyCenter. https://www.babycenter.com/pregnancy/your-body/pregnancy-brain-why-it-happens-and-how-to-be-less-forgetful_236

de Souza, A. C., Carbonera, L. A., & Rocha, E. (2022). *Paid parental leave: Different scenarios around the world. Stroke, 53*(1). https://doi.org/10.1161/strokeaha.121.035919

Dean, J., & Kendall, P. (2012). *Food safety during pregnancy.* Colorado State University Extension. https://extension.colostate.edu/topic-areas/nutrition-food-safety-health/food-safety-during-pregnancy-9-372/

Dellner, A. (2020, January 8). *7 of the most common new mom fears (and how to feel better about them).* PureWow. https://www.purewow.com/family/new-mom-fears

DerSarkissian, C., & WebMD Editorial Contributors. (2022, February 20). *Should you screen your genes before you conceive?* WebMD. https://www.webmd.com/baby/genetic-tests-before-pregnancy

Devi, S. (2022, June 17). *What every dad should know about navigating his rights in the workplace.* A Better Balance. https://www.abetterbalance.org/what-every-dad-should-know-about-navigating-his-rights-in-the-workplace/

Dlugosz, S. (2013). *Fathers at birth: Women's experiences of their partner's presence during childbirth.* https://ro.ecu.edu.au/cgi/viewcontent.cgi?referer=&httpsredir=1&article=1105&context=theses_hons

Do, S. (2019, October 30). *6 things you didn't know about water birth.* The Birth Center. https://www.sactobirth.com/blog/2019/10/30/we-bet-you-didnt-know-these-6-things-about-water-birth

DrKumo Incorporated. (2022, March 26). *5 ways to help your wife cope with postpartum depression.* DrKumo. https://drkumo.com/5-ways-to-help-your-wife-cope-with-postpartum-depression/

Dungan, J. S. (2022, October). *Genetic screening before pregnancy.* MSD Manual Consumer Version. https://www.msdmanuals.com/home/women-s-health-issues/detection-of-genetic-disorders-before-and-during-pregnancy/genetic-screening-before-pregnancy

Emma's Diary Editorial Team. (2014, May 29). *Babyproofing your house: Your complete checklist.* Emma's Diary. https://www.emmasdiary.co.uk/baby/baby-milestones/babyproofing-house-checklist

Erickson, H. (2022, October 12). *Should you use a doula?* Pulling Curls. https://www.pullingcurls.com/should-you-hire-a-doula/

Eunice Kennedy Shriver National Institute of Child Health and Human Development. (2017, January 31). *What are some common complications of pregnancy?* National Institutes for Health. https://www.nichd.nih.gov/health/topics/pregnancy/conditioninfo/complications

Facing your new dad fears. (2015, May 21). Beyond Blue - Healthy Families. https://healthyfamilies.beyondblue.org.au/pregnancy-and-new-parents/dadvice-for-new-dads/facing-your-new-dad-fears

Felton, K. (2021, August 31). *How to install a rear-facing infant car seat.* What to Expect. https://www.whattoexpect.com/first-year/safety-and-childproofing/car-seat-installation

Fields, L. (2023, April 23). *8 early warning signs of postpartum depression.* WebMD. https://www.webmd.com/depression/postpartum-depression/early-warning-signs-postpartum-depression

Fleming, L. (2023, June 13). *Dad's mental health is often overlooked—this needs to change.* Verywell Mind. https://www.verywellmind.com/dads-mental-health-matters-5409299

Foods to avoid when pregnant. (2020, October 1). American Pregnancy Association. https://americanpregnancy.org/healthy-pregnancy/pregnancy-health-wellness/foods-to-avoid-during-pregnancy/

Freutel, N. (2016, November 14). *Sciatica pregnancy: Stretches for pain.* Healthline. https://www.healthline.com/health/pregnancy/sciatica-pain-stretches

Frost, A. (2020, April 21). *Myth or fact: Babies can cry in the womb.* Healthline. https://www.healthline.com/health/pregnancy/do-babies-cry-in-the-womb

5 tips to ease new dad fears. (2019, May 7). Women's Medical Center - Brookwood. https://www.brookwoodwomensmedicalcenter.com/home/stories/5-tips-to-ease-new-dad-fears

5 worries for new moms and ways to resolve it. Health One Medicine. (2023). https://www.healthonemedicine.com/blog/5-worries-for-new-moms-and-how-to-resolve-it

Galla, S. (2020). *Father support groups - a guide to support groups for dads*. Men's Group. https://mensgroup.com/father-support-groups/

Garoo, R. (2014, August 18). *How to hold a baby: 8 safe positions with pictures*. MomJunction. https://www.momjunction.com/articles/ways-hold-new-born-child_0085453/

Gavin, M. L. (2018, February). *What is the Apgar score?* Nemours KidsHealth. https://kidshealth.org/en/parents/apgar0.html

Gavin, M. L. (2021, November). *Formula feeding FAQs: How much and how often (for parents)*. Nemours KidsHealth. https://kidshealth.org/en/parents/formulafeed-often.html

Geddes, J. K. (2022, August 12). *Your guide to prenatal appointments*. What to Expect. https://www.whattoexpect.com/pregnancy/pregnancy-health/prenatal-appointments/

Geddes, J. K. (2023, April 7). *Hospital bag checklist*. What to Expect. https://www.whattoexpect.com/pregnancy/checklist/hospital-packing.aspx

Gingras, J. L., Mitchell, E. A., & Grattan, K. E. (2005). *Fetal homologue of infant crying*. Archives of Disease in Childhood - Fetal and Neonatal Edition, 90(5), F415–F418. https://doi.org/10.1136/adc.2004.062257

Graves, G., & Immergut, D. J. (2020, July 22). *How to create your birth plan: A checklist for parents*. Parents. https://www.parents.com/pregnancy/giving-birth/labor-and-delivery/checklist-how-to-write-a-birth-plan/

GreatDad Writers. (2011, August 31). *Questions you can ask to look smart at your next OB/GYN visit*. GreatDad.com.

https://www.greatdad.com/dad/questions-you-can-ask-to-look-smart-at-your-next-ob-gyn-visit

Greenlaw, E. (2012, June 16). *Foods to avoid in pregnancy.* WebMD. https://www.webmd.com/baby/foods-avoid-pregnancy

Hallowes, L. (2017, November 17). *Bloody brilliant! 11 awesome dad hacks you need to see to believe.* Babyology. https://babyology.com.au/parenting/family/bloody-brilliant-11-of-the-best-dad-hacks/

Hanawalt, Z. (2023, July 19). *Doula vs midwife: These are the differences and how to choose.* Parents. https://www.parents.com/pregnancy/giving-birth/labor-and-delivery/doula-vs-midwife-these-are-the-differences-and-how-to-choose/

Happiest Baby Staff. (2022, June 16). *6 simple ways for dad to bond with baby.* Happiest Baby. https://www.happiestbaby.com/blogs/parents/ways-for-dad-to-bond-with-baby

Harnish, A. (2023, January 5). *Midwives vs doulas: What's the difference?* What to Expect. https://www.whattoexpect.com/pregnancy/labor-and-delivery/midwives-vs-doulas

Harris, N. (2022, October 23). *Your pregnancy symptoms week by week.* Parents. https://www.parents.com/pregnancy/signs/symptoms/a-pregnancy-symptom-timeline/

Harris, N. (2023, June 24). *The ultimate baby poop color chart.* Parents. https://www.parents.com/baby/diapers/dirty/baby-poop-guide/

Haviland, M. (2021, April 19). *Why you should join a single father support group.* All pro Dad. https://www.allprodad.com/join-single-father-support-group/

Health Resources and Services Administration. (2022, December). *Newborn screening process.* HRSA Newborn Screening. https://newbornscreening.hrsa.gov/newborn-screening-process

Healthdirect Australia. (2019). *The role of a birth support partner.* Pregnancy Birth and Baby. https://www.pregnancybirthbaby.org.au/being-a-birth-support-partner

Healthdirect Australia. (2021, October). *Antenatal classes.* Pregnancy Birth and Baby. https://www.pregnancybirthbaby.org.au/antenatal-classes

Healthdirect Australia. (2022, May 6). *Making a birth plan.* Pregnancy Birth and Baby. https://www.pregnancybirthbaby.org.au/making-a-birth-plan#:~:text=A%20birth%20plan%20is%20a

Healthdirect Australia. (2023a, June). *Checkups, tests and scans available during your pregnancy.* Pregnancy Birth and Baby. https://www.pregnancybirthbaby.org.au/checkups-and-scans-during-your-pregnancy

Healthdirect Australia. (2023b, July 17). *Foods to avoid when pregnant.* Pregnancy Birth and Baby. https://www.pregnancybirthbaby.org.au/foods-to-avoid-when-pregnant#backToTop

Healthdirect Australia. (2023c, September 12). *Fathers and miscarriage.* Pregnancy Birth and Baby. https://www.pregnancybirthbaby.org.au/fathers-and-miscarriage

Healthline Australia. (2019). *Apgar score.* Pregnancy Birth and Baby. https://www.pregnancybirthbaby.org.au/apgar-score

HealthPartners. (2019, August 15). *How to help a partner with postpartum depression or anxiety.* HealthPartners Blog.

https://www.healthpartners.com/blog/postpartum-depression-or-anxiety/

Healthwise Staff. (2022, February 23). *Learning about prenatal visits.* MyHealth Alberta. https://myhealth.alberta.ca/health/AfterCareInformation/pages/conditions.aspx?hwid=uh5006

Heid, M. (2016, May 25). *5 parenting hacks for new dads that you won't find in baby books.* Men's Health. https://www.menshealth.com/trending-news/a19521477/easy-parenting-hacks/

Heppleston, S. (2019, September 2). *Father's day: The importance of support groups for dads.* The House of Wellness. https://www.houseofwellness.com.au/lifestyle/parenting/fathers-groups-important-groups-for-dads

Herr, L. (2015, July 14). *22 healthy pregnancy tips for the whole nine months.* Parents. https://www.parents.com/pregnancy/my-body/pregnancy-health/healthy-pregnancy-tips/

Hewlett, B. S. (1991). *The cultural nexus of Aka father-infant bonding.* https://anthro.vancouver.wsu.edu/documents/94/cultural_nexus_fathers_zkdjyPt.pdf

Hicks, T. (2022, October 6). *"Dad brain" and why first-time fathers develop it.* Healthline. https://www.healthline.com/health-news/what-is-dad-brain-and-why-do-first-time-fathers-experience-it

Hochwald, L. (2019, June 5). *How to burp a baby: Baby burping techniques.* The Bump. https://www.thebump.com/a/how-to-burp-a-baby

Horsager-Boehrer, R. (2021, August 17). *1 in 10 dads experience postpartum depression, anxiety: How to spot the signs.* UT Southwestern Medical Center. https://utswmed.org/medblog/paternal-postpartum-depression/

Hosley Stewart, D. (2022). *Top tips for dads on bonding with your baby.* BabyCenter.

https://www.babycenter.com/family/fatherhood/top-tips-for-dads-on-bonding-with-your-baby_3692

Huie Harrison, K. (2019, October 25). *Miscarriage grief: Fathers struggle through loss too.* Undefining Motherhood. https://undefiningmotherhood.com/partners-and-miscarriage/

Hylton-Schaub, A., & Bryant, D. D. (2021, June 17). *The crisis of masculinity and fatherhood.* Project Good Work. https://www.projectgood.work/blog/2021/6/9/the-crisis-of-masculinity-and-fatherhood

Iftikhar, N. (2020, June 27). *How to know when to go to the hospital for labor.* Healthline. https://www.healthline.com/health/pregnancy/when-to-go-to-the-hospital-for-labor

Importance of fathers & statistics. (2019). South Carolina Center for Fathers and Families. https://www.scfathersandfamilies.com/why-it-matters/fathers/

Institute for Quality and Efficiency in Health Care. (2008, September 24). *Pregnancy and birth: When your baby's due date has passed.* National Library of Medicine. https://www.ncbi.nlm.nih.gov/books/NBK279571/

Interesting childbirth and delivery facts. (2006). Unique Ultrasound. https://uniqueultrasound.com/interesting-childbirth-and-delivery-facts

Jhaveri, S., & Cleveland Clinic. (2022, January 14). *Pregnant? Here's how often you'll likely see your doctor.* Cleveland Clinic. https://health.clevelandclinic.org/prenatal-appointment-schedule/

Jones-Choi, A. (2022, March 4). *12 tips for when dad feeds a newborn.* Mom.com. https://mom.com/baby/12-tips-for-when-dad-feeds-a-newborn/get-a-schedule-when-to-feed-baby

Kam, K. (2012, June 7). *How often do I need prenatal visits?* WebMD. https://www.webmd.com/baby/how-often-do-i-need-prenatal-visits

Kashtan, P. (2023, March 13). *Hospital bag checklist: What to pack in hospital bag.* The Bump. https://www.thebump.com/a/checklist-packing-a-hospital-bag?vers=1

Kelly, K. (2022, November 17). *10 labor and delivery support tips for partners.* Parents. https://www.parents.com/pregnancy/giving-birth/labor-support/labor-delivery-advice-dads/

Khandwala, Y. S., Zhang, C. A., Lu, Y., & Eisenberg, M. L. (2017). *The age of fathers in the USA is rising: An analysis of 168 867 480 births from 1972 to 2015. Human Reproduction, 32*(10), 2110–2116. https://doi.org/10.1093/humrep/dex267

Kleiman, K. (2011, March 20). *For dads: What to do, what not to do when your wife has PPD.* Psychology Today. https://www.psychologytoday.com/us/blog/isnt-what-i-expected/201103/dads-what-do-what-not-do-when-your-wife-has-ppd

Kreidman, J. (2023, January 20). *New dad anxiety - How to overcome the fear of fatherhood.* Dad University. https://www.daduniversity.com/blog/new-dad-anxiety-how-to-overcome-the-fear-of-fatherhood

Kull, J. C. (2018, November 16). *15 ways to support a partner after a miscarriage.* Marriage.com. https://www.marriage.com/advice/mental-health/support-a-partner-after-a-miscarriage/

LaBracio, J. (2023, June 14). *Ultimate hospital bag checklist for mom and baby.* Babylist. https://www.babylist.com/hello-baby/what-to-pack-in-your-hospital-bag

Lagudu, S. (2017, June 30). *How to be a good father: Top 9 qualities.* MomJunction. https://www.momjunction.com/articles/how-to-be-a-good-father_00427023/

Lamott, A. (2015). *Anne Lamott quotes.* Goodreads. https://www.goodreads.com/quotes/6830146-almost-everything-will-work-again-if-you-unplug-it-for

Lee, S. (2010, September 22). *Which antenatal class is best for you?* MadeForMums. https://www.madeformums.com/pregnancy/which-antenatal-class-is-best-for-you/

Levine, H. (2022, July 15). *Sex drive changes during pregnancy.* What to Expect. https://www.whattoexpect.com/pregnancy/sex-and-relationships/decreased-sex-drive-during-pregnancy/

Lioi, J. (2015, May 6). *Figuring out fatherhood: What kind of dad do you want to be?* GoodTherapy. https://www.goodtherapy.org/blog/figuring-out-fatherhood-what-kind-of-dad-do-you-want-to-be-0506155

Logan-Banks, P. (2016). *15 surprising newborn baby facts: Photos.* BabyCentre UK. https://www.babycentre.co.uk/l25019371/15-surprising-newborn-baby-facts-photos

LoMonaco, J. L. (2022, June 17). *How your body and brain change when you become a dad.* Cradlewise. https://cradlewise.com/blog/how-fatherhood-changes-your-body-and-brain

Loneragan, D. (2018, August 16). *Father's day: A dad's guide to truly excellent swaddling.* Citizens of the World. https://citizensoftheworld.cc/sheridan-fathers-day-dads-guide-excellent-swaddling/

MacBride, K. (2021, June 18). *Are you ready to be a dad? 8 questions you need to answer first.* Inverse. https://www.inverse.com/mind-body/are-you-ready-to-be-a-father

Majumdar, R. (2017, November 21). *Body changes during pregnancy - week by week*. FirstCry.com. https://parenting.firstcry.com/articles/body-changes-during-pregnancy-week-by-week/

Marcin, A. (2016, August 3). *How to hold a baby: Step by step*. Healthline. https://www.healthline.com/health/parenting/how-to-hold-a-newborn

Marcin, A. (2022, July 21). *What genetic testing is available during pregnancy?* Healthline. https://www.healthline.com/health/pregnancy/genetic-testing-during-pregnancy

Marple, K. (2019, May 22). *Fetal development week by week*. BabyCenter. https://www.babycenter.com/pregnancy/your-baby/fetal-development-week-by-week_10406730

Masters, M. (2022, December 19). *What parents need to know about genetic carrier screening*. What to Expect. https://www.whattoexpect.com/getting-pregnant/health-and-wellness/carrier-genetic-screenings/

Mayo Clinic Staff. (2017). *Help your baby sleep through the night*. Mayo Clinic. https://www.mayoclinic.org/healthy-lifestyle/infant-and-toddler-health/in-depth/baby-sleep/art-20045014

Mayo Clinic Staff. (2018a). *Home birth: Know the pros and cons*. Mayo Clinic. https://www.mayoclinic.org/healthy-lifestyle/labor-and-delivery/in-depth/home-birth/art-20046878

Mayo Clinic Staff. (2018b). *Prenatal care: 1st trimester visits*. Mayo Clinic. https://www.mayoclinic.org/healthy-lifestyle/pregnancy-week-by-week/in-depth/prenatal-care/art-20044882

Mayo Clinic Staff. (2018c). *Sex during pregnancy: What's OK, what's not*. Mayo Clinic. https://www.mayoclinic.org/healthy-lifestyle/pregnancy-week-by-week/in-depth/sex-during-pregnancy/art-20045318

Mayo Clinic Staff. (2021, October 16). *Miscarriage - symptoms and causes.* Mayo Clinic. https://www.mayoclinic.org/diseases-conditions/pregnancy-loss-miscarriage/symptoms-causes/syc-20354298

McDuffey, T. (2023, May 25). *Fathers' rights and FMLA.* Findlaw. https://www.findlaw.com/family/paternity/fathers-rights-and-fmla.html

McTigue, S. (2020, March 27). *Preparing for fatherhood: 16 ways to get ready.* Healthline. https://www.healthline.com/health/preparing-for-fatherhood

Meffert, A. (2021, June 2). *Paternal mental health: The importance of fathers' emotional well-being.* Crossroads Family Counseling Center. https://crossroadsfamilycounselingcenter.com/paternal-mental-health-the-importance-of-fathers-emotional-well-being/

Men get postnatal depression too — here's how to spot it. (2022, June 13). ForWhen. https://forwhenhelpline.org.au/parent-resources/male-postnatal-depression/

Metland, D. (2021, December). *Dads: 10 ways to be the perfect birth partner.* BabyCentre UK. https://www.babycentre.co.uk/a1072/dads-10-ways-to-be-the-perfect-birth-partner

Milbrand, L. (2023, May 30). *Everything you've wanted to know about taking care of a newborn baby.* Parents. https://www.parents.com/baby/care/american-baby-how-tos/newborn-baby-boot-camp/

Miles, K. (2022, November 29). *Growth chart: Fetal length and weight, week by week.* BabyCenter. https://www.babycenter.com/pregnancy/your-body/growth-chart-fetal-length-and-weight-week-by-week_1290794

More than just a birth plan: Crucial questions to discuss with your partner. (2017, April 6). ParentCo. https://www.parent.com/blogs/conversations/more-than-a-birth-plan-45-crucial-questions-to-discuss-with-partner

Morse, J. (2022, March 1). *10 tips for handling and holding a newborn*. UT Southwestern Medical Center. https://utswmed.org/medblog/newborn-holding-tips/

National Childbirth Trust . (2022, August 18). *Choosing your birth partners*. NCT (National Childbirth Trust). https://www.nct.org.uk/labour-birth/dads-and-partners/choosing-your-birth-partners

National Childbirth Trust. (2019, July 25). *Sex during pregnancy: Dads' questions answered*. NCT (National Childbirth Trust). https://www.nct.org.uk/pregnancy/dads-be/sex-during-pregnancy-dads-questions-answered

National Childbirth Trust. (2020a, February 14). *Spotting signs of postnatal depression in your partner*. NCT (National Childbirth Trust). https://www.nct.org.uk/life-parent/how-you-might-be-feeling/spotting-signs-postnatal-depression-your-partner

National Childbirth Trust. (2020b, December 2). *Writing a birth plan and deciding about pain relief*. NCT (National Childbirth Trust). https://www.nct.org.uk/pregnancy/dads-be/writing-birth-plan-and-deciding-about-pain-relief

National Childbirth Trust. (2022a, July 28). *Pampering in pregnancy: Massages, facials and spas*. NCT (National Childbirth Trust). https://www.nct.org.uk/pregnancy/exercise-and-fitness/pampering-pregnancy-massages-facials-and-spas

National Childbirth Trust. (2022b, August 18). *Sex in trimester one, two and three of pregnancy*. NCT (National Childbirth Trust). https://www.nct.org.uk/pregnancy/relationships-sex/sex-trimester-one-two-and-three-pregnancy

National Childbirth Trust. (2022c, November 14). *Postnatal depression in dads and co-parents: 10 things you should know*. NCT (National Childbirth Trust). https://www.nct.org.uk/life-parent/emotions/postnatal-depression-dads-and-co-parents-10-things-you-should-know

Newborn screening tests for your baby. (2015). March of Dimes. https://www.marchofdimes.org/find-support/topics/parenthood/newborn-screening-tests-your-baby

Newman, T. (2023, April 25). *Which foods to eat and avoid during pregnancy.* Medical News Today. https://www.medicalnewstoday.com/articles/246404

Nierenberg, C. (2015, January 29). *What is a midwife? | Weighing pros and cons.* Live Science. https://www.livescience.com/45552-midwife-definition.html

Nightingale Baby Team. (2022, February 25). *Everything you need to know about birthing classes.* Nightingale. https://nightingale.baby/blogs/news/everything-you-need-to-know-about-birthing-classes

Nutricia's Medical and Scientific Affairs Team. (2019, June 11). *Birthing partners & doulas — what are they?* C&G Baby Club. https://www.cgbabyclub.co.uk/pregnancy/labour-and-birth/do-i-need-to-choose-a-birth-partner.html

Nyenbrink, S. (2021, February 22). *Pros and cons of different delivery locations.* Ovia Health. https://www.oviahealth.com/guide/105048/pregnancy-pros-cons-delivery-locations/

Oglesby, P. (2022, July 18). *Instinct - are we born with a protective instinct?* HubPages. https://discover.hubpages.com/health/Instinct-Are-We-Born-With-a-Protective-Instinct

Orth, T. (2022, June 17). *Americans believe the role of fathers has changed over time, but disagree on how.* YouGov. https://today.yougov.com/topics/society/articles-reports/2022/06/17/americans-believe-role-fathers-has-changed-poll

Outten, L. (2017, September 13). *Comparing birth options: The pros and cons of hospital, birth center and home births.* Big City Moms.

https://www.bigcitymoms.com/uncategorized/comparing-birth-options-look-pros-cons-hospital-birth-centers-home-births/

Overfelt, M. (2020, May 15). *How to spot postpartum depression in loved ones.* The Bump. https://www.thebump.com/a/postpartum-depression-partner-friend

Owlet Blog Team. (2022, June 15). *10 ways for dads to bond with their newborns.* Owlet. https://www.owletcare.com/blog/10-ways-for-dads-to-bond-with-their-newborns

Palmer, C. (2022, February 10). *Is hiring a birth doula right for me?* GoodRx Health. https://www.goodrx.com/conditions/pregnancy/birth-doula-pros-cons

Palmer, L. (2021, October 15). *How to support a mother who receives a prenatal diagnosis during pregnancy.* Children's Hospital of Philadelphia. https://www.chop.edu/news/how-support-mother-who-receives-prenatal-diagnosis-during-pregnancy

Pampers. (2018, May 7). *Learn how to change a nappy.* Pampers. https://www.pampers.ph/newborn-baby/care/article/how-to-change-a-nappy

Pampers. (2022a, March 28). *Couvade syndrome: All about men's pregnancy symptoms.* Pampers. https://www.pampers.com/en-us/pregnancy/pregnancy-symptoms/article/couvade-syndrome

Pampers. (2022b, June 20). *How to put your baby to sleep.* Pampers. https://www.pampers.com/en-us/baby/sleep/article/how-to-put-a-baby-to-sleep

Parker, W. (2021, September 13). *Tips for men whose partner has had a miscarriage.* Verywell Family. https://www.verywellfamily.com/dealing-with-miscarriage-1270770

Paternal instinct: What is it (and why is it important). (2020, June 22). Know Your Archetypes. https://knowyourarchetypes.com/paternal-instinct/

Perez, R. (2017, May 24). *5 very good reasons why dads need to be there during childbirth*. Smart Parenting. https://www.smartparenting.com.ph/pregnancy/labor-and-childbirth/5-reasons-why-dads-need-to-be-present-during-childbirth-a00041-20170524

Perkins, S., Korn, S., Lancaster, S., & Mooij, E. (2016, October 28). *Dad's guide to baby-proofing your home*. Dummies. https://www.dummies.com/article/body-mind-spirit/relationships-family/parenting/dads-guide-baby-proofing-home-227984/

Perumalla, M. K. (2020, March 16). *Relationship problems and pregnancy: How to solve relationship stress during pregnancy*. Sprint Medical. https://sprintmedical.in/blog/couple-relationship-during-pregnancy

Pike, A. (2022, May 5). *5 nutrition and food safety pregnancy myths*. Food Insight. https://foodinsight.org/5-nutrition-and-food-safety-pregnancy-myths/

Postpartum preeclampsia. (2023, April 27). Preeclampsia Foundation. https://www.preeclampsia.org/postpartum-preeclampsia

Pregnancy appointments, scans and tests - for dads and partners. (2022, June 16). Tommy's. https://www.tommys.org/pregnancy-information/dads-and-partners/pregnancy-scans-and-appointments

Pregnancy Editors. (2015, January 4). *Dads' guide to swaddling babies*. Pregnancy Magazine. https://www.pregnancymagazine.com/baby/dads-guide-to-swaddling-babies

Promundo. (2019, July 17). *What we know about masculinity, fatherhood, and caregiving*. Equimundo. https://www.equimundo.org/what-we-know-about-masculinity-fatherhood-and-caregiving/

Raising Children Network (Australia). (2022a, January 31). *When your baby is overdue*. Raising Children Network. https://raisingchildren.net.au/pregnancy/week-by-week/third-trimester/baby-is-overdue

Raising Children Network (Australia). (2022b, February 23). *Pregnancy, sex drive and your relationship: Pregnant women*. Raising Children Network. https://raisingchildren.net.au/pregnancy/preparing-for-a-baby/relationships/pregnancy-sex-drive-your-relationship-women

Raising Children Network (Australia). (2022c, November 10). *Sex and intimacy when your partner is pregnant and after your baby is born*. Raising Children Network. https://raisingchildren.net.au/pregnancy/pregnancy-for-partners/relationships-and-feelings/sex-when-your-partner-is-pregnant

Raising Children Network (Australia). (2022d, November 10). *When your partner is pregnant: Your feelings*. Raising Children Network. https://raisingchildren.net.au/pregnancy/pregnancy-for-partners/relationships-and-feelings/partner-is-pregnant-your-feelings

Raising Children Network (Australia). (2023a, February 8). *Appointments during pregnancy*. Raising Children Network. https://raisingchildren.net.au/pregnancy/health-wellbeing/tests-appointments/appointments-during-pregnancy

Raising Children Network (Australia). (2023b, May 3). *How to hold a newborn: In pictures*. Raising Children Network. https://raisingchildren.net.au/newborns/health-daily-care/holding-newborns/how-to-hold-your-newborn

Redshaw, M., & Henderson, J. (2013). *Fathers' engagement in pregnancy and childbirth: Evidence from a national survey.* BMC Pregnancy and Childbirth, 13(1). https://doi.org/10.1186/1471-2393-13-70

Relationship problems and pregnancy. (2018, October 12). Tommy's. https://www.tommys.org/pregnancy-information/im-pregnant/mental-wellbeing/relationship-problems-and-pregnancy

Relationships Australia Victoria. (2019, August 22). *7 types of dad.* Support for Fathers. https://supportforfathers.com.au/resources/resources/7-types-of-dad/

Renter, E. (2020, July 1). *Budgeting for new parents: How to budget for baby.* NerdWallet. https://www.nerdwallet.com/article/finance/baby-budget-new-parents

Reyerson-Warren, D. (2019, March 6). *Miscarriage: A father's grief.* Cherokee Women's Health. https://cherokeewomenshealth.com/2019/03/miscarriage-a-fathers-grief/

Rice, A. (2017, January 17). *Birthing classes - choosing a class.* Familydoctor.org. https://familydoctor.org/birthing-classes/

Rogers, L. (2022, June 13). *Week-by-week pregnancy advice for expecting dads and partners.* What to Expect. https://www.whattoexpect.com/pregnancy/for-dad/week-by-week-pregnancy-advice-dads-partners/

Rothstein, A. (2022, July 20). *Types of birth: Pros and cons of five common delivery methods.* The Mother Baby Center. https://www.themotherbabycenter.org/blog/2022/07/types-of-birth-pros-and-cons-of-common-delivery-methods/

Russ, B. (2017, September 1). *The average age for new U.S. dads has passed 30.* Science. https://www.science.org/content/article/average-age-new-us-dads-has-passed-30

Salyer, J. (2018, January 5). *Sex drive during pregnancy: 5 things that happen.* Healthline. https://www.healthline.com/health/pregnancy/sex-drive

Sanders, L. (2022, July 27). *5 pregnancy nutrition myths to ignore.* The Bump. https://www.thebump.com/news/5-pregnancy-nutrition-myths

Saxe, D., & Martínez García, M. (2022, November 30). *Fatherhood changes men's brains, according to before-and-after MRI scans.* USC Dornsife. https://dornsife.usc.edu/news/stories/fatherhood-changes-mens-brains/

Scheid, V. L. (2014, August 23). *What are newborn screening tests?* Children's Hospital of Philadelphia. https://www.chop.edu/conditions-diseases/newborn-screening-tests

Sen, V. (2008, August). *Common fears about fatherhood.* Region of Peel. https://www.peelregion.ca/health/family-health/before-pregnancy/dads/fathers-emotional-prep/fears-about-fatherhood.htm

Sharpe McCollum, B. (2018, March 1). *Hospital-based vs. independent childbirth education.* Pathways to Family Wellness. https://pathwaystofamilywellness.org/holistic-healthcare/choosing-a-birth-class-hospital-based-vs-independent-childbirth-education.html

Shatzman, C. (2023, February 17). *Spa treatments you can (and can't) enjoy while pregnant.* The Bump. https://www.thebump.com/a/spa-safety-while-pregnant

Sparks, D. (2021, June 17). *New dad: Tips to help manage stress.* Mayo Clinic News Network. https://newsnetwork.mayoclinic.org/discussion/new-dad-tips-to-help-manage-stress/

Spears, N. (2015, June 17). *7 tips for dads during labor and delivery.* Baby Chick. https://www.baby-chick.com/labor-day-for-dads/

Stenson, J. B. (2023). *The father as protector.* Fathers for Good. http://www.fathersforgood.org/ffg/en/flashitems/protector/father.html

Sun, A. (2022, December 8). *Becoming a father can shrink your brain, new study says.* Scienceline. https://scienceline.org/2022/12/becoming-a-father-can-shrink-your-brain/

Tapp, F. (2017, April 17). *12 dads' reactions to finding out they were going to be fathers.* Romper. https://www.romper.com/p/12-dads-share-their-reactions-to-finding-out-they-were-going-to-be-fathers-51644

Terreri, C. (2018, May 18). *Top 3 common pregnancy-related relationship conflicts — and what to do.* Lamaze International. https://www.lamaze.org/Giving-Birth-with-Confidence/GBWC-Post/top-3-common-pregnancy-related-relationship-conflicts-and-what-to-do

Terreri, C. (2019, June 14). *11 ways dads can bond with baby right away.* Lamaze International. https://www.lamaze.org/Giving-Birth-with-Confidence/GBWC-Post/11-ways-dads-can-bond-with-baby-right-away

Tete, S. (2021, August 2). *Relationship stress during pregnancy: What can you do?* Stylecraze. https://www.stylecraze.com/articles/relationship-problems-during-pregnancy/

The American College of Obstetricians and Gynecologists. (2021, January). *Sample birth plan.* ACOG. https://www.acog.org/womens-health/health-tools/sample-birth-plan

The American College of Obstetricians and Gynecologists. (2021, November). *The Rh factor: How it can affect your pregnancy.* ACOG. https://www.acog.org/womens-health/faqs/the-rh-factor-how-it-can-affect-your-pregnancy#:~:text=The%20Rh%20factor%20is%20a

The Bump Editors. (2014, August 19). *Baby proofing checklist: Before baby comes home.* The Bump. https://www.thebump.com/a/checklist-babyproofing-part-1

The Bump Editors. (2023, May 22). *The Bump birth plan tool.* The Bump. https://www.thebump.com/a/tool-birth-plan

The changing role of the modern day father. (2009). American Psychological Association. https://www.apa.org/pi/families/resources/changing-father

The Healthline Editorial Team. (2019, March 5). *What's the difference between a doula and a midwife?* Healthline. https://www.healthline.com/health/pregnancy/doula-vs-midwife

The Honest Company. (2013, March 5). *7 tips for bringing home baby (from a dad!).* Honest. https://www.honest.com/blog/baby/0-to-3-months/7-tips-for-bringing-home-baby-(from-a-dad)/4044.html

The science of fatherhood: How your body and brain change when you become a dad. (2023, June 1). BBC Tiny Happy People. https://www.bbc.co.uk/tiny-happy-people/science-of-fatherhood/zvnhjsg

The ultimate baby proofing checklist: +100 safety tips. (2021, April 15). Watchful Dad. https://www.watchfuldad.com/baby-proofing-checklist/

Tigar, L. (2023, June 6). *How big is my baby? Size comparisons that aren't fruit.* Parents. https://www.parents.com/pregnancy/week-by-week/baby-size-by-week-not-fruit/

Tiller, L. (2023). *Dads' mental health.* Plunket New Zealand. https://www.plunket.org.nz/being-a-parent/being-a-dad/your-mental-health/

Timmons, J. (2022, February 1). *Home birth: Pros and cons.* Healthline. https://www.healthline.com/health/pregnancy/home-birth-vs-hospital-birth

Tips for managing stress as a new dad. (2013). Northwest Primary Care. https://www.nwpc.com/tips-for-managing-stress-as-a-new-dad/

Top 10 financial tips for new dads this father's day? (2021, June 18). RL360. https://www.rl360.com/top10/financial-tips-for-new-dads.htm

Trent, S. (2022, May 23). *Postpartum depression: How to help your wife.* MyCounselor.Online. https://mycounselor.online/supporting-wife-postpartum-depression/

10 tips for new fathers. (2018, March 28). Canopy Health. https://www.canopyhealth.com/10-tips-for-new-fathers/

12 newborn hacks for new dads. (2019, June 20). Dad Life Lessons. https://dadlifelessons.com/newborn-hacks-for-new-dads/

UNICEF. (2021, June 10). *Baby basics: How to burp your baby.* UNICEF. https://www.unicef.org/parenting/child-care/how-to-burp-baby

UNICEF. (2023, March 7). *What to eat before, during and after pregnancy.* UNICEF South Asia. https://www.unicef.org/rosa/stories/what-eat-during-and-after-pregnancy?gad=1&gclid=CjwKCAjw-IWkBhBTEiwA2exyOx6rOtC-fLXrTpxkUIImMrrvilcd4gWc6H3oBeJCw5Mdnb6UgMy4nBoC9jkQAvD_BwE

University of California San Diego Health. (2015). *When to go to the hospital for childbirth.* UC San Diego Health. https://health.ucsd.edu/care/pregnancy-birth/hospital-stay/when-to-go/

van Vuuren, E. (2017, March 2). *Top 10 new dad fears.* The Bump. https://www.thebump.com/a/top-10-new-dad-fears

Victoria State Government Department of Health. (2012). *Childbirth - pain relief options.* Better Health Channel.

https://www.betterhealth.vic.gov.au/health/HealthyLiving/childbirth-pain-relief-options

Wahlberg, R. (2021). *Is it safe to change cat litter during pregnancy?* BabyCenter. https://www.babycenter.com/pregnancy/health-and-safety/is-it-safe-to-change-the-cats-litter-box-when-im-pregnant_1246885

WebMD Editorial Contributors. (2022, August 8). *Taking medicine during pregnancy*. Grow by WebMD. https://www.webmd.com/baby/taking-medicine-during-pregnancy

Weiss, N. (2022, March 18). *How to support your wife after a miscarriage: 6 tips*. Cake. https://www.joincake.com/blog/my-wife-had-a-miscarriage/

Weiss, R. E. (2022, August 26). *When to go to the hospital for labor*. Verywell Family. https://www.verywellfamily.com/when-should-i-go-to-the-hospital-to-have-my-baby-2759045

Whiten, S. R. (2022, March 26). *10 ways to help your wife through a miscarriage*. Dr. Psych Mom. https://www.drpsychmom.com/2022/03/26/10-ways-to-help-your-wife-through-a-miscarriage/

Why do some men experience pregnancy symptoms such as vomiting and nausea when their wives are pregnant? (2004, June 28). Scientific American. https://www.scientificamerican.com/article/why-do-some-men-experienc/

Williams, D. (2004). *Giving birth "in place": A guide to emergency preparedness for childbirth*. Journal of Midwifery & Women's Health, 49(4), 48–52. https://doi.org/10.1016/j.jmwh.2004.04.030

Wilson, J. (2019, May 7). *How to bottle feed a baby: A guide for dads*. Minbie. https://minbie.co.uk/blogs/news/how-to-bottle-feed-a-baby-a-guide-for-dads

Winder, K. (2015, March 26). *Dads-to-be: A guide to labour and how to support her*. BellyBelly.

https://www.bellybelly.com.au/men/supporting-her-in-labour/

Wisner, W. (2021, June 14). *How to support your partner during pregnancy.* Verywell Family. https://www.verywellfamily.com/partner-support-during-pregnancy-4797874

Wisner, W. (2022, December 13). *Do I have postpartum blues or postpartum depression?* Verywell Family. https://www.verywellfamily.com/postpartum-blues-vs-postpartum-depression-4770580

Wooll, M. (2022, April 6). *Paternity leave in the US: A guide to getting it right.* Www.betterup.com. https://www.betterup.com/blog/paternity-leave-in-the-us

Wright, K. (2021, May 3). *The pros and cons of birthing centers, and why I ultimately chose a hospital birth.* Growing Serendipity. https://theexperiencedmama.com/pros-and-cons-of-birthing-centers/

Writes, S. (2022, March 4). *Baby formula 101.* Mom.com. https://mom.com/baby/baby-formula-101

Wu, K. (2020, December 27). *Top 17 fears of new fathers during pregnancy.* Psychology Today. https://www.psychologytoday.com/intl/blog/the-modern-heart/202012/top-17-fears-new-fathers-during-pregnancy

Wu, K. J. (2018, July 16). *This is your brain on fatherhood.* Smithsonian Magazine. https://www.smithsonianmag.com/science-nature/neurochemistry-fatherhood-180969635/

Yang, S. (2017, September 22). *Top 10 fears of new moms.* The Bump. https://www.thebump.com/a/new-mom-fears

Your pregnancy hospital bag checklist and birth plan template. (2023, June 2). Sassy Mama. https://www.sassymamahk.com/pregnancy/hospital-packing-checklist/

Zalewski, P. (2021, April 30). *The ultimate pregnancy guide - week by week pregnancy for dads.* Fathercraft. https://fathercraft.com/pregnancy-for-dads-weekly/

Zammett Ruddy, E. (2022, July 16). *How to put a baby to sleep.* Parents. https://www.parents.com/baby/sleep/tips/five-ways-to-help-baby-sleep/

Image References

Free vector hand drawn fetal development infographic. (2020). Freepik. https://www.freepik.com/free-vector/hand-drawn-fetal-development-infographic_21077197.htm#query=fetal%20development&position=2&from_view=keyword&track=ais

Printed in Great Britain
by Amazon